Managed Care and Public Health

Paul K. Halverson, DrPH, FACHE
School of Public Health
University of North Carolina at Chapel Hill
Chapel Hill, North Carolina

Arnold D. Kaluzny, PhD, MHA
School of Public Health
Cecil G. Sheps Center for Health Services Research
Lineberger Comprehensive Cancer Center
University of North Carolina at Chapel Hill
Chapel Hill, North Carolina

Curtis P. McLaughlin, DBA
School of Public Health
Kenan-Flagler Business School
University of North Carolina at Chapel Hill
Chapel Hill, North Carolina

with

Glen P. Mays, MPH
School of Public Health
University of North Carolina at Chapel Hill
Chapel Hill, North Carolina

AN ASPEN PUBLICATION®
Aspen Publishers, Inc.
Gaithersburg, Maryland
1998

Library of Congress Cataloging-in-Publication Data

Managed care and public health/[edited by] Paul K. Halverson,
Arnold D. Kaluzny, Curtis P. McLaughlin; with Glen P. Mays.
p. cm.
Includes bibliographical references and index.
ISBN 0-8342-0897-0
1. Public health—United States.
2. Managed care plans (Medical care)—United States.
3. Privatization—United States.
I. Halverson, Paul K.   II. Kaluzny, Arnold D.
III. McLaughlin, Curtis P.   IV. Mays, Glen P.
RA395.A3M356   1998
362.1'04258'0973—dc21
97-26357
CIP

Orders: (800) 638-8437
Customer Service: (800) 234-1660

About Aspen Publishers • For more than 35 years, Aspen has been a leading professional
publisher in a variety of disciplines. Aspen's vast information resources are available in both
print and electronic formats. We are committed to providing the highest quality information
available in the most appropriate format for our customers. Visit Aspen's Internet site for
more information resources, directories, articles, and a searchable version of Aspen's full
catalog, including the most recent publications: **http://www.aspenpub.com**
Aspen Publishers, Inc. • The hallmark of quality in publishing
Member of the worldwide Wolters Kluwer group.

Editorial Resources: Jane Colilla
Library of Congress Catalog Card Number: 97-26357
ISBN: 0-8342-0897-0

Printed in the United States of America

1 2 3 4 5

To C. Arden Miller, MD, whose values and commitment to public health have set a standard against which future public health activities within a changing health care system must be judged.

TABLE OF CONTENTS

CONTRIBUTORS

John W. Baker, MD
Vice President
Community Health
Carolinas HealthCare System
Charlotte, North Carolina

Dan Beauchamp, PhD
Professor
Department of Health Policy and
  Management
University at Albany
  State University of New York
Albany, New York

**Montague Brown, DrPH, JD,
  MBA**
Editor
Health Care Management Review
Arizona State University
Tucson, Arizona

Linda L. Bultman, PhD
Director
Research and Public Health
  Assessment Division
Bureau of Community Oriented
  Primary Care

Texas Department of Health
Austin, Texas

Mady Chalk, PhD
Director
Office of Managed Care
Center for Substance Abuse
  Treatment
Substance Abuse and Mental Health
  Service Administration
U.S. Department of Health and
  Human Services
Rockville, Maryland

Robbie J. Davis, PhD
Planning Manager
Bureau of Women and Children
Texas Department of Health
Austin, Texas

Debra A. Draper, MSHA
Research Assistant
Department of Health
  Administration
Medical College of Virginia
Virginia Commonwealth University
Richmond, Virginia

Bruce J. Fried, PhD
Associate Professor
Department of Health Policy and
    Administration
School of Public Health
University of North Carolina at
    Chapel Hill
Chapel Hill, North Carolina

Donald R. Haley, MBA, MHS
Research Assistant
Department of Health Policy and
    Administration
School of Public Health
University of North Carolina at
    Chapel Hill
Chapel Hill, North Carolina

**Paul K. Halverson, DrPH,
    FACHE**
Assistant Professor
Department of Health Policy and
    Administration
Associate Director
Public Health Leadership Doctoral
    Program
School of Public Health
University of North Carolina at
    Chapel Hill
Chapel Hill, North Carolina

Robert E. Hurley, PhD
Associate Professor
Department of Health
    Administration
Medical College of Virginia
Virginia Commonwealth University
Richmond, Virginia

Anne Y. Ilinitch, PhD
Assistant Professor
Kenan-Flagler Business School

University of North Carolina at
    Chapel Hill
Chapel Hill, North Carolina

Matthew C. Johnsen, PhD
Research Director
R.O.W. Sciences, Inc.
Rockville, Maryland

Arnold D. Kaluzny, PhD, MHA
Professor
Department of Health Policy and
    Administration
Director
Public Health Leadership Doctoral
    Program
School of Public Health
Senior Fellow
Cecil G. Sheps Center for Health
    Services Research
Lineberger Comprehensive Cancer
    Center
University of North Carolina at
    Chapel Hill
Chapel Hill, North Carolina

Stephen R. Keener, MPH, MD
Director
Department of Public Health
Carolinas HealthCare System
Charlotte, North Carolina

Donald Malafronte
Director
Urban Health Institute
Roseland, New Jersey

Artemis H. Malekpour, MHA
Research Assistant
Department of Health Policy and
    Administration

School of Public Health
University of North Carolina at
  Chapel Hill
Chapel Hill, North Carolina

Glen P. Mays, MPH
Research Assistant
Department of Health Policy and
  Administration
Interdisciplinary Curriculum in
  Practice and Leadership
School of Public Health
University of North Carolina at
  Chapel Hill
Chapel Hill, North Carolina

Curtis P. McLaughlin, DBA
Professor
Kenan-Flagler Business School
Professor
Department of Health Policy and
  Administration
School of Public Health
University of North Carolina at
  Chapel Hill
Chapel Hill, North Carolina

Jonathan M. Metsch, DrPH
President and CEO
Liberty HealthCare System, Inc.
President and CEO
Jersey City Medical Center, Inc.
Jersey City, New Jersey

Patti J. Patterson, MD, MPH
Commissioner of Health

Texas Department of Health
Austin, Texas

Pam Silberman, JD, DrPH
Fellow
Cecil G. Sheps Center for Health
  Services Research
University of North Carolina at
  Chapel Hill
Chapel Hill, North Carolina

J. Scott Simpson, MD
Medical Director
PCA Health Plans
Austin, Texas

Debra C. Stabeno, BBA
Associate Commissioner for Health
  Care Delivery
Texas Department of Health
Austin, Texas

Gary J. Young, JD, PhD
Senior Researcher
Management Division and Research
  Center
Veterans Affairs Health Services
  Research and Development
  Service
Assistant Professor
Health Services Department
Boston University School of Public
  Health
Boston, Massachusetts

FOREWORD

The premise is really remarkably simple, almost elegant in its simplicity. Public health is *not* just the small cinder-block building financed by Hill-Burton moneys, hard to find behind the county courthouse. It is not merely the clinics for poor people operated in the county hospital—nor even the county hospital itself, no matter how essentially public and health-oriented both are. It is not just the preventive efforts of the health care professions, though prevention is certainly a key part of population-based health efforts. Nor is it solely the indirect, community-level efforts at creating and preserving a healthful environment. It is not even the services of governments at the local, state, and federal levels that have "health" in their titles, and are certainly very public, though these are certainly key pieces of the public health puzzle.

Public health, with all the challenges faced as America approaches the 21st century, can only be understood if it is first understood in its entirety, as the sum of those efforts that society expends to create the context in which people—the public—can be healthy. It represents a collectivity of efforts by all those who identify themselves as professionally involved in health and health care, and many who are unaware that theirs is part of the aggregate effort but who contribute because they take care in separating raw from cooked food, help kids to wash their hands before they return to class, or properly package their waste oil when they drain the crankcase.

In this context, governmental public health can be understood as all of those agencies and government-sponsored or financed interventions that contribute to this sum—even when they do not have "health" in the name of the agency or on the services brochure, or when they, for bureaucratic or clout reasons, have been separated from the body of public health efforts. This fragmentation has characterized many governmental office shuffles over the past two centuries since government's role in creating a healthy environment was first understood and approached in America through the creation of hospitals for the Merchant Marines, quarantine to protect against importation of disease, and environmental restrictions to protect property against infringement from irresponsible neighbors—a true public health service. America has always wanted government to secure individual rights and property and to assure equitable distribution of common goods. To this end, governments at all levels of organization have created offices to look after the public health—to create or stimulate the context in which the community could be healthy, or, when necessary, to become the agent that provided interventions to assure that context. Elegantly simple, not so?

But as a pluralistic, free-market, capitalistic society, America has also emphasized the *laissez-faire* approach to all of its service elements, including medicine and related health services. Thus we have achieved one of the greatest, if also one of the most expensive, levels of private, nongovernmental health care in the world. And like the government agencies that have emerged to fulfill our notions of what government should do, the private offices and institutions addressing and promoting the health of the public have served most of us well most of the time.

The great, failed health care reform debates of the 1930s, 1950s, 1970s, and now 1990s have, however, recognized and emphasized the imperfections of such a division of labor, permitting as it does much heterogeneity, waste, and inequity, and leaving many of our most vulnerable and needy unattended. In response to these gaps and conflicts, governments have created networks of public hospitals and large clinical, outreach, home health, and extended care facilities, varying in their comprehensiveness (and quality) as much as the crazy-quilt of our varied nation has varied from community to community. Constitutionally, and by the constitution, deploring large government and big centralized systems, the nation has resisted centralizing or consolidating its approach to health and health care, including its recent rejection of proposed nationwide health care reforms.

It was with this perspective that the landmark 1988 report of the Institute of Medicine (IOM) found America's public health system to be in disarray and unable to deliver on the guarantees that society had the right to expect of government—to create and assure the context in which people can be healthy. That report has had a revolutionizing effect on our approaches to public health, stimulating major nationwide agencies, institutions, associations, and professional groups to concerted action to review our approaches, coordinate our efforts, and review the bidding. The result has been an unprecedented alignment around the core concepts of what public health is all about—the core elements of the IOM report: assessment, policy development, and assurance. The concept is, once again, elegant in its simplicity. As America views its governance, we want our governmental institutions, including official public health agencies, to keep the system in balance, to be sure that things are working right in every community, without a heavy-handed policing or government takeover. Thus, the assessment function calls for governments to be sure that the needed accountabilities are in place by which all can know whether things needing remedy are being addressed. Based on our ongoing vigilance, we determine what needs to be done, and we govern through the development of agreed policies to fix things in the right order of priority. Finally, we want our government to ensure that the right efforts are in place to protect us against health hazards and that we can have the services we need where and when we need them, in accordance with our agreed policies and plans.

The IOM has recently re-addressed these concepts in the face of a remarkable decade of progress since the first report, and found them to be useful and evergreen, warranting re-emphasis and refocus in the light of this decade of change, particularly to recognize the managed care revolution. Recognizing that even after a decade of progress, there is still continuing evidence of inadequate support for governmental public health in many communities, the 1996 IOM report calls for strong partnerships with community agencies and with managed care organizations to ensure that the vital public health infrastructure is recognized, valued, and supported.

Again, pretty simple! Scarcely the makings of a definitive, lengthy, and scholarly treatise. So why this book?

The answer is the concept of privatization—the incremental restructuring of a system, still not in balance, to merge and consolidate more services within a rapidly evolving system of care management on the private side of the partnership.

As you read this book, you will know the justification for its approach and the need for the extensive analysis and eventual synthesis you will find here. For neither the private partners in public health nor the governmental agencies charged with ensuring that society can create the context in which it can protect its health is without major conflicts of agenda and interest in achieving this balance. From the perspective of the private partners, public health is often viewed as just another vested interest, running clinics or home health agencies in competition with the private sector. From the perspective of the health agencies, the private sector is often seen as moving off in its own direction without regard for the larger public need, accepting patients formerly served by the public agencies without providing the extras that some need because of various barriers erected by stigma, poverty, alienation, mental illness, or other special needs, or the long-term guarantees that were made by a separate public institution.

How simple is the concept—a single mainstream of integrated, seamless, continuous, comprehensive care in the private sector for all, with a strong complementary network of governmental public health agencies protecting the environment, providing the disease surveillance we need to guard against unseen harm, and ensuring that the privatized system functions to meet society's standards and the needs of all of its citizens. How simple in concept . . . how complex in the doing! To achieve this worthy balance, much work will be needed. To get this work done, we will need serious commitment to open, honest, and accountable partnerships. To understand the components of the partnerships, we will need serious, thorough study. This book provides a road map for this arduous but necessary undertaking.

Hugh H. Tilson, MD, DrPH
Clinical Professor
Health Policy and Administration,
Epidemiology, and Interdisciplinary
Curriculum in Practice and Leadership
School of Public Health
University of North Carolina at Chapel Hill
Chapel Hill, North Carolina

PREFACE

As managed care becomes the predominant form of health care delivery in the United States, many people in the public sector have serious doubts about its virtue. Nonetheless, managed care is a reality. Hospitals and other health care providers are forming integrated delivery systems and are moving away from traditional fee-for-service reimbursement toward capitated, per-member, per-month payment systems for service availability. States are rapidly moving toward enrolling their Medicaid population in managed care plans, and many health plans serving the commercial market view the Medicaid patient as a new business opportunity.

All of these groups face new challenges—and perhaps threats—to their current existence. The natural tendency for most of us is to ignore what we don't understand or to oppose what moves us from the comfort zone of the familiar. A quick look at material from many of the health professional associations during the last few years reveals that many regard managed care as something to be avoided or fought like a dreaded disease at the point of infection. Therefore, rather than to explore potentially useful applications within the context of improving health care delivery, a common approach is to emphasize the many reasons why managed care will not work. Likewise, many hospitals and managed care organizations view working with public health as nothing more than moving into the abyss of governmental bureaucracy.

It is time to change this situation. We hope this book will provide a practical examination of the issues and opportunities found at the intersection between public health and managed care. Within this context, we will examine the implications of privatization within the health services environment and look at a few specific examples of how this strategy has played out in practice. There are many good examples of where managed care has provided the motivation to make important improvements to the delivery of public health services. Likewise, some hospitals and managed care organizations have adopted public health principles to the point of greatly enhancing the capacity of public health within their community. Managed care is not the "boogie man" imagined by stalwarts of public health, nor is public health the undefined bureaucratic morass imagined by hospital and managed care executives. Both perspectives deserve careful attention, particularly at the point of intersection. We see stronger and more vibrant communities emerging as a result of collaboration and joint activity between public health and managed care.

This book was designed primarily with the practitioner in mind. Whether you are a hospital administrator interested in understanding public health or a public health director interested in managed care, we hope you will find this work helpful. For the student of health administration or public administration, we hope to provide an appropriate introduction to the various dimensions found within public health, privatization, and managed care.

This work is presented in four parts. Part I examines the principles of public health, managed care, and privatization and how they affect quality in health care. Starting with an explanation of the environment at the intersection of these principles, the first chapter provides a contextual overview for understanding the relationship between managed care and public health. The next three chapters address current trends and issues in public health, managed care, and hospital organization. Chapter 5 offers a critical assessment of privatization initiatives as they occur in all areas of health care.

Part II examines the public health implications of trends in managed care and privatization in a range of settings within health care. These settings include the Medicaid program; state maternal and child health programs; public and private mental health and substance abuse services; and health care quality-assurance bodies.

Part III presents a series of case studies that examine in detail developments in managed care and privatization in individual communities and organizations. Chapter 11 is an explanation of what we see as the typology of relationships between managed care and public health agencies. The chapters that follow describe the experiences of a diverse collection of communities and organizations throughout the country, and provide insight into the decisions and strategies of key stakeholders.

The final part of the book addresses key policy implications created by the growth of managed care and privatization. While the entire book could be entirely devoted to the important issues of ensuring quality and accessibility under these evolving structures, it is our intent in these chapters to encourage the reader to move forward toward entering the debate and seeking answers to the outstanding questions of the day. In this way, our hope is that this discussion of policy issues will provide a point of departure for your own unique circumstances and perspectives.

ACKNOWLEDGMENTS

A large number of individuals and organizations made generous contributions of time and effort to make this book possible. Authors acknowledge many of these contributions at the end of their chapters; however, the editors would like to give special thanks to those who provided critical assistance for major portions of this book. Research for Chapter 11 and many of the case studies (Chapters 12 to 16) was supported through a cooperative agreement grant from the Centers for Disease Control and Prevention (CDC) and the Association of Schools of Public Health (agreement S038-11/13). Thomas B. Richards, MD, a Medical Officer at the CDC, provided invaluable guidance and direction for these case studies. Several other chapters (Chapters 7, 9, 10, 19, 21, and 22) were based in part on a conference entitled "Privatization and Public Health" held during February 1996 by the Interdisciplinary Curriculum in Practice and Leadership, School of Public Health, University of North Carolina at Chapel Hill. Authors wish to thank conference organizers and participants for their helpful comments and support. Additionally, Glen Mays should be recognized for his role in reviewing and editing many of the chapters for this book, as well as his work as an author or coauthor for several chapters. Finally, the editors wish to thank Marleen Strugill, Heidi Ott, Kim Vaughn, and Heather Manning at the University of North Carolina at Chapel Hill for their assistance in the preparation of manuscripts for this book.

Current Themes in Public Health and Managed Care

The common ground between managed care and public health is more expansive than many observers may readily recognize. Nonetheless, caution is needed in traversing this ground because it is still not well explored, and its consistency varies widely across organizations and communities. The chapters in Part I offer an overview of the trends and issues currently emerging among managed care and public health organizations. In Chapter 1, the authors examine the major political and marketplace phenomena that lead public health agencies and managed care plans to interact within a common environment. Chapter 2 describes recent trends in the organization and operation of public health agencies, with a specific focus on the effects of managed care and privatization. Chapter 3 provides an overview of managed care organizations and the numerous roles these entities may assume within public health systems. Chapter 4 summarizes major trends in the privatization of public hospitals and examines the public health implications of these activities. Chapter 5 expands this discussion to address the public health implications of privatization efforts occurring in a variety of health care settings. Collectively, these chapters explore the landscape of public health and managed care issues in order to identify opportunities and challenges facing health care organizations and the populations they serve.

CHAPTER 1

Introduction

Paul K. Halverson, Glen P. Mays, and Arnold D. Kaluzny

Public health and managed care are on a potential collision course. Historically, public health agencies at local, state, and federal levels serve as the primary organizations for sustaining community-wide efforts in health promotion, disease prevention, health assessment, and the provision of medical care to vulnerable population groups without sufficient access to private providers.[1] Under the evolving systems for medical care delivery and financing in the United States, managed care plans now face strong incentives to engage in many of these same activities. Capitated financing arrangements and performance-based reimbursement systems create imperatives for these plans to promote behavior that reduces health risks and to emphasize utilization of preventive services that may forestall costly medical treatment in the populations they serve.[2] These plans face a growing need to collect population-based information on health status and health risks in order to anticipate service needs and financial obligations. Further, public sector cost-containment initiatives create opportunities for managed care plans to serve vulnerable population groups traditionally served in the public sector under the fee-for-service model, such as Medicaid and Medicare beneficiaries.

Both public health and managed care organizations now claim responsibility for activities in health promotion, disease prevention, health assessment, and care for vulnerable population groups. This recent development raises two important questions:

1. Can these two types of organizations continue to coexist in the current environment of cost containment, privatization, and competition?

Source: Adapted with permission from P.K. Halverson et al., Not-So-Strange Bedfellows: Models of Interaction between Managed Care Plans and Public Health Agencies, *Milbank Quarterly*, Vol. 75, No. 1, pp. 113–138, © 1997, Blackwell Publishers.

2. Are there opportunities for both types of organizations to fulfill their missions while also assuring the health of the public?

This chapter provides an introduction and overview of the issues facing public health agencies and managed care plans as these organizations interact within an evolving health care environment. First, we examine the underlying economic, political, and organizational trends that create opportunities for interaction between the managed care and public health fields. We describe these opportunities from the perspectives of both public health agencies and managed care organizations. Next, we explore the challenges that confront public health agencies and managed care organizations as they struggle to define their respective roles and responsibilities and to identify acceptable mechanisms for interaction. We conclude with several durable themes that characterize the shared ground between managed care and public health.

OPPORTUNITIES FOR MANAGED CARE AND PUBLIC HEALTH

Where is the common ground between managed care and public health? The health promotion and disease prevention objectives that have long been the hallmark of public health agencies are becoming increasingly important to managed care plans seeking long-term cost savings through healthier enrolled populations.[2] Some of the older, nonprofit health maintenance organizations (HMOs) demonstrate a long history of emphasis on prevention and community wellness.[3,4,5] However, many of the newer and largely for-profit managed care plans have only recently begun to place emphasis in these areas[6,7] in response to such pressures as consumer and purchaser demands for quality, the National Commission for Quality Assurance (NCQA) accreditation standards, and consolidation in local health care markets, which is allowing plans to assume responsibility and risk for a growing proportion of a community's total population. Data from a survey of 63 public health jurisdictions seem to reflect this trend, indicating that for-profit managed care plans are significantly less likely to engage in alliances with public health agencies as compared with nonprofit plans, even after controlling for other factors.[8]

A common need for population-based data on health status, disease incidence, and risk factor prevalence may help spark alliances between public health agencies and managed care plans. Public health agencies face an urgent need for these types of data as they face new and resurgent public health threats and increasing demands for accountability from policy makers and taxpayers. Managed care plans desire this population-based information as they move to expand their presence in health care markets and therefore attempt to anticipate health service needs and demands within current and potential enrolled groups. Data-sharing agreements and joint surveillance efforts may allow public health agencies and managed care plans to pursue their individual and collective interests in population-based information more efficiently and effectively.

In addition, many local health departments have both the expertise and the infrastructure necessary to provide preventive and primary health care services to vulnerable population groups, such as Medicaid beneficiaries. Under Medicaid managed care programs, which are now operational in 41 states, managed care organizations may seek to expand their market penetration by contracting to serve these beneficiaries. As a result, managed care plans—especially those with little or no experience with serving the often complex needs of vulnerable populations—face compelling reasons to establish cooperative relationships with public health agencies.

Finally, local health departments in many areas of the nation are facing uncertainty regarding the availability of public funds to sustain many of the population-based and personal health services they provide.[9,10] Federal Medicaid-waiver programs operating in many parts of the country are forcing local health departments to compete with managed care plans that enroll Medicaid beneficiaries, or to negotiate subcontracting arrangements with these plans, if they are to maintain fee-based revenues.[11] Additionally, many local and state governments are confronting budgetary difficulties that may constrain their financial contributions to local public health activities. Limited governmental appropriations threaten to force local health departments to grow even more financially dependent upon fee-generating activities such as clinical services provision and environmental permitting, at the expense of population-based activities such as health promotion, health assessment, and surveillance.[11–13] Public health agencies face an urgent need to forge partnerships with other community organizations to sustain and expand health promotion and disease prevention efforts even in the face of funding uncertainties.[14,15] The growing presence of managed care plans in local communities—and their connections with large numbers of enrollees and affiliated health care providers—make these organizations ideal partners for community health improvement initiatives.

CHALLENGES FOR PUBLIC HEALTH AND MANAGED CARE

Managed care plans and public health agencies are engaging in a wide range of interorganizational arrangements to capitalize on their common interests and shared environments (see Chapter 11). These arrangements may take various forms, ranging from loosely structured alliances to contractual agreements and consolidation.[16] Important differences may exist among these arrangements regarding their impact upon community health. Particularly compelling are the ways in which these models affect how the community is defined and which population groups are targeted for intervention; the overall quality and accessibility of health services in the community and how these attributes are monitored; and the respective roles of public and private organizations and individuals in shaping health resources, policies, and plans within the community.

Defining the Community and Targeting Interventions

Relationships between managed care plans and public health agencies may focus on population groups that do not correspond directly to the traditional ways of defining communities from a public health perspective. Rather than focusing on the entire population of a city or county, interorganizational arrangements may target interventions to specific groups of health plan enrollees or to a "target audience" of potential enrollees that extends beyond the boundaries of the local jurisdiction. Defining the community in relation to enrollees or potential enrollees may result in fewer resources available for addressing the health concerns of groups falling outside managed care target populations. The directors of several local health departments participating in alliances with Medicaid managed care plans, for example, report that fewer resources are now available for serving uninsured individuals not eligible for Medicaid. Public health agencies may encounter difficulties in maintaining a broad, community-wide focus under some arrangements with managed care plans.

Clearly, public health agencies need policies and strategies to ensure that they maintain and expand their efforts in addressing the health needs of groups that fall outside the target populations of managed care plans. Several organizational and financial strategies hold promise for addressing this potential problem in managed care–public health relationships: assembling community governing boards formed specifically to provide oversight and governance to these alliances; segregating alliance activities in public health agency divisions that are organizationally and administratively distinct from other agency operations; using contract provisions that require managed care plans engaged in public health alliances to contribute specified levels of funding or resources to community-wide public health practices; and developing public health performance measurement systems at local or state levels for ensuring that the performance of public health practices in local communities remains adequate for serving vulnerable populations after managed care alliances are developed. For this last policy option, a number of validated instruments and methodologies are now available for assessing public health performance, many of which are being used in state-wide public health report card initiatives.[17–21] These policy options may be used separately or collectively to ensure that public health agencies maintain a community-wide focus in their alliances with managed care plans.

Ensuring Health Care Availability, Accessibility, and Quality

A core function of public health agencies at federal, state, and local levels involves ensuring the availability, accessibility, and quality of health services in a community.[1] Local public agencies carry out this assurance function through direct provision of services and through cooperative relationships with other health care providers in the community. Relationships with managed care plans contribute to this function, but they may also detract from this function by creating difficulties in maintaining relationships with the full spectrum of health care providers in a community. Public health agencies that are allied with a particular managed care plan may encounter resistance in establishing relationships with competing health plans or with the physicians, hospitals, and health centers affiliated with these other plans. A county health department in Tennessee, for example, reports a diminished ability to collaborate with the county hospital in areas such as patient referral because of alliances that the organizations maintain with competing health plans (see Chapter 15). Resistance may be even greater when the public health agency operates its own competing plan. A health department in Oregon reports such resistance in establishing referral relationships with hospitals that are allied with competitors of its own Medicaid HMO (see Chapter 14). In addition to the competitive nature of local managed care markets, the tendency toward closed-panel provider networks within these markets may pose problems for public health agencies seeking to participate in them while still working with the complete range of the community's health care providers.

The problems public health agencies face in maintaining broad-based, community-wide partnerships with health care providers alongside organization-specific alliances with managed care plans are substantial. Actions public health policy makers and practitioners may take to reduce these problems include: avoiding exclusive relationships in the contracts and agreements established between public health agencies and managed care plans, wherever possible; allowing outside agencies and community groups to participate in reviewing and advising the structure and function of managed care–public health alliances; and structuring alliances within divisions of the public health agencies that are organizationally and administratively distinct from community-wide public health operations. This last policy option may also be achieved by establishing a separate, not-for-profit corporation to administer the alliance, especially in cases where organizations may have concerns about the release of proprietary information to public health agencies that maintain relationships with their competitors.

Shaping Health Resources, Policies, and Plans within the Community

As local health care markets mature under managed care, successful health plans are acquiring greater numbers of enrollees and larger networks of providers and health care facilities. In this environment, public health agencies face daunting challenges in maintaining positions of influence and leadership regarding local health resources, policies, and plans that may affect community health. These challenges are heightened as health plans begin to assume responsibility for the care of populations traditionally served in the public sector, such as Medicaid beneficiaries. Public health agencies in these communities risk losing their visibility and authority in the community as they surrender their responsibilities in delivering personal health services to private sector providers. This loss of visibility and authority may have severe consequences for the ability of public health agencies to successfully perform population-based activities in health promotion and disease prevention, and to significantly influence health planning and policy development activities for the community.

Several models of interaction may assist public health agencies in securing a continued role in shaping the landscape of community health services, policies, and plans. Cooperative planning and policy development groups may allow public health agencies to inform and influence the decisions and actions of managed care plans as they relate to community health. By contrast, contractual arrangements may have either positive or negative effects upon the influence of public health agencies, depending upon the nature of the contract. Under subcontracting arrangements, poorly structured contracts have the potential to further subject the public health agency to the decisions and actions of the managed care plan, or, alternatively, to subject the health plan to the decisions of the agency. Another policy option beginning to appear in some public health jurisdictions involves establishing a competitive managed care plan within the local public health agency. In the few jurisdictions where this strategy is pursued, public health agencies report having the ability to maintain and expand their influence and leadership among health care providers and the public in general. "Leading by example" is the approach taken by these agencies (see Chapter 14).

The need to maintain visibility and influence in the community should not exist as the primary policy justification for a continued or expanded role in medical services delivery by public health agencies. Public health leadership can be maintained and expanded in the presence of alliances that transfer responsibility for public health services to managed care plans and other private providers.[22] The contracts and agreements supporting managed care–public health alliances need to be structured so that responsibility for direct service provision is exchanged for heightened public health agency roles in alliance governance, management, oversight, and evaluation. These types of arrangements potentially may allow public health agencies to maintain their visibility and influence in the community while also realizing improvements in the effectiveness and efficiency of public health practice through collaboration with managed care plans.

CONCLUSION

Collaboration between managed care plans and public health agencies is a natural product of the health promotion and disease prevention objectives shared by both types of organizations. Strong and enduring relationships between these organizations may prove to be a critical step in establishing broadly defined community health partnerships that have been characterized as essential elements of health system reform and improvement.[14,15,23,24] Indeed, relationships between public health agencies and managed care plans create linkages not only between the two parent organizations but also among the network of physicians, hospitals, and clinics that are affiliated with health plans, as well as the collection of governmental and private organizations that are allied with public health agencies.

Recognizing the potential value of these relationships, the Institute of Medicine's recently released report on public health calls upon policy makers and practitioners to clarify roles and responsibilities among public health agencies and managed care organizations, and to explore successful models of integration between these organizations.[15] Increasingly, communities are moving beyond the state of speculating about and anticipating these types of relationships and are confronting a need for action.

Clearly, important differences exist among the types of relationships that are possible between managed care plans and local public health agencies and among the outcomes that may reasonably be expected from these efforts. Nevertheless, the continued growth of managed care and the continued vulnerability of the nation's local public health systems create unique and compelling opportunities for exploring the boundaries of collaboration. Although there is much yet to be learned, collaborative alliances between managed care and public health hold clear potential for improving health system performance in an environment where health care costs, quality, and accessibility are of profound importance.

REFERENCES

1. Institute of Medicine. *The Future of Public Health.* Washington, DC: National Academy Press; 1988.
2. Centers for Disease Control and Prevention. Prevention and managed care: opportunities for managed care organizations, purchasers of health care, and public health agencies. *MMWR.* 1995;44:1–12.
3. Thompson RS, Taplin SH, McAfee TA, Mandelson MT, et al. Primary and secondary prevention services in clinical practice: twenty years' experience in development, implementation, and evaluation. *JAMA.* 1995;273:1130–1135.

4. Nudelman PM, Andrews LM. The 'value added' of not-for-profit health plans. *N Engl J Med.* 1996;334:1057–1059.

5. Claxton G, Feder J, Shactman D, Altman S. Public policy issues in nonprofit conversions: an overview. *Health Affairs.* 1997;16:9–28.

6. Hasan MH. Let's end the nonprofit charade. *N Engl J Med.* 1996;334:1055–1057.

7. Hurley RE. Approaching the slippery slope: managed care as industrial rationalization of medical practice. In: Boyle P, ed. *Rationing Sanity: The Ethics of Mental Health.* Washington, DC: Georgetown University Press; 1997.

8. Halverson PK, Mays GP, Miller CA. The determinants of interaction between managed care plans and public health agencies: implications for quality, accessibility, and efficiency in health care delivery. *Association for Health Services Research 13th Annual Meeting Abstracts.* Washington, DC: Association for Health Services Research; 1996. Abstract.

9. Gerzoff RB, Gordon RL, Richards TB. Recent changes in local health department spending. *J Public Health Policy.* 1996;17:170–180.

10. Miller CA, Moore KS, Richards TB, Kotelchuck M, et al. Longitudinal observations on a selected group of local health departments: a preliminary report. *J Public Health Policy.* 1993;14:34–50.

11. Koeze JS. Paying for public health services in North Carolina. *Popular Government.* 1994;60:11–20.

12. Allen NK. A national program to restructure local public health agencies in the United States. *J Public Health Policy.* 1993;14:393, 397–401.

13. Larry G. Public health is more important than health care. *J Public Health Policy.* 1993;14:261–264.

14. Baker EL, Melton RJ, Strange PV, Fields ML, et al. Health reform and the health of the public. *JAMA.* 1994;272:1276–1282.

15. Institute of Medicine. *Healthy Communities: A New Look at the Future of Public Health.* Washington, DC: National Academy Press; 1996.

16. Halverson PK, Mays GP, Kaluzny AD, Richards TB. Not-so-strange bedfellows: models of interaction between managed care plans and public health agencies. *Milbank Q.* 1997;75:113–138.

17. Halverson PK, Miller CA, Kaluzny AD, Fried BJ, et al. Performing public health functions: the perceived contribution of public health and other community agencies. *J Health Hum Serv.* 1996; 18:288–303.

18. Miller CA, Moore KS, Richards TB, Monk JD. A proposed method for assessing the performance of local public health functions and practices. *Am J Public Health.* 1994;84:1743–1749.

19. Richards TB, Rogers JJ, Christenson GM, Miller CA, et al. Evaluating local public health performance at a community level on a statewide basis. *J Public Health Manage Pract.* 1995;1:70–83.

20. Speake DL, Mason KP, Broadway TM, Sylvester M, et al. Integrating indicators into a public health quality improvement system. *Am J Public Health.* 1995;85:1441–1448.

21. Nelson DE, Fleming DW, Grant-Worley J, Houchen T. Outcome-based management and public health; the Oregon Benchmarks experience. *J Public Health Manage Pract.* 1995;1:8–17.

22. Halverson PK, Mays GP, Kaluzny AD, House RM. Developing leaders in public health: the role of executive training programs. *J Health Adm Educ.* In press.

23. Fielding J, Halfon N. Where is the health in health system reform? *JAMA.* 1994;272:1292–1296.

24. Gamm LD, Benson, KJ. The influence of governmental policy on community health partnerships and community care networks: an analysis of three cases. *J Health Politics Policy Law.* In press.

CHAPTER 2

Current Practice and Evolving Roles in Public Health

Paul K. Halverson, Donald R. Haley, and Glen P. Mays

The domain of public health is often ill-defined and, as a consequence, not well understood. Certainly, measures to ensure clean water and safe food, and to control infectious disease, are easily recognized examples of public health initiatives. Public health activities extend beyond these often visible functions to include more basic efforts such as: health promotion and disease prevention initiatives; community health needs assessment; programs to ensure the quality and accessibility of personal health services; and the development of plans and policies for addressing health needs. The wide array of services and activities contained within the domain of public health, and the broad spectrum of public and private organizations that contribute to these activities, may pose problems for individuals and organizations seeking a clear understanding of the nature and value of public health. Further, it is often said that public health functions are transparent when they are carried out effectively.[1] This chapter provides an overview of the structure and operation of the public health system in the United States. In doing so, it explores the often-transparent value added by public health to the larger health care environment comprised of providers, purchasers, and consumers of health services.

BACKGROUND

Over the last decade, the Institute of Medicine (IOM) has published two landmark reports on public health that have helped shape current practice in the field. The first of these reports, released in 1988, endeavored to define the field, describe its current state, and articulate a vision for its future.[2] IOM defined the mission of public health as "fulfilling society's interest in assuring conditions in which people can be healthy."[2(p7)] This broad definition extended the scope of public health to include environmental, economic, and political as well as medical aspects that affect the health of society. By many accounts, the IOM report had a substantial impact on how public health is conceptualized, organized, and delivered by the many organizations and individuals who are engaged in this field. In the years since this report was released, significant changes have occurred in the organization and delivery of public health services and in the public health issues facing individuals and communities. In light of these changes, the IOM recently assembled a committee to re-examine the state of public health practice. This committee identified two issues of overriding importance in determining the ability of public health agencies to ensure health in society: the relationships maintained between managed care organizations and public health agencies, and the roles played by public health agencies in communities.[3] Using the IOM work as a foundation, we provide a brief review of public health's history in the United States in order to foster an understanding of its current challenges and opportunities.

The modern public health system has been shaped by the growth of scientific knowledge and the understanding of how to control disease. With the recognition of bacteriology in the late 19th century, state and local health departments were established to improve sanitation and to control disease transmission. Local health departments played critical roles in the diffusion and integration of effective new disease control methods with public health practice. As a result, the incidence of many communicable diseases, such as typhoid fever and bubonic plague, was dramatically reduced. At the same time that local health departments and state agencies grew, the federal government also expanded its involvement in public health. For example, in 1906, "Congress passes the Food and Drug Act, which initiated controls on the manufacture, labeling, and sale of food. In 1912, the Marine Hospital Service was renamed the U.S. Public Health Service, and its director, the surgeon general, was granted more authority."[2(p67)] Federal agencies gradually expanded their capacities and roles to become major players in public health along with their state and local counterparts.

The federal government's expansion into the field of public health accelerated during the 20th century. Many new health-related agencies and programs began during this century, most focusing on personal health care. The National Institutes of Health, the Centers for Disease Control and Prevention, the National Institute of Mental Health, Institute for Child Health and Human Development, Institute for Environmental Health, Medicare, and Medicaid are just a few examples of major health programs instituted in the past century. Some of these federal programs were established primarily to support state and local public health initiatives, such as maternal and child health services, immunizations, venereal disease control, and tuberculosis (TB) control. As a result, state and local health initiatives began to mirror the structure of federal categorical aid programs for public health services.

Despite tremendous growth in health-related programs and services, the nation's public health system has faced severe challenges in addressing emerging health threats during recent years. The IOM's 1988 report on public health[2] observed that the public health system was in disarray—confused about its central mission and therefore often unable to respond effectively to emerging biological, environmental, economic, and political threats to health. During the 1980s, public health agencies confronted the emergence of human immunodeficiency virus (HIV) and acquired immune deficiency syndrome (AIDS), the resurgence of tuberculosis and other communicable diseases, growing morbidity and mortality associated with chronic disease, and the escalation of a host of behavioral and societal problems ranging from teen pregnancy to domestic and community violence. Many public health agencies offering personal health services also faced the challenges of serving the growing number of individuals who did not have adequate access to services from private health care providers. At the same time, many state and local governments began to face budget shortfalls, which created funding uncertainties, if not outright reductions, for many public health agencies.

The IOM report helped to motivate a host of efforts at federal, state, and local levels to improve public health agency performance in addressing these emerging issues. These efforts include the identification of essential practices and services that enable agencies to achieve the core public health functions identified in the report;[4,5] the reorganization of public health agencies around the core public health functions identified in the report; the development of systems and tools for evaluating the performance of public health agencies;[6-8] and education and training interventions designed to improve the leadership capacities of public health professionals.[9,10] A new report by the IOM suggests that substantial progress has been made in strengthening the nation's public health system since the 1988 report appeared.[3] Nevertheless, the field of public health continues to confront challenges posed by emerging diseases, behavioral and social problems, and resource constraints. Public health agencies must now address these challenges within the context of a health care environment that is rapidly moving toward managed health care, privatization, and marketplace competition.

ORGANIZATION OF PUBLIC HEALTH

Public health is a global issue; it is in the best interest of all countries to ensure that their citizens are healthy. In 1978, the World Health Organization and the United Nations adopted a declaration that is endorsed by most countries. This declaration contends that individuals' health is a human right to be preserved by their governments, rather than a privilege.[11] The United States has adopted this philosophy, but many would not agree that it has been fully achieved in practice.

The United States endeavors to ensure the health of its citizenry through a public health system that is composed of a wide range of organizational contributors. Public health services are provided by a variety of governmental and private sector organizations. Governmental public health agencies exist at the federal, state, and local levels.

Federal Agencies

The federal public health system is composed of various government agencies with one common mission: assuring the health of a population. Collectively, these agencies implement a wide variety of services that address preventable health outcomes. In his recent book on public health practice, Bernard Turnock notes that, "Since public health represents collective decisions and actions rather than purely personal ones, it is often governmental forums that make decisions, and establish priorities for action."[12(p41)] Federal public health agencies play a large role in this priority-setting and decision-making process.

Department of Health and Human Services and the Public Health Service

The U.S. Public Health Service (PHS) has a long history of providing health care services for the American people. The agency was established in 1798 as the Marine Hospital Service, which had evolved to include a variety of diversified public health services. The PHS grew into the predominant federal agency in charge of creating public health programs, subagencies, and services at a federal level. These services were designed to assess the health status and to meet the identified health needs of the nation. In 1993, after Vice President Al Gore began the National Performance Review, Health and Human Services Secretary Donna E. Shalala established a Continuous Improvement Program at the Department of Health and Human Services (DHHS). In response to the Vice President's goal to create a more efficient and customer service-oriented government, the PHS was reorganized and placed under the domain of the DHHS in 1996. Figure 2–1 shows the present organization of the DHHS. The department is directed by the Office of the Secretary and the Deputy Secretary, who oversee the Assistant Secretary of Health, Assistant Secretary of Management and Budget, Assistant Secretary of Planning and Evaluation, Assistant Secretary of Legislation, and the Assistant Secretary of Public Affairs. The Office of the Secretary also directs the following key public health agencies.

Administration for Children and Families

The Administration for Children and Families (ACF) is just one part of the DHHS that brings together an extensive range of federal programs and services.

U.S. Department of Health and Human Services

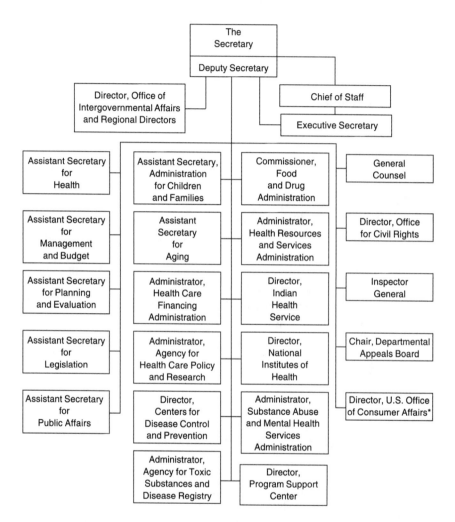

*Located administratively in DHHS; reports to the President

Figure 2–1 Organization Chart of the U.S. Department of Health and Human Services. *Source:* Reprinted from U.S. Department of Health and Human Services.

The purpose of these services is to address the needs of the nation's children and families. Several key ACF programs include the following:

- The Administration on Children, Youth, and Families administers the major federal programs that support social services, promotes growth and development, provides shelter for at-risk children and youths, and provides access to child care for working families.
- The Administration on Developmental Disabilities is an agency that funds state, local, and private sector efforts that safeguard the rights of people with developmental disabilities.
- The Administration for Native Americans promotes the self-sufficiency of Native American, Native Hawaiian, and Pacific Basin Tribes and their communities.
- Aid to Families with Dependent Children provides financial assistance based on need to families with children.
- The At-Risk Child Care program finances child care to working families with low incomes.
- The Children's Bureau provides grants to states, tribes, and communities to operate child welfare services.
- The Child Care and Development Block Grant provides financial support for state programs to establish child care services for working families.
- Job Opportunities and Basic Skills Training helps people on welfare to become self-sufficient by providing education, training, transportation, and child care services.

Administration on Aging

The Administration on Aging (AOA) is a federal agency that has worked to develop a network of state and community agencies focusing on aging-related and tribal organizations. Through this network, the AOA provides a diversity of needed services to the elderly population in either their own homes or in their communities. These agencies develop and support comprehensive in-home and community services for the elderly, including those at risk of losing their independence. The AOA also sponsors programs that provide the elderly with access to resources relevant to this age group, job and volunteer opportunities, senior center and day-care center programs, transportation, home delivery of meals, and home assistance services.

Agency for Health Care Policy and Research

The Agency for Health Care Policy and Research (AHCPR) was established in 1989 as the primary agency that supports research on the improvement of health care. Its goal was recently broadened to include research that pertains to the reduction of health care costs and the improvement of access to essential health services. The AHCPR is composed of divisions that are directed by the Office of the Administrator. According to the AHCPR, the following describes the primary function of each of these divisions:

- The Office of Policy Analysis furnishes technical assistance to health services researchers in the public and private sectors.
- The Office of Planning and Evaluation provides strategic planning and program evaluation for the AHCPR and coordinates efforts related to issues such as HIV and AIDS and minority and women's health.
- The Office of Management directs the administrative activities of AHCPR. These activities include financial management, human resources, and information resources management.
- The Office of Scientific Affairs directs the scientific review process for grants and contracts. This division allocates projects to agency centers and assesses the medical and scientific contribution of proposed and ongoing research.
- The Office of the Forum for Quality and Effectiveness in Health Care, which is also known as the Forum, facilitates the development and evaluation of clinical practice guidelines. The guidelines are designed to assist practitioners in providing quality care to their patients. These guidelines are also used to educate patients by increasing their understanding of health care decisions.
- The Center for Health Care Technology conducts and studies health care technology assessment. These studies include the safety and effectiveness, as well as cost-effectiveness, of health technologies.
- The Center for Outcomes and Effectiveness Research conducts studies of the effectiveness of diagnostic, therapeutic, and preventive health care services.
- The Center for Primary Care Research conducts studies pertaining to primary care, preventive medicine, and public health policies.
- The Center for Organization and Delivery Studies conducts research on the characteristics and structure of the health care system and its providers.
- The Center for Cost and Financing Studies conducts research pertaining to the cost and financing of health care. This division also develops data sets to support policy and behavioral research and analyses.
- The Center for Quality Measurement and Improvement studies the measurement and improvement of the quality of health care through patient satisfaction surveys of their health services and systems.
- The Center for Information Technology conducts studies on health information systems, including computerized patient record systems, data standards, automated medical records, and decision support systems.

- The Center for Health Information Dissemination plans and manages programs for distributing the results of agency activities.

Agency for Toxic Substances and Disease Registry

The mission of the Agency for Toxic Substances and Disease Registry (ATSDR) is to prevent "adverse human health effects and diminished quality of life associated with exposure to hazardous substances from waste sites, unplanned releases, and other sources of pollution present in the environment." Core functions of the ATSDR include public health assessments of waste sites, health surveillance and registries, and support of research in public health assessment. It also develops and distributes data pertaining to toxic substances and educational programs on hazardous substances. This agency is organized into three administrative offices, five program support offices, and four program-specific divisions. According to the ATSDR, these offices support and implement 10 program areas, including:

- public health assessments
- toxicological profiles
- emergency response
- exposure and disease registries
- health effects research
- health education
- literature inventory/dissemination
- health and safety of workers
- listing of areas closed to the public
- special initiatives, including the Childhood Lead Report and the Medical Waste Tracking Act

The ATSDR has 10 regional offices located throughout the United States.

Centers for Disease Control and Prevention

The Centers for Disease Control and Prevention (CDC) is an agency whose mission is to promote health and quality of life by preventing and controlling disease, injury, and disability. The CDC currently employs more than 6900 employees in 170 occupations. According to the CDC, the following describes the missions of its 11 centers:

- The National Center for Chronic Disease Prevention and Health Promotion was established to prevent death and disability from chronic diseases; to promote maternal, infant, and adolescent health; and to promote healthy personal behaviors.

- The National Center for Environmental Health was established to prevent and control disease, birth defects, disability, and death resulting from interactions between people and their environment.
- The National Center for Health Statistics is a division of the CDC that provides statistical information to guide actions and policy to promote the health of the population.
- The National Center for HIV, STD, and TB Prevention provides surveillance, prevention research, and programs to prevent and control HIV infection, AIDS, other sexually transmitted diseases (STDs), and tuberculosis (TB).
- The National Center for Infectious Diseases is charged with controlling and preventing infectious disease in the United States.
- The National Center for Injury Prevention and Control establishes programs to reduce injury, disability, death, and costs associated with injuries outside the workplace.
- The National Institute for Occupational Safety and Health is responsible for conducting research and making recommendations for the prevention of work-related illness and injuries.
- The Epidemiology Program Office was established to coordinate public health surveillance at the CDC. It also provides domestic and international support through scientific communications, statistical and epidemiologic consultation, and training of experts in surveillance, epidemiology, applied public health, and prevention effectiveness.
- The International Health Program Office is responsible for collaborating with other nations to promote healthy lifestyles.
- The Public Health Practice Program Office was established to strengthen the community practice of public health through information networks, ensuring laboratory quality, and through conducting practice research.
- The National Immunization Program coordinates immunization programs nationwide.

Food and Drug Administration

The Food and Drug Administration (FDA) is responsible for ensuring that foods are safe for consumption by the general population. In addition, the FDA is responsible for the safety and efficacy of human and veterinary drugs, biological products, and medical devices, and the safety of cosmetics and electronic products that emit radiation. With its 9000 employees and 1100 inspectors, the FDA ensures that regulated products are "honestly, accurately and informatively represented" or else are removed from the marketplace.

Health Care Financing Administration

The Health Care Financing Administration (HCFA) was created in 1977 to administer the two national health care funding programs: Medicare and Medicaid. Medicare is a federally funded program and Medicaid is a federal- and state-funded program. HCFA purchases health services for those who qualify for Medicare and Medicaid and ensures that these programs are properly administered. This agency also establishes policies for the reimbursement of health care providers; conducts research on the effectiveness of various methods of health care management, treatment, and financing; and assesses the quality of health care facilities and services.

Health Resources and Services Administration

The mission of the Health Resources and Services Administration (HRSA) is to provide programs designed to improve the health of the nation by ensuring that quality health care is available to underserved and vulnerable populations. Programs established to support this effort focus on issues such as AIDS, minority health, rural health policy, and public health practice.

Indian Health Service

The Indian Health Service (IHS) was established in 1921 to provide federal health services to American Indians and Alaska Natives. The IHS is the principal federal health care provider for Indian people, with a goal to improve the health status of this population. According to the IHS, the agency currently provides health services to approximately 1.4 million American Indians and Alaska Natives who belong to more than 545 federally recognized tribes in 34 states. IHS establishes programs to assist Indian tribes in developing health programs and in coordinating health planning and program evaluation. It provides comprehensive health care resources for American Indian and Alaska Native people.

National Institutes of Health

The primary mission of the National Institutes of Health (NIH) is the acquisition of new knowledge through research that will help prevent, detect, diagnose, and treat all forms of morbidity. The NIH conducts its own research as well as supports the studies of researchers in universities, medical schools, and health care and research institutions throughout the country and abroad. It is located in Bethesda, Maryland, with 75 buildings and an annual budget of more than $12 billion in 1996.

Substance Abuse and Mental Health Services Administration

The Substance Abuse and Mental Health Services Administration (SAMHSA) was established to reduce morbidity, mortality, and societal cost resulting from substance abuse and mental illnesses. This goal is accomplished in partnership with substance abuse and mental illness agencies and centers located throughout the United States. SAMHSA develops preventive and treatment programs and funds programs that improve the delivery of services associated with substance abuse and mental health.

Office of Public Health and Science

With the 1996 reorganization of the PHS, many PHS program offices were placed into the DHHS's Office of Public Health and Science (OPHS). This newly formed office is under the direction of the Assistant Secretary for Health, who serves as the Secretary's Senior Advisor for Public Health and Science. OPHS provides direction, advice, and counsel on public health and science issues to the offices within OPHS and to the Secretary. The following describes the offices within OPHS and their missions:

- The Office of Disease Prevention and Health Promotion is responsible for improving the health of the population through prevention of premature death, disability, and disease.
- The Office of Emergency Preparedness provides federal health, medical, and health-related social service response and recovery to federally declared disaster areas.
- The Office of HIV/AIDS Policy establishes policies, programs, and activities related to this disease across OPHS agencies.
- The Office of International and Refugee Health promotes the achievement of U.S. goals through participation in the Pan American Health Organization, United Nations Children's Fund, United Nations, and the World Health Organization.
- The Office of Minority Health coordinates activities to promote disease prevention and research-related activities for racial and ethnic populations across all OPHS Offices.
- The Office of Population Affairs provides comprehensive family planning services and conducts family planning and program research.
- The President's Council on Physical Fitness and Sports coordinates and promotes opportunities in physical activity, fitness, and sports.

- The Office of Research Integrity responds to allegations of scientific miscon-
  duct and promotes research integrity.
- The Office of the Surgeon General is appointed by the President of the United
  States to serve as a figure to promote and protect the health of the nation. The
  major functions of this office are to provide leadership and awareness in
  promoting disease prevention and health promotion and articulating research
  in health policy analysis and advice to the President. Current initiatives
  include the continuation of efforts to reduce tobacco use among Americans
  through the release of surgeon general reports and promoting effective
  disease prevention strategies through surgeon general policy statements on
  public health issues.
- The Office of Women's Health's mission is to serve as the focal point for
  women's health activities within the U.S. Department of Health and Human
  Services.

Federal Categorical Programs

Federal health agencies administer a variety of special programs designed to
support the provision of health services to designated populations. These special
programs—referred to as categorical programs because of their focus on specific
types of services and target populations—often take the form of grants-in-aid to
states and local government agencies as well as private service providers. Historically, categorical programs have been dominated by two specific types of services: the provision of health services for women and children, and the eradication
of disease. Programs such as the Special Supplemental Food Program for Women,
Infants, and Children and the Title V Maternal and Child Health Program are both
examples of federal programs that aim specifically to improve the health of the
nation's children. Other categorical programs, such as those targeting chronic
disease, HIV/AIDS, infectious diseases, and tuberculosis, emphasize the prevention and control of diseases. Many of these categorical programs are specified (or
"mandated") by federal legislation created by Congress. Although funding for
these categorical health programs is administered by federal agencies, the implementation of many occurs at state and local levels. The organizational structures
of state and local public health agencies often reflect the categorical nature of the
funds they receive from federal agencies. Federal categorical programs address a
wide range of public health issues; some of the most influential programs are
described below.

Women, Infants, and Children Program

The Special Supplemental Food Program for Women, Infants, and Children
(WIC) provides nutrition as well as nutritional education services to participants,

their parents, or caregivers. WIC is administered through state and local agencies targeting pregnant women as well as infants and children. Food items and infant formula are provided to program participants. The impetus is that early intervention programs for children and their families can help avert illnesses such as low birth weight and preventable diseases. In addition to food products, this program also offers educational services that focus on improved nutrition for this population and finances programs that put a greater emphasis on breastfeeding.

In 1990, the Department of Agriculture's Food and Nutritional Services Division conducted a study to assess the characteristics of WIC participants. It found that approximately 4.5 million people were enrolled in this program, of whom 46% were children, 30% were infants, and 24% were women. The average annual income of the women who participated in WIC in 1990 was $9002, with nearly 75% having recorded annual incomes under the federal poverty level. More than 82% of all local WIC programs are operated through a public health agency, with most programs being sponsored by the county or the state health department. Other services provided by local WIC agencies may include access to Medicaid, Aid to Families with Dependent Children (AFDC), food stamps, and general assistance programs.[13]

Maternal and Child Health Services

Categorical grants to support maternal and child health (MCH) services were established under Title V of Franklin D. Roosevelt's 1935 Social Security Act. Federal legislation passed in 1981 consolidated these categorical grants into a single block grant administered to states, thereby giving state agencies broad discretion in the use of these funds. The MCH block grant supports a wide array of state and local programs that are designed to meet changing family structures and needs. Programs include comprehensive child health and reproductive health care for low-income women and children; promoting greater access to care for pregnant women and infants; child health clinics; programs for crippled children; and other services for children with special health care needs (CSHCN). Other programs focus on areas such as training in pediatric and adolescent AIDS, injury and violence prevention, health and safety in child care, immunization of children, and substance abuse services. Under the block grant, states are responsible for the following functions: needs assessment; program planning and development; service delivery, coordination, and financing; standard setting and monitoring; technical assistance, information, and education; and reporting. MCH departments in each state are also required to coordinate with other related federal health, education, and social service programs. For example, MCH programs have participated in efforts to expand Medicaid eligibility and benefits for pregnant women and children. Chapter 7 provides an in-depth look at one state's approach to public health service delivery under the MCH block grant.

Chronic Disease

Federal categorical programs for chronic disease support state and local initiatives that provide education and screening for chronic diseases and services for kidney dialysis. Chronic disease programs, such as those for the prevention and control of cancer and heart disease, are provided in many communities across the country. Many of these programs supply morbidity and survival rate information for chronic diseases to state registries. Programs may also take the form of community workshops designed to teach individuals the risk factors and warning signs of chronic diseases. Screening programs are also supported in many communities. Preventive services such as screening for cholesterol, high blood pressure, and melanoma are part of many community programs. These services assist in the early detection and treatment of diseases, and in the process of informing and educating the public about preventable diseases.

HIV/AIDS

A number of federal categorical programs support HIV testing and counseling in public health departments and other settings. Over the past decade, publicly funded HIV testing and counseling have dramatically expanded. In 1991, for example, more than 2 million HIV tests were performed, compared to only 85000 in 1985.[14] Publicly funded HIV services often include counseling, testing, and education. Such services are designed to inform people about the mode of transmission of HIV, help to change patients' behavior to reduce their risk of infection, identify those with HIV and AIDS, and refer them to or provide them with appropriate resources. Publicly funded HIV counseling and testing are provided in many free-standing public health clinics in all 50 states. These services are provided in addition to those provided by the CDC.

Tuberculosis

TB is another infectious disease receiving a substantial amount of attention through federal programming and funding. TB was one of the leading causes of death in the United States in the 19th century. This highly contagious communicable disease was most prevalent in populations of lower socioeconomic classes that were more likely to have poor living or working conditions and poor nutrition. The development of antibiotics led to an effective cure and treatment of TB. As a result, the incidence of TB dramatically declined in most regions of the world. More recently, a resurgence in TB case rates in certain areas of the United States and in certain populations (such as recent immigrants from less-developed countries, HIV-infected individuals, homeless individuals, and other impoverished individuals) has triggered renewed concern about the spread of the disease. The emergence of drug-resistant strains of TB has also escalated this concern.

In 1989, the CDC announced a goal of eliminating TB in the United States by the year 2010. The responsibility to achieve this goal and to monitor the number of TB cases belongs to state and local agencies, which provide services to treat, monitor, and support the eradication of the disease. Local agencies also provide the CDC with vital statistics on the incidence of cases and ensure that a curative regime is being followed by the patient.

Other Infectious Diseases

With changes in human behavior and technology, and with advances in the accessibility of transporting systems, infectious diseases remain a significant public health hazard for many population groups. Newly emerging diseases such as Legionnaires disease, Lyme disease, hantavirus, toxic shock syndrome, and HIV/AIDS are of increasing concern in the United States. These emergent infectious diseases—together with historically problematic conditions such as cholera, dengue, and measles—are now a global concern. Adding to the concern is the discovery that some diseases that were previously controllable by antibiotics, such as tuberculosis and common bacterial infections, are now mutating into drug-resistant strains.

The CDC defines infectious diseases as those that are caused by microscopic organisms and spread from person to person. According to the DHHS, infectious diseases are the leading cause of death worldwide, with direct costs attributable to this morbidity of $30 billion a year in the United States alone. State and local agencies are working with the CDC, as well as with international organizations, to improve early detection and find new ways to prevent the spread of infectious disease. In addition, the NIH is directing new research efforts to understand and develop technology to diagnosis, treat, and prevent new diseases.[15]

State Agencies

While a myriad of federal agencies fund and promote public health initiatives, a strong block of state-level public health agencies assumes much of the responsibility for developing and implementing policies and programs that impact health. Historically, state health agencies "developed the structure and organizations needed to use their police powers to protect citizens from communicable diseases and environmental hazards, primarily from wastes, water, and food."[12(p42)] Police power refers to a state's authority to enforce laws to protect the health and general welfare of its population. As a result of this authority, state health agencies were established to conduct a wide variety of public health functions and services. These include collecting health information, providing health inspections, enforcing environmental regulations, and establishing policies focusing on individual and community health.

In the early 1980s, the Reagan administration promoted the concept of decentralization of government services. This concept introduced a change in government that affected the financing and delivery of many community health services, because public health and prevention were certainly components in this effort. With decentralization, the federal government gave state and local governments the directive to provide community health services that were previously offered through federal programs. Each state was given greater flexibility to meet the diverse needs of its population. The Reagan administration believed that state and local agencies were more sensitive to the needs of their community than those at the federal level.

Currently, most state public health systems are composed of official health agencies and voluntary agencies. Official health agencies are supported by government tax funds, and their employees are government officials. Voluntary health or nonofficial agencies are those programs supported by contributions instead of tax funds. Examples of voluntary agencies are the American Lung Association and the American Cancer Society.

Generally, each official state agency is supervised by an administrative health commissioner or a state health officer who may or may not be a physician. Some states have adopted a board of health commission that is responsible for the development of policies and the allocation or administration of state public health funds. The membership of these boards is primarily composed of health care professionals. The health officer either reports to or is a member of this board. Official state health agencies are either independent agencies that report to the board of health commission or directly to the governor, or they may be a component of a superagency. A superagency is a large, multipurpose human services organization with the goal of improving the continuity of health and social services. A superagency may be made up of several subagencies that are responsible for environmental health, population health, and regulation. While specific programs, staffing levels, and organization of official public health agencies vary among states, there is some uniformity in activities of state public health agencies. Activities associated with vital statistics, planning, epidemiology, personal health services, water quality, and sanitation are performed in almost all states.

Local Public Health Agencies

Local health departments (LHDs) have traditionally served as focal points for identifying and providing solutions to the health needs of communities. Generally, LHDs directly implement public health services and programs that are tailored to community needs. Many LHDs are accountable to local political structures through their organization as departments of county or city governments, or as regional districts that are operated by the municipalities. Many LHDs also receive administrative oversight and direction from state health agencies. Researchers at Johns Hopkins University developed a typology of local health department administrative relationships that has been widely used to study these organizations.[16] In states with decentralized local health departments, local agencies and officials maintain primary responsibility for governing the operations of local health departments. Other states operate a centralized system in which local health departments operate as administrative units of the state health agency. In shared systems, local entities may hold administrative authority for some activities performed by the local health department, while the state health agency retains responsibility for other activities carried out through local departments. Finally, some states have mixed administrative systems in that some local departments within the state may be decentralized and others centralized.

In many local public health jurisdictions, local boards of health provide oversight, governance, and/or advice to local health departments and their administrators. A 1992–1993 survey of local health departments suggests that 73% of departments operate under local boards of health.[17] Boards may hold statutory authority for such responsibilities as establishing local health policies, fees, and regulations; recommending budgetary appropriations; approving budgets; setting community health priorities; and hiring the local health director. Board members are often appointed by local political representatives and may include representatives from local government, public and private health care organizations, and community members at large. These boards may work in cooperation with other entities, such as boards of county commissioners or city councils, or with the governing and advisory boards of other public agencies.

Local health departments vary widely in organization, size, staffing, and services. Depending on state and local priorities and the availability of private health care providers, the structure of a local public health system may be characterized by a diversity of regulatory, planning, assessment, and service provision units. Much of this diversity reflects the priorities of local and state governments, the values and needs of community members, the capacities of private providers, and the economic realities of the community. The local organization of public health services can be viewed as representing the changing pattern of human activity in a local community. Some LHDs are divisions of larger "umbrella" agencies, while others operate as distinct organizational units.

LHDs are often managed by both an administrative director and a health officer—positions that may be filled by a single individual with both clinical and managerial experience. Health officers are typically physicians, while administrative directors often have advanced training in public health administration. The administrator is appointed to supervise a salaried professional staff that varies in size depending on population and resources. State legislatures delegate activities to these local agencies in the interest of the state, including responsibilities in enforcing state public health codes and in developing specified policies, plans, and regulations relevant to health.[2(p 184)]

LHDs provide health care services to their communities through professional staff members who may serve more than one local department. In some communities, staffing may consist of as many as several hundred people, while in other communities staffing may consist of as few as two people. Depending on LHD staffing and local community need, there is a large variation of services provided by these agencies. Some may offer only a few community health services while others may offer a wide variety. Generally, LHDs provide health education, conduct health inspections, and collect community vital statistics such as births, morbidity, mortality, and marriages. In addition, many LHDs provide personal health services. In some communities, LHD involvement in personal health care delivery is limited to categorical services that are not adequately accessible to all community members, such as childhood immunizations, screening and treatment for sexually transmitted diseases, adult and child preventive health screenings, family planning, and prenatal care. Many of these categorical services are supported by established federal and state funding streams that local health departments receive for this purpose. In other communities, LHDs provide a full range of primary care to children and/or adults, including treatment services and preventive services. These "full-service" LHDs support their primary care delivery systems through funding sources that may include: patient fees; federal grants for the provision of indigent care through designation as federally qualified health centers; state and local government grants for indigent care; and patient billings to Medicaid, Medicare, and private health insurers.

Figure 2–2 shows the organization of one North Carolina local health department. The governing body for this LHD, the Board of Health (BOH), is the overall policy-making body and is accountable to the County Commissioners. The board supervises a Health Director, who is the chief executive officer of the local health department and serves as the Secretary of the BOH. An Assistant Health Director manages the operating units of the LHD and reports to the Health Director. The operating units are Budget and Finance, Human Resources, and Staff Development and Training, in addition to four provider divisions. These provider divisions are Adult Health/Central Services; Child Health; Environmental Health; and Family Planning/Maternity. The Adult Health/Central Services Division provides community health services pertaining to communicable and infectious disease, child and adult immunization, sexually transmitted disease, tuberculosis, and refugee health services. In addition, this division also provides such corporate-level services as laboratory, pharmacy, and radiology. The Child Health Division provides clinical and preventive services to children, including dental care, nutrition, speech and hearing, social work, health education, community nursing,

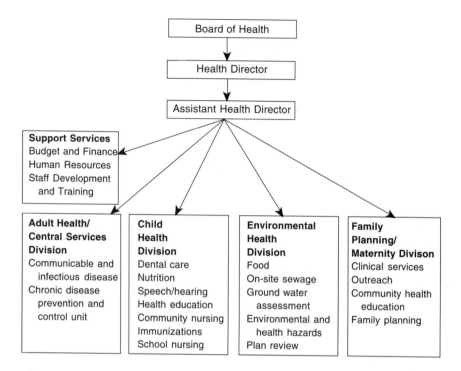

Figure 2–2 Organizational Structure of a County Health Department in North Carolina.

immunizations, and school nursing. The Environmental Health Division provides programs pertaining to food and lodging, on-site sewage, ground water assessment, environmental and health hazards assessment, and plan review. Finally, the Family Planning/Maternity Division provides clinical services, outreach services, community health education, care coordination, and postpartum visits for this population.

Due to the changing health care environment, many local health departments are being reorganized. For example, Figure 2–3 shows the organizational design of the Marion County Health Department (MCHD) of Indianapolis, Indiana.[18] MCHD underwent a major reorganization in 1994. This new structure was created to improve the efficiency and effectiveness of providing public health services in a changing health care environment. MCHD is the public division of the Health and Hospital Corporation, a municipal corporation created by the Indiana legislature in 1954. A seven-member Board of Trustees guides the direction of the local health department. Three members of this board are appointed by the Mayor, two members are appointed by the City Council, and two members are appointed by the County Commissioners. The Director of MCHD is a physician who oversees

Marion County Health Department Director
Health status and research
Fiscal, grants, and materials management
Health policy and planning
Health education, promotion, and training
Public relations
Maternal and child health

Population Health
Public health laboratory
Community-based care
Maternal and child health
Acute and chronic disease
Adolescent and school-based health
Women, Infants, and Children Program
Dental health

Environmental Health
Housing and neighborhood health
Hazardous materials management
Water/indoor air quality
Occupational health
Mosquito, rodent, and environmental control
Foodborne disease prevention
Geographic information systems

Figure 2–3 Marion County Health Department Organizational Structure. *Source:* Reprinted from *Marion County Health Department: A Brighter Tommorow*, 1994–1995 Report to the Community, 1996.

the two provider divisions: Population Health and Environmental Health. Population health maintains community programs in vital statistics, maternal and child health, acute and chronic disease, and WIC. Environmental health implements programs in hazardous materials management and water quality, environmental control, and foodborne disease prevention.[18]

Private Organizations

Public health services in the United States are provided both by governmental agencies and by private organizations including hospitals, private clinics, and voluntary agencies. The role of private organizations in public health practice is often overlooked by observers from both inside and outside the field.[12] While there are differences between the roles played by governmental agencies and those played by private organizations, they usually have a common mission of community health improvement. One study of 63 diverse local public health jurisdictions found that, on average, more than 26 percent of total community effort in public health activities was performed by organizations other than the official local health department.[19] Clearly, both public and private organizations are vitally important to the public health infrastructure of many communities.

At the national level, a variety of voluntary agencies are organized to respond to community health needs by providing services or taking action on a specific health-related issue. The American Diabetes Association, the American Cancer Society, The American Red Cross, and the American Lung Association are examples of national voluntary public health agencies. These organizations are generally focused around one central morbidity and provide education and resources to the public. They may also advocate for new government policies associated with their cause. In addition to this type of voluntary organization, citizen groups provide education and resources on community health issues. Examples of these groups are Alcoholics Anonymous, Mothers Against Drunk Driving, and Gay Men's Health Crisis.[2]

Professional societies, such as the American Medical Association, the American Nurses Association, the American Hospital Association, the Society for Public Health Education, and the American Public Health Association, are examples of expert organizations that promote public health policies. Professional associations are composed of people who are certified in the organization's professional field. Members promote their professional interest as well as community health needs.

Organizations that promote community health through the provision of funds are referred to as philanthropic foundations. These foundations promote public health by funding research and services. Examples of national foundations are the Robert Wood Johnson Foundation, the Milbank Memorial Fund, and the W.K. Kellogg Foundation. The Robert Wood Johnson Foundation, established in 1972, provides support for research programs that emphasize the improvement of access to primary medical and dental care. The Milbank Memorial Fund was established in 1905 and awards grants and fellowships furthering research in preventive medicine. The W.K. Kellogg Foundation was established in 1930 to promote the health and education of the public by providing financial assistance to institutions for a variety of public health issues.

At the state level, there are a variety of voluntary agencies that usually parallel the efforts of the national voluntary organizations. Professional associations organized at the state level represent the medical, nursing, social work, and public health professions, for example. There are also state health coalitions involved in promoting the health of certain populations or groups. At the local level, private practitioners, community hospitals, or media may draw attention to a local public health cause. These groups, as well as consumers and the media, are nonofficial agencies that can educate a community on public health issues and influence local government to make changes in policy.[2] Additionally, many private hospitals, clinics, and community and migrant health centers are critical providers of personal health services to uninsured and underinsured individuals. As such, these organizations participate in the vital public health function of ensuring access to health care services for vulnerable and disadvantaged population groups.

ROLE OF PUBLIC HEALTH

The IOM's 1988 report, *The Future of Public Health*, was a landmark document because it stated what many people feared: the health of the public was unnecessarily threatened because current capabilities for effective public health actions were inadequate. IOM recommended that public health agencies focus on their core functions of assessment, policy development, and assurance as a means to regain its capabilities to maintain conditions in which people can be healthy.[2]

Assessment

Public health departments are responsible for assessing the health care needs of their population. While there is no universal systematic framework for the assessment of community health status, community health agencies generally analyze health care statistics in an effort to evaluate the public health needs of their population. IOM recommends that at all levels, public health agencies "regularly and systematically collect, assemble, analyze and make available information on the health of the community, including statistics on health status, community health needs, and epidemiologic and other studies of health problems."[2(p7)] The core function of assessment concerns the evaluation of the health status of a community or population. Through the assessment process, information will be regularly and systematically collected for analysis and dissemination. Practices in public health that support the assessment process include assessing the health needs of a community, investigating the occurrence of health effects and hazards within the community, and analyzing the determinants of identified health needs.

Increasingly, a community-needs assessment is developed at the local level to describe the health status and needs of the community. Generally, needs assessments encompass the morbidity and mortality data of the community in an effort to identify potential risk factors. Through this process, community health agencies can identify and assess trends of potential health problems in a community. Once the identification process is complete, public health agencies usually assess the existing programs and practices to establish why these needs are not being adequately addressed.[4]

Policy Development

Through the initial assessment process, community health agencies can develop strategies and policies to address the identified health care needs of a population. These strategies include setting priorities and goals in an effort to create an effective intervention. Public health agencies also build constituencies with political leaders as a means to propose policy and create legislation to ensure a healthier community.

The policy development function in public health encompasses the development of policies that promote the health of a population. According to IOM, these policies should promote the use of the scientific knowledge base in policy development. Public health practices supporting the development of policy include advocating for public health through the establishment of constituencies and the identification of resources; prioritizing the health needs of a community; and planning policies to address these priorities.[4]

Assurance

The final essential function of public health agencies is to ensure that the health care needs of the population are being addressed. The assurance process may take the form of managing resources to establish programs that will address priority health care needs of the community. Assurance may also lead to the development of programs that will maximize the efforts of local community agencies to deliver needed public health services. An evaluation or quality assurance process is often incorporated into policy or program development to assess the inadequacies and changes needed in the programming process. As part of the assurance process, agencies may also inform and educate the public on community health issues of concern that will contribute toward a healthier community.[4]

Assurance of public health also involves making sure services are established to meet the health care needs of a community. Public health agencies may provide these needed services directly to the community or encourage the actions of other entities to provide identified services, which may include regulation. Practices in public health supporting assurance include: the management of resources and the development of organizational structure; the implementation of programs; the evaluation of the quality of programs; and informing and educating the public on matters associated with public health.[4]

NEW DEVELOPMENTS IN PUBLIC HEALTH PRACTICE

The 1988 IOM report was written to convey an urgent message that the American public health system was in disarray. Challenges such as HIV/AIDS, substance abuse, and access to care for the indigent were identified as crises that could only be solved by collective action. Since the publication of this landmark report, the public health environment has been reshaped by the challenges and potential opportunities associated with health care reform. In 1995, managed care plans covered approximately 1 in 5 Americans, and this number continues to grow. Medicaid, and the once sacred Medicare program, are being threatened by budget cuts and the reduction of services. Public distrust of government and its representative agencies is growing at a time when taxes are increasing and community health services are being reduced. These issues will undoubtedly affect the effectiveness of public health delivery in future generations.

Public Distrust of Government

One of the benefits of living in the United States is being a part of a democratic society. Unfortunately, the democratic policy-making process is not necessarily rational. "Sometimes this process is disjointed and incremental, other times it is more erratic and random."[20(p79)] Many community health problems require the assistance of a variety of governmental public health agencies. It is often a challenge to coordinate several bureaucratic organizations in an effort to quickly provide comprehensive health care to populations within a community. The growing distrust of the government bureaucracy was readily apparent during the elections of the 104th Congress in 1994. With their rubric of devolution, or less federal government, and more power to local communities, the Republicans gained majority power in the House and in the Senate. Clearly, voters have high expectations for services provided by their tax dollars. However, in a society where taxes are rising and services are being reduced, expectations are often higher than what the government can provide.

The Republican philosophy of devolution, in theory, is expected to increase efficiency and save money by giving states and local governments more authority in allocating resources. With this transfer of authority, the expectation is to significantly decrease the federal bureaucracy in terms of providing services and programs. While society emphasizes the need for less government, devolution of responsibility is often linked to a reduction in funds.[21] As funding for public health diminishes and as federal standards loosen, society's distrust of government will continue to grow.

Medicaid

The theory of devolution may also be applied to the federal- and state-funded Medicaid program. As Congress identifies ways to balance the budget, Medicare and Medicaid have become targets of debate. In 1995, the Republican Congress proposed reducing the Medicaid budget by 17% over seven years by turning the Medicaid program into a block grant to the states. Under a block grant program, the federal government would allocate a set amount of funds to the states to be used for Medicaid. Each state would have the latitude to use these funds to create its own Medicaid system, with few federal strings attached. It is believed that with the advent of Medicaid block grants, some savings would be achieved through a reduction in federal bureaucracy.

Clearly, Medicaid block grants would be designed to provide less money to the states and to the local governments than the current Medicaid system. With more flexibility, states may have the choice to increase taxes to fund current programs or eliminate needed services. Patients could be dropped from coverage and local health departments would be responsible for providing for the health needs of these individuals. "Medicaid reforms could worsen pressures on departments that already must cannibalize core population-wide programs to provide direct medical care to the indigent."[21(p 8)]

Collaboration

Faced with limited funds, public health must collaborate with unofficial agencies to clearly define and delineate roles in order to efficiently provide cost-effective services. With this delineation of authority, public health can implement a strategy to ensure that the health care needs of the community are being met. The assurance that the health care system operates to benefit the community is one of the core functions of public health. With a definition of roles, these stakeholders may also be held accountable for community health services provided to the community. Sophisticated and specialized organizations, such as those that focus on HIV/AIDS, substance abuse, or issues with the elderly, may more adequately meet the needs of the population when compared to the services provided by official agencies. Through partnerships and alliances with unofficial, specialized agencies, public health can diffuse and integrate its tools of assurance through its collaborations.

A health care environment that is driven by market forces will mean a very different organization of public health. Health care delivery is undergoing a rapid and turbulent transition as managed care changes the way health care is financed. As a mechanism to cope with this environmental change, strategic alliances are being created between public health agencies and other health care providers. "Strategic Alliances are defined as any formal arrangements between two or more organizations for purposes of mutual gain."[22] Alliances in public health allow organizations to work together as a means to share risks and costs, to share knowledge and capabilities, and to reach common objectives. Strategic alliances also allow an organization to enhance its ability to manage uncertainty and solve complex problems, develop opportunities to learn and adapt new competencies, gain mutual support, and respond to rapidly changing markets.[23]

Increasingly, as managed care plans become more prevalent in many communities, public health agencies are forming strategic alliances with managed care corporations. A local public health department may contract to provide primary and preventive services for a managed care plan that serves Medicaid enrollees, for example. In most cases, the local health department will continue to provide health services to members of the community who are not enrolled with the contracting managed care agency, as well as case-manage plan enrollees. As alliances between public health departments and managed care organizations evolve, clearly there is a potential to establish a more integrated health care delivery system for the community. With this more integrated system, public health departments may continue to provide education, policy development, and assurance initiatives to the community as well as to plan enrollees. There is the potential to invest the cost savings generated by the managed care component to improve and expand services provided by the public health component.[24]

Medicine and public health are also strengthening their collaboration at a time when both professions are experiencing extensive change. These alliances are being created because of changes in the public and private health finance system, the need to improve health system access, and the prevalence of behavioral diseases. "Both sectors face fiscal constraints that make collaboration essential: for medicine, the growth of managed care, with an emphasis on cost containment; and for public health, the dwindling budgets that threaten programs at all levels of government."[25] Alliances may involve informal relationships between public health clinics and community hospitals as a strategy to exchange patient referrals, for example. In some communities, local medicine societies are forming alliances to provide volunteer physicians and leadership to public health clinics.

However, quality public health care may be lost to cost containment. Clearly, the new health care environment requires that clinicians focus on the promotion of wellness and the prevention of disease. Thus, both professions must emphasize population-based intervention, as well as patient care. For example, a large Minnesota integrated delivery system is working with local public health authorities to identify populations at risk for diabetes in an effort to intervene before the onset of disease.[25]

Similar to those being formed between physicians and public health agencies, alliances are also being created between hospitals and public health groups. Hospitals are forced to provide a continuum of care as a criterion to contract with managed care organizations. Alliances with public health systems are allowing hospitals to provide community care as well as intervention programs. Thus, these systems are more "attractive" to contracting managed care organizations. In some communities, these alliances have evolved into an organization in which the hospital has fully integrated the public health agency into its system.

Privatization

"Traditionally, public health was seen as the province of the public health department; but increasingly, government agencies are contracting with private community-based providers to carry out service programs."[3(p34),5] As public health is being forced to reduce budgets, local governments are either privatizing or pairing up with private groups to reduce their financial risk of providing health care services. For example, in 1995 New York City and Los Angeles turned over the management of several of their community health care facilities to private providers. "Privatization shifts the authority and financial responsibility from the public governmental sectors to the private sector, offering advantages in a competitive environment. The bureaucracy that characterizes public institutions often prevents government owned health care organizations from responding to competition."[26(p20)]

It is believed that privatization of some official public health programs will save money and salvage programs that would otherwise be abandoned due to fiscal constraints. The near-bankruptcy of the Los Angeles public health system could have left hundreds of thousands of people without ambulatory medical care services. The privatization of the management and staffing of Los Angeles' ambulatory care clinics is expected to save the local government at least $1 million in salaries and benefits.[27] Public health agencies may then concentrate their funds on core population–based services for the entire population. For example, one agency in California no longer provides comprehensive personal health services for its community, but it continues to manage essential services aimed at water safety, education, and other community-wide concerns (Exhibit 2–1).[5]

Managed Care

Since the publication of the IOM's 1988 report on public health, the growth of managed care has provided new challenges and opportunities for governmental public health agencies in interacting with private organizations. Recognizing these changes, a new IOM report on public health calls attention to the need for greater collaboration with the evolving health care organizations in the private sector.[3] A managed care organization provides health benefits for its enrollees or "covered lives." These benefits are provided through its network of health care providers. The managed care organization usually manages the practices of its providers as a means to reduce the cost of unnecessary procedures and improve efficiency. With this paradigm shift to reduce expensive inpatient admissions and to reduce health care costs, marketplace trends have advanced the goals of

Exhibit 2–1 Essential Public Health Services

- monitor health status to identify and solve community health problems
- diagnose and investigate health problems and health hazards in the community
- inform, educate, and empower people about health issues
- mobilize community partnerships and action to solve health problems
- develop policies and plans to support individual and community health efforts
- enforce laws and regulations that protect health and assure safety
- link people to needed personal health services and assure the provision of health care when otherwise unavailable
- assure a competent workforce in public health and personal care
- evaluate effectiveness, accessibility, and quality of personal and population-based health services
- research new insights and innovative solutions to health problems

Source: Reprinted with permission from *Journal of the American Medical Association*, 1994, Vol. 272, pp. 1276–1282.

---

wellness and prevention and created opportunities for innovative partnerships between public health agencies and private providers.

As health reform proceeds and as governments reduce their funding for community health services, some public health agencies are transferring their role of providing direct personal health care for indigent populations to managed care organizations and other private providers. Managed care organizations have proliferated in the United States due to the belief that they can deliver services to their enrollees more efficiently and cost-effectively than traditional fee-for-service plans. With this belief, public health agencies are opting to contract with managed care organizations to provide personal health services to those enrolled in such programs as Medicaid. In 1996, there were an estimated 90 million Americans enrolled in managed care plans. Included in this number were more than 25% of the nation's Medicaid beneficiaries and 10% of the nation's Medicare beneficiaries.[28,3]

"Managed care's population-based approach and emphasis on prevention are more in step with public health than medicine's traditional, diagnose and cure focus."[29(p18)] Both sectors share the same approaches of emphasizing disease prevention and managing the care of individuals based on a population approach. Also, a collaboration with managed care may furnish an opportunity for public health to contribute and acquire innovative methods of assurance. Some managed care organizations have been monitoring the health outcomes of enrollees and their utilization of services. Clearly, these data collection methods can augment the assessment and assurance of public health. Further, efforts such as the Health Plan Employer Data and Information Set by the National Committee for Quality

Assurance have the potential to systemize accountability measures for those collaborating with managed care.

However, as community health agencies collaborate with managed care, there is a concern that this partnership may force the public health agency to only target plan enrollees instead of the general population. Further, preventive procedures which are not effective in lowering health care costs may not be implemented or embraced under the managed care philosophy. "In actual practice, some managed care organizations seem more concerned about efficiency and controlling short-run costs than about prevention or the health status of their members. Governmental public health agencies have a geographic perspective and are accountable to the people within their jurisdiction while many managed care organizations focus on current enrollees, an ever changing group, who may only be a subset of the population."[3(p 16)] With managed care's emphasis on the bottom-line, there is a clear motivation for plans to shy away from enrolling high-risk patients and to only focus on enrollees rather than providing prevention efforts to the general population.

CONCLUSION

The United States public health system has had a long history of ensuring clean water and safe food, controlling infectious disease, and providing health services for special populations. Public health is organized at the national, state, and local level and may be composed of both governmental and nongovernmental agencies. Public health delivery varies widely at state and local levels, but in virtually all circumstances, public and private agencies share responsibilities for public health functions.

Pressures to contain expenditures at all levels of government have introduced uncertainties into the funding mechanisms for public health services. These uncertainties are emerging at a time when there are new threats of antibiotic-resistant infections, chronic disease, and new and re-emerging infectious disease. In addition, managed care is changing the health care delivery systems with which public health agencies must interact. Public health agencies may experience both opportunities and challenges in establishing partnerships with these emerging organizations.[3] Recognizing the opportunities and anticipating the challenges created by these new developments requires strong and effective leadership in public health. Otherwise, public health is likely to continue as its own worst enemy in striving to influence and manage the changes brought about through such developments as privatization and managed care.[30] As public health agencies confront their changing environments, strategic alliances and partnerships with the private sector may allow them to maintain a focus on the core functions of assessment, assurance, and policy development.

REFERENCES

1. Elders J. The future of U.S. public health. *JAMA*. 1995;269:2293–2294.
2. Institute of Medicine. *The Future of Public Health*. Washington, DC: National Academy Press; 1988.
3. Institute of Medicine. *Healthy Communities: New Partnerships for the Future of Public Health*. Washington, DC: National Academy of Sciences; 1996.
4. Dyal WW. Ten organizational practices of public health: a historical perspective. *Am J Prev Med*. 1995;11:6–8.
5. Baker EL, Melton RJ, Strange PV, Fields ML, et al. Health reform and the health of the public: forging community health partnerships. *JAMA*. 1994;272:1276–1282.
6. National Association of County and City Health Officials. *Assessment Protocol for Excellence in Public Health*. Washington, DC: NACCHO; 1991.
7. Turnock B, Handler A. *Surveillance of Effective Public Health Practice: Preliminary and Draft Set of Performance Standards and Performance Indicators*. Chicago: University of Illinois at Chicago; 1992.
8. Miller CA, Moore KS, Richards TB, Monk JD. A proposed method for assessing the performance of local public health functions and practices. *Am J Public Health*. 1994;84:1743–1749.
9. Scutchfield FD, Spain C, Pointer DD, Hafey JM. The public health leadership institute: training for state and local health officers. *J Public Health Policy*. 1993;16:304–323.
10. Halverson PK, Mays GP, Kaluzny AD, House RM. Developing leaders in public health: the role of executive training programs. *J Health Adm Educ*. In press.
11. Greene L, Ottoson J. *Community Health*. 7th ed. St. Louis, Mo: Mosby–Year Book Publishing; 1994.
12. Turnock BJ. *Public Health: What It Is and How It Works*. Gaithersburg, Md: Aspen Publishers; 1997.
13. Lazere EP, Porter KH, Summer L. *How Many People Are Eligible for WIC?* Washington, DC: Center on Budget and Policy Practices; 1991.
14. Publicly funded HIV counseling and testing—United States, 1991. *MMWR*. 1992;41:613.
15. *HHS Initiatives To Combat Emerging Infectious Diseases*. Centers for Disease Control and Prevention; June 12, 1996. Press release.
16. Mullan F, Smith J. *Characteristics of State and Local Health Agencies*. Baltimore, Md: Johns Hopkins School of Hygiene and Public Health; 1988.
17. National Association of County and City Health Officials. *1992–1993 National Profile of Local Health Departments*. Washington, DC: NACCHO; 1995.
18. Marion County Health Department. *Marion County Health Department: A Brighter Tomorrow. 1994–1995 Report to the Community*. Indianapolis, Ind: MCHD; 1996.
19. Halverson PK, Miller CA, Kuluzny AD, Fried BJ, et al. Performing public health functions: the perceived contribution of public health and other community agencies. *J Health Hum Serv Adm*. 1996;18:288–303.
20. Lindblom CE. The science of muddling through. *Public Adm Rev*. 1959;19:79–88.
21. Kent C. Feds act to shed role as guardian of nation's health. *Am Med News*. 1996;39:5–8.
22. Zajac EJ, D'Aunno TA. Managing strategic alliances. In: Shortell S, Kaluzny AD, eds. *Health Care Management: Organizational Design and Behavior*. 3rd ed. Albany, NY: Delmar Publishers; 1994:355–391.

23. Zuckerman HS, Kaluzny AD, Ricketts TC. Alliances in health care: what we know, what we think we know, and what we should know. *Health Care Manage Rev.* 1995;201:54–64.

24. Halverson PK, Mays GP, Kaluzny AD, Richards TB. Not-so-strange bedfellows: models of interaction between care plans and public health agencies. *Milbank Q.* 1997;75:113–138.

25. Hearn W. Time for medicine, public health to join forces. *Am Med News.* 1996;39:3–4.

26. Metsch JM, Haley DR, Malafronte D. Privatization of a public hospital: a quality improvement strategy. *Qual Manage Health Care.* 1997;5:19–24.

27. Shelton D. Agencies short on cash are turning to the private sector. *Am Med News.* 1996;39:14.

28. Rosenbaum S, Richards TB. Medicaid managed care and public health policy. *J Public Health Manage Pract.* 1996;2:76–82.

29. Hearn W. Health agencies pursue partnerships with 'bottom-line' medicine. *Am Med News.* 1996;39:18–19.

30. Coye MJ, Roper WL, Saege W. *Leadership in Public Health.* Boston, Mass: Milbank Memorial Fund; 1994.

CHAPTER 3

Managed Care and Its Relationship to Public Health: Barriers and Opportunities

Curtis P. McLaughlin

Managed health care is

> a regrettably nebulous term. At the very least, [it] is a system of health care delivery that tries to manage the cost of health care, the quality of health care, and access to that care. Common denominators include a panel of contracted providers that is less than the entire universe of available providers, some type of limitations on benefits to subscribers who use noncontracted providers (unless authorized to do so), and some type of authorization system. Managed health care is a spectrum of systems from so-called managed indemnity, through PPOs, POS, open panel HMOs, and closed panel HMOs.[1]

In other words, it is the broad set of alternatives to traditional, fee-for-service medicine in which a rational management other than an individual provider is assumed to be in charge of trading off between cost, quality, and access over some time horizon. Issues of cost, quality, and access have long been concerns in the public health arena. Therefore, there is a common set of interests between managed care and public health, although the approaches may differ widely.

One might even suggest that managed care organizations, public health decision makers, and governmental leaders have three different orderings of these performance criteria. A characteristic ordering among these sectors by priority is:

Managed Care	Public Health	Legislators
Cost	Access	Cost
Quality	Quality	Access
Access	Cost	Quality

The time horizons also differ with for-profit organizations that have publicly held stock and are concerned with periods of 3 to 12 months; entrepreneurial nonprofits concerned with periods of one to two years; legislatures with periods of two to four years; and public health officials with periods of one to 20 years. (The distinction between donative, entrepreneurial, and membership nonprofits is discussed in more detail in Chapter 5.)

MANAGED CARE IN THE PUBLIC SECTOR

Federal and state governments have not been passive spectators in the development of managed care. As their share of the U.S. health care dollar has increased, so has their buying power and their willingness to use the bargaining leverage that this implies. Although they were relative latecomers to the health insurance business, governments quickly became major players once they were involved.

HISTORY OF HEALTH CARE FINANCING

Prepayment for health care in the United States dates back at least to the 1930s Blue Cross plans, if not the 1880s Mayo Clinic practices.[2] The first major efforts were the attempts of hospitals to have their bills prepaid, which resulted in the then hospital-owned Blue Cross associations and later the Blue Shield programs for physician bills. Before World War II, relatively few Americans had health insurance. For the most part, physicians took whatever people could pay. The urban indigent went to the teaching hospitals, where care was free because learners and volunteers were delivering it.

Things started to change during World War II, when the government instituted wage and price controls and developments such as sulfa drugs and antibiotics gave providers the tools to do much more for their patients. Workers were heavily unionized, and collective bargaining was the norm in the heavy industries that produced wartime weaponry. The Office of Price Administration insisted on holding the line on wages, but placated a restless workforce by allowing workers and management to expand fringe benefit payments through collective bargaining. Health insurance expanded rapidly during that period. It was soon accepted as part of the employment package in the collective bargaining process. Most of these employer-financed programs were indemnity contracts involving fee-for-service medicine. They set the stage for a national policy of health care that was employer-financed and involved dependents as well as workers. That is how U.S. health care financing became associated with the workplace.

Since it was part of the collective bargaining process, the elected union leadership wanted a package allowing most union members to experience benefit payments. Employers were indifferent to its terms, since it was part of a fixed-wage payment package. Union leadership was free to allocate this benefit as they saw fit. This led to the system of first dollar coverage rather than one focused on catastrophic illness. In fact, lifetime payments to enrollees were capped at relatively low levels. But there was very little concern about those who did not participate in the collective bargaining process and about the cost of health care.

Cost-Shifting Starts

The Blue Cross/Blue Shield (BC/BS) associations, owned by hospitals and medical societies, represented the primary point of departure from published fee schedules (charges) as the basis for payment. Since what was involved for Blue Cross and the hospitals was essentially transferring money from one nonprofit pocket to another, they agreed that the basis for transfer would be a fair share of the costs. These fair shares were established using a relatively complicated cost-finding (step-down) system based on activities performed on the patient, such as the number of X-rays, bed-days, and operating room hours.

With BC/BS associations paying costs and some patients being unable to pay at all, the other payers were asked to pay "charges," which hospital boards increased above costs sufficiently to cover uncompensated care. Thus began the practice of cost-shifting. At first, other insurers, representing employer and labor groups, did not object too strongly to this price discrimination. This is because other mechanisms were available to cover the needs of uninsured patients, such as free care at the teaching hospitals provided by faculty, many of whom donated their clinical time.

Enter Medicare and Medicaid

In 1965, part of the excluded population's needs were addressed through the establishment of Medicare. At this point, millions of individuals achieved access to paid health care. The new law, however, contained a phrase (the result of last-minute compromise) requiring that all physicians, including hospital-based physicians (anesthesiologists, pathologists, and radiologists) be paid directly for their services. This guaranteed a fee-for-service system for many years. Physician incomes rose rapidly, since no new capacity was generated by the program. However, there was little concern about the ability of the trust fund to pay for these services. The Medicare program followed the pattern established in collective bargaining, except that only hospital costs were covered. Physician bills could be covered by a separate, privately funded premium. Long-term care and drugs were not covered.

Several years later, Medicaid was introduced as part of the Great Society's programs. This was an add-on paid for by a combination of federal, state, and local monies. One had to be below the poverty line and even lower in many cases, low enough to be eligible for public assistance. Here there was concern for specific underserved groups—pregnant mothers, children on welfare, elderly in nursing homes, and care for the mentally retarded. The latter in many cases actually represented the transfer of a state liability to the federal government. Medicaid, like other programs, was a fee-for-service plan, but with heavily discounted fees. In some states, less than half the eligible physicians participated. There has always been an access problem despite the availability of payment.

With Medicare and Medicaid, hospitals and medical school faculties stopped focusing on charity care and began maximizing departmental clinical revenues in response to these stimuli. Patients who had been unable to pay had a charge card and were empowered to shop around for care. Many charity wards and teaching clinics, with their volunteer faculty, disappeared. Indigent patients wanted the same care as other Americans, and the institutions could bill the government for the services that once had been provided free. For a while, there was an income bonanza among providers.

Expanding Eligibilities

One must have been associated with the social security system to be eligible for Medicare. Therefore, one had to have been healthy and working at one time or currently be indigent in order to be able to get government-financed health care. However, some programs such as MediCal (California's Medicaid program) did provide categorical coverage for some chronic, catastrophic illnesses, such as hemophilia. The federal government added kidney dialysis to Medicare as a categorical eligibility, and many patients, such as the mentally ill, also became eligible for Medicare.

Most states continued to expand coverages for pregnant women as a cost-effective measure to control the skyrocketing costs of neonatal care. As time went on, the Medicaid program began to expand to include older children and raise the barrier for some services to as much as 185% of the poverty level. However, local and state governments became increasingly concerned about the costs of the Medicaid program.

Privatization

Most municipalities are averse to the open-ended payment requirements of Medicaid. If they rely on real estate taxes, these are set early in the fiscal year and cannot be revised once set. They also often lack the means to borrow efficiently. Further, many local governments also have owned or subsidized hospitals to meet local needs, including the indigent population. However, these institutions and their ability to spend and lose money have grown rapidly and, in the absence of cross-subsidization from other programs, represent a potential source of financial embarrassment to the local government. Recently, for-profit entities have come forward offering to buy these institutions, thereby relieving the local government of that underwriting risk and of future capital requirements for modernization and improvements, and to put the property onto the tax rolls and pay property taxes.

The federal government and the states and municipalities began to exert their buying power, demanding the same advantage that BC/BS patients had and paying "costs." With much of the former charity care being compensated, earlier mechanisms for delivering care to the uninsured were virtually dismantled. Teaching clinics, once free, became major revenue sources for hospitals and for the compensation of medical school faculty.[3] Full-time clinical faculty were added to service this demand and generate additional revenue. The remainder of the uncompensated care became a cost to be shifted to the indemnity insurers other than BC/BS and the governments. Charges as a percentage of costs rose to 125% to 133% to cover the costs not covered or disallowed by the privileged providers, especially the federal and state governments who were paying for 30% to 60% of the care.

An Expanding Federal Role

Because of their accountability requirements as public programs, Medicare and Medicaid and then the Civilian Health and Medical Program of the Uniformed Services began to manage their costs more closely, adopting developing systems of prospective payment such as diagnosis-related groups, which were first field tested by the state of New Jersey. These public programs began incorporating more and more of the methods used by private managed care plans, such as prior certification requirements for hospital admissions (called "preadmission certification"); uniform payment schedules for physicians; incentives for physicians to charge patients no more than the fees specified in the uniform payment schedules (called "accepting assignment"); and contracts that give public programs discounts on the standard fees charged by hospitals and other providers.

Management Responds

Labor and management saw the costs of indemnity premiums soar and recognized that this was one factor involved in competing with manufacturing based in countries without comparable health services. In the late 1980s and throughout the early 1990s, they turned to managed care as their way of dealing with cost-shifting and cost-inflation issues. They turned to health maintenance organizations (HMOs) as their answer to the need for negotiated rates.

HMOs were not new. The United States has had managed care for more than 60 years, but it was long confined to a limited arena within the health care sector. It was cost-effective, but ran contrary to the ideology that defined the way that health care had been organized and financed in the United States since World War II. Some plans, such as Kaiser-Permanente, had long proven that premium costs could be cut sharply with managed care that included closed panels of physicians and integration of primary care, hospital care, and specialist care into a single economic and decision-making system. However, these early HMOs remained a small proportion of the industry, operating with a self-selected population of physicians willing to work for a salary or a salary plus very limited incentives.[4] Most physicians chose to operate in the fee-for-service environment where the influx of money, the idiosyncrasies of legislation, and the ensuing regulation had rapidly inflated physician income.

Managed care, except in the areas where it has grown up organically as an alternative means of delivery, has been stimulated by the desire of employers to reduce the skyrocketing costs of health care. Large industrial firms with heavily unionized work forces began to observe that the health care bill was rising faster than most other wage costs and putting them at a competitive disadvantage domestically and internationally. Unions also became concerned, because health care issues were dominating the bargaining and also dividing the interests of the workers in the packages contracted for. Young workers wanted more take-home pay, while older workers and retirees preferred tax-sheltered health care benefits. Therefore, union officers also became concerned about controlling the costs of health care. A significant number of strikes in recent years have centered on issues of constraining health care benefits.

Managed care options mostly involving group or staff model HMOs, already proven to save about one-third of the premium dollar, were available in many areas. In response, companies offered their employees managed care options and began to reduce the attractiveness of indemnity plan options with higher premiums and greater copayments and deductibles. Companies have been reluctant to force their employees into any one plan; they have continued to offer a series of choices, some of which are attractive and some of which are not.

Since insurance contracts with these employers have been large and potentially lucrative, a number of organizations have sprung up to compete for their business on the basis of reduced costs and acceptable employee satisfaction. Most of the cost reduction has come in the form of constraints on the use of expensive resources such as hospital days and specialist visits. Practice guidelines have been developed and gradually enforced. High-cost providers have been culled out. More recently, individuals, practices, and institutions have merged to provide greater and greater control of methods of care delivery and to industrialize what has long been accepted as a cottage industry—albeit one with technology replacing some of the craft involved.[5] Note the system that has been left by this process. It is one with no attention paid to capacity, especially capacity to provide access for the indigent, except in a limited number of communities. Likewise, it has no funding for indigent care except through Medicaid. It is also important to note that there has been no attempt to determine how to support the costs of medical education, a substantial portion of which has been financed through the clinical incomes of specialists and subspecialists on the clinical faculty.

STAGES OF MANAGED CARE MARKET MATURITY

Managed care is different in each medical market, depending on the power of the players in the equation of payers, patients, providers, and planners. Shortell and colleagues[6] suggest a four-stage model of maturation of managed care markets. Stage 1, of unstructured access markets with relatively little market penetration (managed < 20%) and relatively independent players, is followed by stage 2, a loose cost market with alliances being forged and 20–40% managed care penetration. In stage 3, the consolidated advanced cost arenas, inpatient bed numbers are significantly reduced following mergers and consolidations, managed care penetration is 40–60%, and the majority of physicians move into groups. By stage 4, the strict managed care value market, the consolidation has reached 3–5 dominant providers in major metropolitan markets, capitation emerges as a force, managed care penetration exceeds 60%, and 75% or more of physicians are in groups. Shortell suggests that it is in stage 3 that one sees concern with disease prevention and health promotion developing among the providers, and in stage 4 that they become concerned with planning for a population and with stronger partnerships with public health and other community agencies. That is borne out by the cases reported in this book and is consistent with the reasoning in several chapters.

THE LIMITED ROLE OF HEALTH DEPARTMENTS

Health departments have been very inconsistent from state to state in the levels of care offered, ranging along a spectrum of primary care to preventive care only. There is no consensus in the country that the public health system has any responsibility for the provision of acute care to any population in the community, except for specific situations involving communicable diseases such as tuberculosis and sexually transmitted diseases as noted in Chapter 2. They do seem to get involved in the stage 3 and stage 4 markets once they can deal with provider networks, which have developed considerable political and economic clout.

However, it is yet to be determined what will happen in those markets that do not progress to stages 3 and 4 and how the public health establishment can take a leadership role in the more fragmented markets of stage 1 and stage 2 communities.

ACCESS, COST, AND QUALITY UNDER MANAGED CARE

Much has been written about the potential impact of managed care on access, cost, and quality. These three aspects of managed care for public health are discussed next.

Access

Access often is the first issue that arises in the public health context. Many populations, such as Medicaid recipients, have experienced restricted access in markets dominated by fee-for-service medicine. One right that a vendor (i.e., provider) has in the U.S. legal system is not to accept business. This, however, can be limited by constraints on discrimination against specific classes of customers on unacceptable grounds, such as race or religion. Yet it is not unusual under fee-for-service medicine to find areas in which less than half of the physicians take Medicaid patients. The grounds cited are many, including low payment scales, bureaucratic red tape and slow payment, adequate demand from other populations yielding more net income, and nonacceptance of Medicaid patients by other patient groups. There is little doubt, however, that much of the reluctance, especially as expressed in the last point, represents racial and ethnic discrimination.

Therefore, it has been access as well as cost control that has motivated the use of managed care delivered through HMOs to public sector dependents. A good indicator of the access problem is the level of usage of emergency departments by disadvantaged populations. This is also a source of excess costs, but one closely linked to alternative means of access. The development of HMOs designed to serve that population or their integration into the delivery network of existing HMOs has had a startling impact on this indicator of access. For example, when Group Health of Puget Sound acquired a contract with the state of Washington in the Olympia, Washington, area to enroll a Medicaid population, Group Health, which does have clinics open from 7 AM to 9 PM, saw the emergency department utilization in this population drop by 90%. Tennessee's TennCare program experienced similar changes in the utilization of emergency departments once patients were given access to care through an HMO.

This emphasis on access represents a departure from health care industry practice. Restricting access (underwriting) has been a primary way that insurers have kept costs down. Underwriting is a process that analyzes the expected costs associated with a potential or renewing client. It accepts people who are expected to be profitable and rejects or increases premiums for people who represent a history of or exhibit a potential for losses. One of the most distressing practices has been the cancellation of policies, particularly those of small employers when one or more enrollees is identified as having a chronic or catastrophic illness.

Cost

In the private sector, cost is the primary concern of employers selecting group health insurance programs. "Efficiency can serve quality, so long as the judgments are truly made in the patient's interest. But you can't be sure that's always the case. Employers pick health plans based on service and price. They get *assurances* of quality but no proof."[7] There is an accreditation process, administered by the National Commission for Quality Assurance (NCQA), managed on behalf of the insurers. However, as of early 1997 only 35% of the country's HMOs had full or partial accreditation. This process does not yet include clinical outcomes, and certainly is far away from looking at population-specific outcomes.

Cost information is of interest to corporate health care purchasers. Historically, inflation in medical care motivated a corporate push away from indemnity care. Rates of inflation in managed care have been brought back into line with the general economy by the intervention of managed care for more than two-thirds of insured Americans. Physicians' incomes have been constrained sufficiently to cause an actual decline in their average income in 1994 and since. The physician group most affected has been the specialists, especially those that are hospital based. The incomes of gatekeeper primary care physicians have actually risen during the same period. So HMOs have shown to corporate America that they can deliver the goods cost-wise, and they have been taking the same arguments to the public sector.

Quality

Assessing the quality of managed care organizations is still an infant science. There are some measures available, but they seem to have little influence on the industry or on consumer choices.[7] A new initiative launched by the Joint Commission on Accreditation of Healthcare Organizations (Joint Commission) requires that health care organizations select a set of quality indicators for implementation over the period 1997–1999 and implement them. The initiative, termed Project ORYX to emphasize its uniqueness, identifies some 60 systems of assessment that an organization might choose to use. Possibly, these systems may lead to performance-based reimbursement similar to those linked to immunization rates in the United Kingdom and to multiple health status indicators in U.S. HMOs.[8-10] Halverson and colleagues[11] suggest that performance-based reimbursement might be more effective than formal accountability systems.

For the interim, the key control mechanism in privatization will be the contracting mechanism. State and local public health agencies will have to develop specific skills to manage such contracts. To do so, the contract administrators will have to specify the service packages and practices that private organizations should provide; be able to monitor and evaluate compliance with these specifications; and mobilize the political power to enforce those specifications. These specifications should be for clinical services *and* for support services such as transportation and language translation. They should also apply to collecting and analyzing quality assurance data, limiting disenrollment of clients, acceptable marketing practices involving Medicaid enrollees, and involving public health departments and community health centers as providers under these contracts. Performance monitoring of both in-house and contract providers should include measurements of health outcomes, levels of service activity, cost, access and the makeup of the enrollee populations, and customer satisfaction. With this information, the contract administrators and contractors must be able to continue to improve the process through periodic process and outcome reviews.[12]

Even with an effective contracting process, the design and implementation of these new delivery relationships must still provide for a number of functions still in the public domain. This might involve restructuring the public providers, providing funds for key functions, and preserving the availability and quality of population-based services. It also means realigning service jurisdictions and geographical boundaries to match up better with regional health care markets.

There is a danger that overall quality measures may not apply to the population segment being served. It has been shown that in three urban HMOs, the elderly, the chronically ill, and the sickest patients did worse compared to similar patients in traditional plans, whereas younger, working adults appeared to do equally well under either circumstance.[7] This is an especially important concern, since there is already some evidence that managed care will have trouble maintaining the service levels provided to subpopulations with significant special needs. For example, a study of services to children with special needs enrolled in Medicaid managed care shows that, while their traditional medical needs were met equally well, the managed care servers did not do as well as fee-for-service plans at early identification and treatment of behavioral, development, and emotional problems.[13]

There are three types of measures of quality that should be considered: perceived quality, technical quality, and outcomes. Perceived quality exists in the eye of the beholder, the customer, the patient. It is measured through surveys of customer satisfaction and through questions about intent to use the service in the future as well as whether one would recommend it to a friend. Technical quality is the perception of quality as concluded by technical experts after examining the process through observation, chart review, process review, and asking questions of care deliverers and patients. The decision as to whether or not to keep mothers in the hospital more than 24 hours after a normal delivery is a technical decision, although it is one about which patients and their families also have perceptions of quality in mind. Outcomes are just that, objective measures of what the health care system achieved for its participants. Such measures include the percentage of depressed patients readmitted within 365 days and rates of communicable diseases among school-aged children. All three sets of quality measures are valid for specific purposes and are typically gathered in the managed care arena.

A SAMPLE CONTRACT: THE CASE OF NORTH CAROLINA

North Carolina's model contract with managed care plans serving Medicaid beneficiaries illustrates many of the salient issues that must be addressed through arrangements between purchasers and health plans. This contract, shown in full in Appendix A, was established in 1996 for managed care plans participating in a mandatory enrollment, capitated-reimbursement demonstration program for Medicaid beneficiaries in Mecklenburg County, which includes the state's largest city (Charlotte). This program operates under a 1915(b) demonstration waiver from the federal Health Care Financing Administration, also granted in 1996. Note the amount of detail involved in this contract by a relative latecomer to this type of contracting. The state is not buying a standard product from an HMO, but had decided to deliver a product for parts of its covered populations. The matters of concern to the state include:

- Length of contract. Contract is three years with a possible extension of three years. This gives the HMO a chance to be concerned about prevention and reduces the administrative costs to both parties.
- Enrollment eligibles. Eligibility is defined carefully. Note that this does not include the medically needy as the Washington State mental health plan did.
- Provider choice within plan. This allows the enrollees to select among the possible providers belonging to this HMO.
- Plan composition. The plan must strive for a 25% composition of non-Medicaid enrollees.

- Independent health benefit manager. This prohibits the plan from doing its own enrolling and presumably limits the possibility for adverse selection against the state. This means that the plan must assume the underwriting risk controlled by someone else.
- Plan transfers. The participants in a plan can move to another plan throughout the year.
- Marketing. Note that the plan may advertise its services, but must have its media materials approved by the state. The plan may not solicit door-to-door nor offer financial inducements to potential enrollees.
- Covered services. The plan must offer or cover a wide range of services, including emergency medical care. Exclusion does not mean that these services are not provided under other contracts to the same population, so that these patients may still be getting mental health services, prescription drugs, and nursing home care.
- Accessibility of services. The plan must have adequate numbers of providers for all of the covered services, including 24-hour, seven-days-per-week toll-free telephone contact. It outlines in Section 6.5 specific maximum waiting times for various levels of service urgency. Patients with appointments must not wait more than one hour, while emergencies must be seen immediately and other walk-ins within two hours.
- Provider choices. The plan may not assign more than 2000 clients to any one full-time-equivalent provider. A weaker provision is that the Plan is "encouraged" to continue to use the providers that currently serve this population, including federally qualified health centers, school-based health services, and county health departments. However, it is interesting to note that Mecklenburg County is one area where the clinical delivery role of the county health department has since been absorbed by one of the city's integrated delivery systems. Section 6.10 also insists that the plan have or contract for hospital beds (one per 727 enrollees), specialists, a medical director, data processing, and quality assurance. The plan also must have the capacity to provide member orientations as detailed in Section 6.10 and provide an initial health assessment visit within 90 days of enrollment. It must also deliver a range of preventive services, including early and periodic screening, diagnosis, and treatment, childbirth education and parenting, smoking cessation, self-care for diabetics, and nutrition assessment, education, and counseling.
- Support services. This contract includes specific support services, including transportation, interpreter services, and referral services to community resources, including WIC and out-of-plan services.
- Payments from members. There are no copayments, deductibles, or other collections from patients allowed.

- Quality assurance/quality improvement. The state can require two focused studies from a list provided and also a series of member satisfaction surveys and retrospective medical records reviews. The plan must also submit to outside audits as required.
- Medical records and data. There are specific requirements for medical records and maintaining a common data set.
- Activity reporting. There are monthly requirements for reporting activity data.
- Rates. The state provides a set of rates of payment that are shown in the rate sheet appendix, including calculated effective discounts off fee-for-service Medicare upper limits. The contract also includes the method by which the state will set rates in future years.
- Grounds for termination. While these sections include the usual reasons to terminate, such as fraud and abuse, one disconcerting provision basically says that the state will not spend more money than is appropriated and can terminate the contract if it runs out of money.

The contract also includes a useful glossary of relevant terms.

North Carolina's Medicaid managed care contract provides a useful example of how states may approach the task of transitioning public beneficiaries into private, capitated managed health care systems. This contract should by no means be interpreted as representative of all state approaches. Recent efforts to compare and evaluate state Medicaid managed care contracts reveal a relatively high degree of variation in contract provisions.[14]

THE VOCABULARY OF MANAGED CARE

Any description of managed care must deal with the array of acronyms that have developed in this field. While presenting the definitions of the various organizational arrangements for delivering managed care, a colleague once noted, "You know, this whole field suffers from TMA—Too Many Acronyms." This alphabet soup can be daunting unless one finds a structure for mapping alternative ways of looking at the relationships and the risks and incentives involved. Because of the potential for organizational arrangements between the public sector and the health care industry, ways of looking at risks and relationships will be examined first, rather than the acronyms.

MAPPING THE RELATIONSHIP OF MANAGED CARE AND PUBLIC HEALTH

In order to ensure the delivery of health care to a population, the system (or nonsystem) providing the care must deal with five generic sources of risk:

- Underwriting risk—identifying correctly the population involved and its likely utilization of resources so that an appropriate charge can be assessed. Underwriting has been a primary tool for insurers in controlling costs by restricting the access of the chronically ill and at-risk enrollees.
- Marketing risk—being able to sell sufficient individuals on the program offered to make it operationally and financially viable, given effective handling of the other risks.
- Financial risk—avoiding financial collapse due to lack of revenue, excess costs, or both, as well as the effective management of cash flows to avoid default and/or bankruptcy.
- Operational risk—being able to deliver the quantity and quality of services required to meet the perceived needs and the technically defined needs of the patient and payer population involved.
- Regulatory risk—meeting the requirements of various regulatory agencies such as the state insurance regulators, the Health Care Financing Administration (HCFA), the National Institutes of Health, and the Occupational Safety and Health Administration. There are also other regulatory risks imposed by specific health care legislation relating to Corporate Practice of Medicine acts, mandatory benefit and anti–managed care laws, requirements of the Employee Retirement Income Security Act (ERISA), Medicare and Medicaid fraud and abuse regulations, and antitrust laws.

Table 3–1 illustrates how one might characterize the allocation of these risks under varying forms of managed health care arrangements. The types of arrangements displayed are fee-for-service (first dollar coverage), fee-for-service with deductibles and coinsurance, preferred provider with negotiated fees, capitation, and point-of-service plans. These are intended to be illustrative only, since other arrangements involving hybrids of these (such as fee-for-service plans with negotiated rates that also involve deductibles and coinsurance).

- Fee-for-service (first dollar coverage). In this system, most of the risk is borne by the insurer. The insurer has to select the population properly and market the policy. However, providers must also compete against each other for the patient's business, since the patient can choose any provider. Providers can set their own prices to ensure profitability, passing the operational risks on to the insurer. The financial risks would therefore be with the insurer. The patients are not sharing these risks, since first dollar coverage is involved. Each would be responsible for a specific set of regulatory risks, which do not change very much with the type of plan involved.
- Fee-for-service with deductibles and coinsurance. The addition of deductibles and coinsurance makes the patient somewhat more aware of the cost of the services. The patient does not assume much financial risk, but the patient's

Table 3–1 Allocations of Risks among Representative Managed Care Arrangements: Primary Bearer of Risk by Type of Service

	Risk type				
Service type	Underwriting	Marketing	Financial	Operational	Regulatory
Fee-for-service	Insurer	Insurer/ provider	Insurer	Insurer	Insurer/ provider
Fee-for-service with deductibles and coinsurance	Insurer	Insurer/ provider	Insurer	Insurer/ provider	Insurer/ provider
Preferred provider with discounted fees	Insurer/ provider	Insurer	Insurer/ provider	Provider/ insurer/ patient	Insurer/ provider
Capitation	Provider	Insurer	Provider	Provider/ patient	Insurer/ provider
Point-of-service plan	Insurer	Insurer/ provider	Insurer/ patient/ provider	Insurer/ provider/ patient	Insurer/ provider

concern about the costs associated with utilization will mean that the provider must get more involved in the marketing of the services and in the effective operation of the practice sufficient to satisfy the patient. The primary bearer of the financial risk, especially of catastrophic illness, is still the insurer under this system.

- Preferred provider organization (PPO) with discounted fees. The insurer demands that the providers offer a substantial discount that is either negotiated or imposed and then limits the patient's access to only those preferred providers. Now more of the operational risks lie with the provider, although utilization is still a concern of the insurer. The patient also begins to share in the operational risks in the sense that the patient is tied to a limited panel of providers who are willing to cut prices and has more limited selection to choose from to adjust for shortfalls in perceived or technical quality.

- Capitation. This method of payment shifts the financial and operational risks to the provider, who receives a set amount per person to cover a package of services. It is analogous to the premium received by the insurer except that now the insurer allocates a portion of that premium as a fixed payment to the provider. The patient assumes some risk, since the patient is locked into that set of providers and cannot opt out for quality reasons.

- Point-of-service (POS) plan. In this arrangement, the patient chooses at the time the health care services are needed which of several options to use. For example, if the patient chooses the services of a plan's HMO physicians or its PPO, then coverage would be higher than when the patient goes outside the plan on the indemnity option. Thus the patient assumes some of the financial risk that might have been the insurer's when choosing the indemnity option, but also takes control (with the attendant risk) of the operational delivery of care. The patient is still at operational risk for the HMO or PPO choices.

Public sector organizations can be both insurers and providers within this context. As an insurer, the public sector has moved through the first four stages cited above. Starting with a fee-for-service model, for example, Medicaid quickly installed coinsurance payments, but found that these were relatively inconsequential for a low-income population. If they were kept low enough that the indigent could pay them, they had relatively little impact on costs.

Public programs have moved toward requiring deep discounts, which, in effect, limited the population of providers (equivalent to an independent practice association [IPA] or PPO). This held down the costs but limited accessibility for patients. Because of the access problem, fees tended to be closest to open market fees for primary care physicians, especially the scarcer ones, such as obstetricians. The discounts to specialists, especially academic-center specialists, tended to be the greatest. However, in recent years, the impact of HMOs and their capitation approaches has caught the eye of the public policy makers. Therefore, they are pushing for the HMO solution, which in effect is competitive bidding for capitation. The POS arrangement is not really a viable one for low-income populations, since they cannot pay the approximately 30% portion of the bill that the indemnity option would entail. However, it is an option for higher-income segments, including much of the Medicare population.

As providers, public health organizations can also participate in managed care, although it may mean the development of many new skills at underwriting, cost-finding, negotiation, cost control, and cash-flow management, which are often lacking in budget-based organizations. They will also have to undertake new types of accountability—economic accountability to the insurer and marketing accountability to the clients. They must provide care at prevailing market prices. This would be possible with a governmental subsidy, but such organizations must be acutely aware that they are subject to scrutiny by the press and the political process and that their competitors will object strongly to such subsidies, real or imagined.

As public policy makers, state and federal governments have high-profile and often conflicting objectives. Often we hear talk that the budget will be balanced by cuts in Medicare and Medicaid and discussions about whether coverage for children above the poverty level is or is not a new entitlement. Entitlements now make up more than 50% of the federal budget, and health care looms as the largest of these after income maintenance programs. In 1995, national health care spending rose by 5.5%. However, spending for the private sector rose 2.9% and for the government sector, largely Medicare, costs rose 8.7%.[15] State and local budgets are also strongly affected by Medicaid, mental retardation, and mental health programs, as well as the types of health problems that also show up in the criminal justice system.

LEGISLATIVE RESPONSES

When the public expresses dissatisfaction with the quality of managed care organizations, state and federal legislators have shown themselves to be ready to act. Where the government is the payer, it also can act to expand the role of managed care in its programs. In those states where initiative petition is easy to utilize, the public can vote directly on managed care issues. In 1996, voters turned down anti–managed care initiative petitions in California and Oregon by reasonable majorities. The laws currently in effect are of three types: anti–managed care laws; quality-of-care laws; and legislation enabling and regulating managed care.

Anti–managed care laws include:

- Any-willing-provider laws. These compel managed care organizations to accept any qualified provider who accepts the terms and conditions of their standard contract. Proponents argue that this legislation is not anticompetitive, since the unwanted providers must abide by standard contract terms. However, managed care companies object because they cannot concentrate their business on a limited number of practices to increase their bargaining power and gain physician compliance. This weakens their ability to select out providers on the basis of their quality of care and service. Stapleton[16] reports that insurers do not believe that physicians pay much attention to them unless the insurer controls at least 100 of that physician's patients, whereas the average IPA or PPO provides only 25.[17] There are only a limited number of states with any-willing-provider laws for physicians, although a majority have them for pharmacists, a group that traditionally has had more legislative influence.

- Freedom-of-choice laws. These laws allow the patient to receive care from any qualified provider regardless of whether or not that provider belongs to the insurer's managed care network. This clearly negates the bargaining power and managerial influence of managed care organizations. Most state legislatures have defeated freedom-of-choice laws for physician services.

- Direct-access laws. A number of states have passed laws that guarantee a patient direct access to a specialist without going through a primary care gatekeeper. Most of these refer to providers of obstetrical/gynecological services. Isolated individual states have also passed laws providing direct access to specific types of providers, arguing that they provide components of primary care, including dermatologists, optometrists and ophthalmologists, chiropractors, nurse practitioners, and nurse midwives.

- Constraining incentives. A number of states have constrained the differential for copayment rates between participating and nonparticipating providers to 20% or 30%. One state also prohibits the withholding of payments to providers who accept capitation, while another forbids financial incentives to motivate provider or patient behaviors.
- Constraining exclusive provider contracts. A few states have passed laws that restrict the ability of managed care organizations to sign exclusive contracts with non-employee providers. This type of law may be used to slow the growth of managed care or to constrain its overconcentration in areas such as Minnesota, where three integrated systems control 80% of the state's managed care and employ or contract with almost 10000 physicians.[18]

Quality-of-care legislative initiatives include:

- Length-of-stay laws. Many states have passed laws requiring that new mothers be allowed to stay in the hospital for 48 hours after a vaginal delivery and 96 hours after a Caesarean section, and similar federal legislation followed in 1996.
- Mandated coverages. Many state regulations require the offering of specific mandated services to achieve state licensure, including mental health, prenatal care, mammograms, and drug and alcohol treatment. As new technology is developed, it may be accepted by a managed care organization, or it may be mandated by legislation after coverage is denied. For example, some states have mandated coverage of bone marrow transplants for treatment of breast cancer.
- Direct-access laws. Hellinger[19] argues that the passage of direct-access laws in states with high managed care market penetration indicates that these laws relate not to hindering managed care, but to improving quality of care.
- Regulating utilization management. State legislation often defines which organizations must provide utilization management and how it is to be implemented, and limits retroactive denials.
- Mandating point-of-service plans. To provide enrollees with some access outside their insurer's network, some states have mandated that available plans include a POS option.
- Anti–gag-rule laws. Many plans have clauses that require loyalty to the insurer and include clauses that prohibit providers from criticizing the plan or from trying to influence the patients to switch to another plan. The public has

been especially concerned about clauses that try to constrain the provider from discussing treatments that are not approved by the plan. These clauses have considerable teeth, since they are paired with clauses that allow contract cancellation without explanation or recourse in 30–90 days.

- Other regulations. The insurance regulations and statutes govern:
    1. issuance of false, misleading, or deceptive materials
    2. providing "adequate" access to facilities and providers
    3. having quality assurance in place and following up on findings
    4. having specific grievance procedures
    5. reporting to the state on enrollment, utilization, and number of grievances
    6. informing enrollees about coverage and exclusions, how to complain, how to obtain services, and enrollee financial responsibilities
    7. having a governance process involving enrollees
    8. ensuring solvency and holding enrollees harmless in case of default, and enforcing such regulations and laws
    9. minimum ratios of providers to patients
    10. maximum travel times or distances[20]

Further, the National Association of Insurance Commissioners has also developed model acts that cover quality assessment and improvement, provider credentialing, utilization review, data collection, and confidentiality.[20] One can see other possibilities in the package considered by the 1997 North Carolina legislature. This included provisions to:

- Force managed care companies to pay for emergency department treatment when patients have good reasons to believe that they are seriously ill.
- Ensure that care managers cannot force patients to travel great distances to specialists when comparable care is available nearby.
- Make sure easy access to providers would be available to patients with expensive chronic illnesses, including acquired immune deficiency syndrome (AIDS).
- Require that when a managed care payer refuses to pay for a treatment, if asked, it must provide the medical reasons for its decision in writing and notice of how to appeal the decision.
- Require that a report card be available to report quality of care, including immunization rates, Caesarean rates, and eye examinations for diabetics.

Most of these requirements are part of the package recommended by the National Association of Insurance Commissioners.[21]

Federally licensed HMOs (an HMO must be federally licensed to enroll Medicare and Medicaid patients) must also have a comprehensive set of benefits; be broadly representative of the age, social, and income groups in their service area; use a modified community rating plan; and report to the federal Health Care Financing Administration as well as the state authorities. Medicaid plans must also have at least 25% enrollees from other populations. Medicare must have at least 50% and offer the same services to the Medicare patients as to the others. Medicare HMOs must also accept Medicare enrollees on a first-come, first-served basis to constrain cherry-picking of patients.[20]

Legislation enabling and supporting managed care includes:

- Licensure. Managed care could not operate without specific legislation that allows managed care organizations to operate in each jurisdiction. Forty-eight states have enacted such legislation. Only Wisconsin and Oregon lack this legislation, preferring to treat the issue under existing insurance laws. In many states, these organizations are regulated by specific legislation, by insurance regulations, and by state health department regulations. Many of these enabling acts also limit the malpractice liability of managed care organizations. ERISA exempts some aspects of self-funded plans from state legislation, although insurance aspects still come under state insurance regulation.
- Requiring managed care alternatives in governmental programs. This constitutes the strongest endorsement of managed care by governments and will be discussed below.

PREVENTION AND MANAGED CARE

Disease prevention and health promotion is one of the fundamental objectives of public health that is frequently linked conceptually with managed care. It has long been understood that prevention of disease was poorly incentivized under fee-for-service medicine. The risk of future illness lay with the insurer and the patient, not with the provider. That is one positive aspect often advanced about managed care. Once the provider begins to bear the risk of the cost of future illness, the provider should be increasingly interested in reducing future costs by preventing disease.

Historically, many HMOs have been concerned with disease prevention and health promotion among their populations and have developed techniques for measuring and improving their performance in this area—one which most fee-for-service plans only paid lip service to, lacking information systems to track the delivery of preventive services.[22,23] A Centers for Disease Control and Prevention

(CDC) report[24] on prevention and managed care cited three reasons why HMOs could play a powerful role in prevention:

1. Size. With the majority of the employed work force in managed care, HMOs can have great impact, especially with the further addition of Medicare and Medicaid populations.
2. Scorecards on HMOs emphasizing prevention. The NCQA, the Joint Commission, and others have been emphasizing performance indicators for institutions and practices that rely heavily on prevention measures as process measures of performance. NCQA has developed its Health Plan Employer Data and Information Set (HEDIS), which is part of its accreditation process and given to employers and sometimes to enrollees. Included in that set of multiple indicators of quality of care are rate-based, population-specific measures of prenatal care, low-weight births, vaccinations, cervical cancer screening, and retinal examinations for diabetics. However, these measures are essentially process and structural measures and do not yet include much in the way of outcome measures. Certainly, these measures are not yet sufficiently sophisticated to identify outcome effects on small subpopulations. Further, there is little effort underway to make sure that the collected information is in comparable formats or disseminated to all potential stakeholders in the service.[20] HEDIS measures are frequently evaluated and revised. The latest version, HEDIS 3.0, is designed for both commercial and public sector health plans. NCQA reported in 1997 that some 330 managed care organizations used their standards. The HEDIS 3.0 Reporting and Testing Set Measures are listed in Exhibit 3–1.
3. System integration. The HMOs are often part of integrated systems and have information systems and procedures that allow them to follow patient status above and beyond the concerns of the individual provider. New information systems that always seem to be just around the corner will enhance that property of integrated organizations.

A fourth reason, not cited directly by the CDC report, is that, as HMOs achieve high market penetration, they can begin to analyze opportunities and take actions on a community-wide basis. Once a successful HMO realizes that it is not going to achieve its vaccination goals by one-on-one interactions with its enrollees, it may begin to think about joint efforts with others—HMOs, health department, and schools to "treat" the community instead, as the Group Health Cooperative of Puget Sound in this case illustrates (see Chapter 13).

This is the encouraging part, and there are many sterling examples of effective prevention plans at HMOs for items such as those mentioned above along with others, such as bicycle head injuries, and numerous patient education programs. However, there is also a dark side to this prevention issue.

BARRIERS TO PREVENTION

While there are many success stories about prevention among HMOs, and there are marketing incentives to have a good report card, there are four factors that must be overcome to have effective and lasting prevention programs in managed care organizations. These include:

- individual provider disinterest
- impact of costs of prevention on short-term earnings and the discount rate
- disenrollment rates
- lack of integration in many organizations

INDIVIDUAL PROVIDER DISINTEREST

Providers do not necessarily change their procedures when serving at an HMO, especially if it is a provider network (e.g., IPA or PPO) in which they are only very loosely affiliated with the insurer. Most of the reported prevention successes have been with physicians employed in either staff-model or group-model HMOs. These are practices where individual physician autonomy is somewhat diminished and where there is likely to be strong central medical direction. However, these two types of practices are not in the majority of the HMO arrangements, and their growth currently seems to be slower than that of networked arrangements. Physician disinterest is not linked as much to economic disincentives as it is to time availability and to resistance to change, and some evidence indicates that many screening techniques have not yet proven effective.[22]

TIME VALUE OF PREVENTION

The cost of prevention occurs in the present, while the benefits and potential cost savings occur quite some time later (except in the case of prenatal care).[25] In a business, prevention would be considered a capital investment, except that it is not possible to capitalize on it for accounting and tax purposes. New prevention initiatives depress current earnings with the hope of improved future earnings. To the extent that many of the integrated systems and HMOs are for-profit companies with newly issued stocks and very high price-earnings multiples, administrators

Exhibit 3–1 HEDIS 3.0® Reporting and Testing Set Measures as of April 1997

EFFECTIVENESS OF CARE

Reporting Set Measures

- advising smokers to quit (in member satisfaction survey)
- beta blocker treatment after a heart attack
- the health of seniors
- eye exams for people with diabetes
- flu shots for older adults
- cervical cancer screening
- breast cancer screening
- childhood immunization status
- adolescent immunization status
- treating children's ear infections
- prenatal care in the first trimester
- low birth-weight babies
- checkups after delivery
- follow-up after hospitalization for mental illness

Testing Set Measures

- number of people in the plan who smoke
- smokers who quit
- flu shots for high-risk adults
- cholesterol management of patients hospitalized after coronary artery disease
- aspirin treatment after a heart attack
- outpatient care of patients hospitalized for heart failure
- controlling high blood pressure
- prevention of stroke in people with atrial fibrillation
- colorectal cancer screening
- follow-up after an abnormal pap smear
- follow-up after an abnormal mammogram
- stage at which breast cancer was detected
- assessment of how breast cancer therapy affects the patient's ability to function
- continuity of care for substance abuse patients
- substance counseling for adolescents
- availability of medication management and psychotherapy for patients with schizophrenia
- patient satisfaction with mental health care
- family visits for children 12 years of age or younger
- failure of substance abuse treatment
- screening for chemical dependency
- appropriate use of psychotherapeutic medications

continues

Exhibit 3–1 continued

- continuation of depression treatment
- monitoring diabetes patients
- chlamydia screening
- prescription of antibiotics for the prevention of human immunodeficiency virus (HIV)-related pneumonia
- use of appropriate medications for people with asthma

ACCESS/AVAILABILITY OF CARE

Reporting Set Measures

- availability of primary care providers
- children's access to primary care providers
- availability of mental health/chemical dependency providers
- annual dental visit
- availability of dentists
- adults' access to preventive/ambulatory health services
- initiation of prenatal care
- availability of obstetrical/prenatal care providers
- low birth-weight deliveries at facilities for high-risk deliveries and neonates
- availability of language interpretation services

Testing Set Measures

- problems with obtaining care

SATISFACTION WITH THE EXPERIENCE OF CARE

Reporting Set

- the member satisfaction survey (numerous measures)
- survey descriptive information

Testing Set

- Consumer Assessments of Health Plans Study
- disenrollment survey
- satisfaction with breast cancer treatment

HEALTH PLAN STABILITY

Reporting Set

- disenrollment
- provider turnover

continues

Exhibit 3–1 continued

- narrative information on rate trends, financial stability, and insolvency protection
- indicators of financial stability
- years in business/total membership

USE OF SERVICES

Reporting Set

- well-child visits in the first 15 months of life
- well-child visits in the third, fourth, fifth, and sixth year of life
- adolescent well-care visit
- frequency of selected procedures
- inpatient utilization—non-acute care
- inpatient utilization—general hospital/acute care
- ambulatory care
- Caesarean section and vaginal birth after Caesarean rate (VBAC-rate)
- discharge and average length of stay for females in maternity care
- births and average length of stay, newborns
- frequency of ongoing prenatal care
- mental health utilization—percentage of members receiving inpatient, day/night care, and ambulatory services
- readmission for selected mental health disorders
- chemical dependency utilization—inpatient discharges and average length of stay
- chemical dependency utilization—percentage of members receiving inpatient, day/night care, and ambulatory services
- mental health utilization—inpatient discharges and average length of stay
- readmission for chemical dependency
- outpatient drug utilization

Testing Set

- use of behavioral services

COST OF CARE

Reporting Set

- high-occurrence/high-cost diagnosis-related groups
- rate trends

Testing Set

- health plan costs per member per month

continues

Exhibit 3–1 continued

INFORMED HEALTH CARE CHOICES

Reporting Set

- language translation services
- new member orientation/education

Testing Set

- counseling women about hormone replacement therapy

HEALTH PLAN DESCRIPTIVE INFORMATION

Reporting Set

- board certification/residency completion
- provider compensation
- physicians under capitation
- recredentialing
- pediatric mental health network
- chemical dependency services
- arrangements with public health, educational, and social service organizations
- weeks of pregnancy at time of enrollment
- family planning services
- preventive care and health promotion
- quality assessment and improvement
- case management
- utilization management
- risk management
- diversity of Medicaid membership
- unduplicated count of Medicaid members
- enrollment by payer (member years/months)
- total enrollment

Source: Reprinted with permission from the National Committee for Quality Assurance (NCQA); HEDIS® 3.0, *Volume I: Narrative—What's in It and Why It Matters*; pp. 30–34, © 1997.

---

are very concerned about maintaining an upward trend in quarterly earnings. Suggestions for new initiatives that run counter to that goal may fall on deaf ears. If the management really believes that its primary responsibility is to the stockholders, then it is not going to invest heavily in prevention, since the stockholder concern is often more in maintaining steady earnings and steady stock price growth rather than in enhancing future earnings. With publicly traded American companies earning at least 12% on investment before taxes, and with many shares outstanding due to the high prices paid during mergers and acquisitions of practices, the value of future earnings is devalued (discounted) very rapidly. Table 3–2 shows the net present value of a stream of income growing for five years with discount rates of 10%, 15%, and 20%, which are not realistic rates in corporate America. It assumes that the money was borrowed at 9%. Even though the savings amount to the initial investment by the end of the fifth year, having to borrow for the investment and the discount rates in effect make prevention a difficult economic choice. In the real world, things are even bleaker, with relatively few preventive programs requiring no continued investment to maintain desired behaviors after the first year or yielding a 30% return starting in the second year.[22] The argument for prevention is best left a quality-of-care argument.

DISENROLLMENT

In the market for managed care, there is fierce competition for each employee's business at the annual re-enrollment date. Changes of plan by enrollees are frequent, often in the range of 15–25% per year, as competition heats up and premium reductions take place. Disenrollment by the patient in three major cities produced an average time of less than three years in the plan. For Medicaid, the average time in the plan was less than a year.[26,27] If the plan's enrollee population is not stable, then the likelihood of a payoff from preventive measures is reduced, unless all the competing plans also undertake the same efforts. Therefore, that is a disincentive for individual plans, but an opportunity for public health policy makers to promote success through community-wide efforts that would offset the disenrollment effect.

LACK OF INTEGRATION

A minority of HMO providers are employees. Most are in loose networks where they are not as much subject to intrusion by medical directors with sufficient authority to induce them to change their methods of practice. Earlier studies found that even having monetary incentives to perform preventive measures did not necessarily result in health care improvement. The providers must first perform the intervention, and if it is a screening measure, act on any findings. We provided a tracking system along with the incentives and still found that a surprisingly small percentage of these screening measures were actually carried through to completion. Lack of integration can be a major factor in slowing down the effect of any prevention interventions.[22]

Table 3–2 Net Present Value in Dollars of Stream of Prevention Investments under Different Rates If $100000 Is Invested in Year 1

Year number	Annual savings	Net present values at rates of		
		10%	15%	20%
1	0	−104500	−104500	−104500
2	10000	−103965	−103994	−104024
3	30000	−87244	−89082	−90816
4	30000	−71098	−75581	−79641
5	30000	−55613	−63472	−70288
6	30000	−40854	−52696	−62531
7	30000	−26864	−43170	−56142
8	30000	−13672	−34798	−50910
9	30000	−1288	−27477	−46646
10	30000	10290	−21101	−43183
11	30000	21073	−15569	−40379
12	30000	31083	−10783	−38118

Note: Assumes that the firm borrows at 9%

CONCLUSION

It appears that the role of the HMO as a vehicle of disease prevention and health promotion is very likely to depend on the mix of organizational forms and ownership incentives operating. Relatively few HMOs are currently using capitated contracts to reimburse physicians, and most primary care physicians are still in relatively loose networks. If one agrees that prevention provides less motivation in networks than in staff and group model HMOs and is less likely to happen in those that are publicly owned and traded, then there is still a great need to mandate prevention in the marketplace—if one believes that it is a critical component for providing good health care.

A CDC conference on prevention and managed care in 1995 suggested a strong role for public health agencies in the motivation of disease prevention and health promotion activities by managed care organizations. The conference report[24] mentioned the following as opportunities:

- To realize the potential of health information systems as a society, concerns about confidentiality and privacy issues and the proprietary nature of the data of medical care organizations (MCOs) must be addressed.
- Public agencies must bring valuable skills and experience to partnerships with MCOs and purchasers (e.g., experience with surveillance and informa-

tion systems, epidemiologic and laboratory skills, health promotion skills, experience in developing and implementing prioritized prevention strategies, experience in using policy and legislation to promote the public's health, and experience in management and providing enabling services to promote access to health services for vulnerable populations).

- Public and private purchasers of health care, particularly large employers, HCFA, and state Medicaid agencies, have a direct interest in promoting quality in managed care and could be natural partners with public health agencies in improving health outcomes.
- MCOs have the opportunity to become active leaders in promoting and protecting the health of the communities in which they are located.
- Partnerships among MCOs and public health agencies will require all entities involved to augment skills through continuing education and training.

The report also mentioned the following "barriers":

- As Medicaid beneficiaries convert to managed care arrangements and no longer receive care from local health departments, those health departments will lose the Medicaid reimbursement that has helped subsidize care to the uninsured. As a result, fewer resources may be available with which to care for the uninsured.
- Some local health departments are electing to become part of an HMO and compete with other HMOs in the delivery of health care. This competition may affect their ability to form partnerships with HMOs.

The same report also suggests a number of research and development activities that the CDC should undertake in response to the new structure of medical care delivery and to support the effective delivery of preventive services throughout the health care sector. This includes research on models for contracting services with HMOs to encourage delivery, measurement, and evaluation of preventive services; on information systems to support public health case-finding activities within HMOs; on using insurance billing and electronic consumer records for public health surveillance; on further development of measures such as HEDIS; and on building and maintaining partnerships between purchasers, public health departments, and HMOs. For example, the CDC has used *Morbidity and Mortality Weekly Report* to publicize methods of improving the delivery of preventive care conducted by Voluntary Hospitals of America. These methods involved hundreds of organizations and significantly improved performance through collaboration with public health departments and other community organizations.[28]

REFERENCES

1. Kongstvedt PR. *Essentials of Managed Health Care.* Gaithersburg, Md: Aspen Publishers; 1995:295.
2. Lau SA. *Blue Cross: What Went Wrong?* New Haven, Conn: Yale University Press; 1976.
3. Wilson MP, McLaughlin CP. *Leadership and Management in Academic Medicine.* San Francisco: Jossey-Bass; 1984.
4. Madison D, Konrad TR. Large medical group-practice organizations and employed physicians: a relationship in transition. *Milbank Q.* 1988;66:240–282.
5. McLaughlin CP, Kaluzny AD. Total quality management issues in managed care. *J Health Care Finance.* In press.
6. Shortell SM, Gillies RM, Anderson DA, Erickson KM, et al. *Remaking Health Care in America: Building Organized Delivery Systems.* San Francisco: Jossey-Bass; 1996.
7. Quinn JB. Is your HMO OK—or not? *Newsweek.* February 10, 1997:52.
8. Lynch ML. The uptake of childhood immunization and financial incentives to general practitioners. *Health Econ.* 1994;3:17–25.
9. Kouides RW, Lewis B, Bennett NM, Bell KM, et al. A performance-based incentive program for influenza immunization in the elderly. *Am J Prev Med.* 1993;9:250–255.
10. Schlackman N. Evolution of a quality-based compensation model: the third generation. *Am J Med Quality.* 1993;8:103–110.
11. Halverson PK, Mays GP, Kaluzny AD, Richards TB. Not-so-strange bedfellows: models of interaction between managed care plans and public health agencies. *Milbank Q.* 1997;75:113–138.
12. Speake DL, Mason KP, Broadway TM, Sylvester M, et al. Integrating indicators into a public health quality improvement system. *Am J Public Health.* 1995;85:1448–1449.
13. Fox HB, McManus P. Preliminary analysis of issues and options in serving children with chronic conditions through Medicaid managed care plans. Presented at the Annual Meeting of the National Academy for State Health Policy; August 1994; Portland, Me.
14. Rosenbaum S, Darnell J. *Medicaid 1115 Demonstration Waivers: Approved and Proposed Activities as of February 1995.* Washington, DC: Henry J. Kaiser Family Foundation; 1995.
15. Levit KR, Lazenby HC, Stewart MW. Dataview: national health expenditures, 1995. *Health Care Financing Rev.* 1996;18:175–214.
16. Stapleton DC. *New Evidence on Savings from Network Models of Managed Care.* Washington, DC: Lewin-VHI Inc; 1994.
17. General Accounting Office. *Managed Health Care: Effect on Employers' Costs Difficult To Measure.* Washington, DC: Government Printing Office; 1993.
18. Winslow R. Employer group rethinks commitment to big HMOs. *Wall Street J.* July 21, 1995: B1–B2.
19. Hellinger FJ. The expanding scope of state legislation. *JAMA.* 1996;276:1065–1070.
20. Silberman P. Ensuring quality and access in managed care: how well are we doing? *Quality Manage Health Care.* 1997;5:44–54.
21. Clabby C. Protection of managed care customers sought. *News and Observer.* February 19, 1997:8A.

22. Morrissey JP, Harris RP, Kincaid-Norburn J, McLaughlin CP, et al. Medicare reimbursement for preventive care: changes in performance of services, quality of life, and health care costs. *Med Care.* 1995;33:315–331.

23. Leininger LS, Harris R, Jackson RS, Strecher VJ, et al. CQI in primary care. In: McLaughlin CP, Kaluzny AD, eds. *Continuous Quality Improvement in Health Care: Theory, Implementation, and Applications.* Gaithersburg, Md: Aspen Publishers; 1994:253–264.

24. Centers for Disease Control and Prevention. Prevention and managed care: opportunities for managed care organizations, purchasers of health care, and public health agencies. *MMWR.* 1995; 44:14.

25. Sisk JE. The cost of prevention: don't expect a free lunch. *JAMA.* 1993;269:1710–1715.

26. Freudenheim M. Managed care empires in the making: companies build networks to stay a step ahead of hard-charging field. *N York Times.* April 2, 1996:D1.

27. Davis K, Collins KS, Morris C. Managed care: promise and concerns. *Health Affairs.* 1994;13:178–185.

28. Increasing pneumococcal vaccination rates among patients of a national health care alliance. *MMWR.* 1995;44:1–2.

CHAPTER 4

Privatization of Public Hospitals: Trends and Strategies

Montague Brown

Health care providers, especially public hospitals, face many pressures to compete with other providers for patients, capital, and other resources. For most hospitals, being able to count on the continued opportunity to provide services to some assigned or traditional group of patients is gone. Today it is essential to secure contracts with managed care organizations, including those operated or contracted with by states to serve the Medicaid population, a mainstay service population for public hospitals. Most hospitals face enormous pressures, with many deciding to merge or even turn over their operations to other institutions perceived to be better positioned to survive in these turbulent times. Public universities and local governments are shedding their hospitals to cut their costs and risk of loss in a volatile marketplace. Privatization of public hospitals is part and parcel of the larger transformation taking place in health care.

BACKGROUND

With the passage of Medicare and Medicaid, the health care field began a series of transformations leading up to today's heavy focus on cost control. Quality, access, and public accountability (*accountability* is used here when one might want to substitute public scrutiny, direct oversight, or control) are falling behind to varying degrees as principal goals (see Chapter 5). With the advent of Medicare and Medicaid, hospitals faced with guaranteed payment for their most vulnerable patients went on a spending spree both to gear up to meet the standards of these new programs and to become more attractive to the specialist whose work would attract patients. Money for this transformation came from Wall Street in the form of tax-exempt financing and then, increasingly, from equity funds fueling the growth of now giant corporations that own and operate hospitals. This growth is reaching proportions sufficient to raise the issue as to whether we are seeing the end of the not-for-profit and public hospitals as two more transformations occur. For a more wide-ranging critique and discussion of these trends, consult Johnson, Brown, and Johnson.[1] A volume edited by Brown (1996)[2] explores a variety of perspectives on integrated systems, which almost always provide for some elements of change in ownership. Indeed, in this book some chapters suggest that the vertical integration that is driving much of the merger activity may not work. Finally, Brown and Lewis[3] provide a historical perspective on the early days of these trends. The purpose of this chapter is to examine the various forms of hospital privatization, their motivating factors, and the strategies being used to guide these processes.

PRIVATIZATION TAKES MANY FORMS

Many terms are used in describing the various transformations occurring. The term *privatization* is used here to indicate a movement away from public ownership, operation, and governance by elected government officials or direct appointees of public bodies. In other words, privatization as used here means a movement away from strict government ownership, control, and operation. Privatization can therefore mean the establishment of an authority to own and operate a hospital (or clusters of related services). McLaughlin[4] discusses distinctions ranging from quasi-governmental organizations to Wall Street–financed firms. Sometimes these authorities have the power to appoint their own boards and successors, some rely on public appointment or confirmation, while some have direct public elections for such posts. These forms of privatization may seem benign and merely a public choice as to how closely or loosely the operation needs to have official public oversight. However, as described below, these changes have long-term implications.

Another form of privatization occurs when a public body or authority establishes a not-for-profit managing corporation. The managing corporation may well be without public official oversight. However, since the public body continues to be the owner of the health facility, there will be some form of accounting for the operation to the public body. One reason for being concerned about even this relatively mild form of privatization is that over time, assets, capital, and expertise accumulate in the not-for-profit managing corporation. While no evil should be assumed from this fact, it is possible, even likely, that over time what was once a public operation with full public accountability is more and more a private operation. If and when further privatization may need to be considered, the public bodies will have long since lost their sense of what is happening and what needs to be done. For these kinds of reasons, it is essential to consider each step toward privatization to be part of a long-term process, each moving toward full privatization.

Another major step in the move toward privatization may be to transfer the hospital assets to a not-for-profit corporation set up or already in place to then assume full responsibility for the hospital. While not-for-profit hospitals are expected to operate in the public interest, their decision processes are essentially private, not public. Once an unambiguous transfer from public to private owner-ship is made, it is possible to make a private decision to go another step and sell or otherwise transfer ownership to for-profit organizations.

Many public hospitals are sold directly to private owners. The public body thus recovers the equity value from the institution and then proceeds to tax the now for-profit organization. How privatization unfolds over time can vary considerably from place to place, making it important to consider all such moves for both their immediate rationale and their possibly longer term consequences.

When considering a partner, whether it be buyer, joint venture, merger, or some other form of consolidation and privatization, it is essential to know how it will affect the mission. If access is critical, then it becomes possible to press the investigation of potential partners by exploring how access will be affected.

REASONS FOR TRANSFORMATION

Most transformation decisions are driven in large part by the need to improve the efficiency and to increase the productivity of institutions. For example, Metsch and colleagues[5] stress that efficiency and productivity provide a major rationale for change, yet the process of change is part of a larger quality improvement effort. Gray[6] contends, however, that the issue of efficiency and productivity is too murky to use as a rationale for the conversion. The all-purpose efficiency argument for transformation is difficult to sustain in practice and should be tested to the greatest extent possible before relying on it for major changes. Of course, the efficiency argument may mask other reasons for a public agency to wish to dispose of a public hospital. In the Jersey City case discussed by Metsch and colleagues in Chapter 19, the public hospital went into bankruptcy before it took on an additional element of its mission to control cost and improve efficiency. With privatization it became possible to gain access to more capital and thus to implement essential strategies for improving the performance of the failed institution. *Health Affairs*[7] contains a number of articles and sources that make it essential reading for anyone who wants to be alert to the many nuances of transformation, especially when transformation might lead to conversion to for-profit status. The reader should know that it is possible to first convert a public institution to a not-for-profit and follow that conversion to a further change to for-profit, possibly leaving any proceeds from a sale to a private foundation instead of the original public owner.

Privatization may involve many goals, including such things as depoliticizing operations, enhancing competitiveness, and reducing financial risk to local governments, according to Camper et al.,[8] who outline a number of reorganization options, some helpful, how-to steps, and case-study examples of how public systems can be organized. While many people applaud such goals, there are others who believe that such moves are part and parcel of an ideology that places markets and market forces as ends more important than the people's welfare.[9] Of course, market advocates argue that protecting the market ultimately produces goods and services more efficiently than in public systems. While both notions have important lessons, some people think that no matter what kind of institutional arrangement is selected, there is a tendency over time for rigidity and unresponsiveness to develop, especially when monopoly control is achieved. This includes the vesting of total control in governments otherwise democratically controlled by elected officials. Public, not-for-profit, and for-profit institutions also can suffer from a loss of focus over time.

BROAD AND ACCELERATING TRENDS

Whatever position one takes on this transformation, the rate of change seems to be accelerating. A number of examples illustrate this. For smaller towns, the need for facility replacement raises the specter of tax increases and the prospects for building hospitals where planning experts see no need. Often such small hospitals are sold to entrepreneurs with a strong economic incentive to make an investment profitable. These firms bring new capital, an aggressive attitude toward physician recruitment and maximizing services provided locally, and instantly the local hospital becomes profitable. Universities with public hospitals see managed care coming fast and find that other area providers are better positioned to offer a regional network of services, so they join the network. In Minneapolis, for example, a not-for-profit, multi-unit hospital system purchased the University of Minnesota teaching hospital and continues to operate it as a teaching institution while making it a linchpin hospital for its system. Similarly, in Charleston, South Carolina, the medical school hospital is being leased to Columbia-HCA in order to link effectively with a regional network of hospitals and physicians. Another neighboring not-for-profit hospital is going to be contract managed by a public authority hospital from Charlotte, North Carolina, a colossus several hundred miles away with growing influence in a two-state region. Some hospitals are sold outright. Some are converted from entities governed nominally by boards beholden directly to public officials. Others submit nominations to public officials for approval, while still others are self-perpetuating boards answerable only to themselves.

For an interesting assessment of how this process of conversion is going, see *Modern Healthcare*.[10] This article also contains a rundown on a number of public and private teaching hospitals undergoing some form of major change. While the nongovernmental and authority hospitals have substantial autonomy, a comment by Lewis Vaughn, a South Carolina legislator, makes the essential point that laws written by one legislative body can be rewritten and changed by another. However, the reader should be forewarned that it is possible to write legislation that gives something away completely, so it is prudent to transfer property with some strings attached, such as, "unless the hospital shall be sold. Under which circumstances the sales proceeds will be returned to. . . ." There are a lot of hospitals in the nation worth millions, even billions, which were once beholden to church groups and governments and now can be sold without any recompense to the founders. Let the giver beware.

Although there are some examples of public hospitals acquiring for-profit and not-for-profit hospitals, most of the conversions (change of ownership status) are going the other way. Much attention has been paid in recent years to the conversion of not-for-profit hospitals to for-profit institutions (110 went for-profit between 1980 and 1990 and 65 went public), while public hospitals accounted for 73 conversions to for-profit and 223 conversions to not-for-profit status.[7]

KEY CONCERNS FOR PRIVATIZATION: SOURCE OF DECISION CRITERIA

Each organization must ultimately develop its own criteria for assessing whether or not it should convert and, if so, with whom. Criteria should be developed around the most important values and goals of an institution. For instance, if access by people in the neighborhood of the hospital is an overarching goal, then one criterion for assessment would be the ability and desire of the new owner to make the hospital successful in its present location. If the overall cost to the community were a value, then some institutions would turn over the hospital to a neighboring facility that could maximize the number and range of services that could be consolidated, even to the point of closing a hospital. Below are some of the key concerns for privatization, which exemplify the sorts of issues that will drive the development of decision criteria.

Mission

Mission is usually the first issue to be considered. The mission of an institution represents its fundamental reason for existence and needs periodic examination and reaffirmation. Most public hospitals exist because there was at some point a need for such an institution and it was determined at the time that public financing and operation was the most desirable solution. This may have been in response to a need for services for all citizens or the need to serve those who could not get care in private facilities. Over time, missions change. For a number of public hospitals, teaching roles become important. In communities where public hospitals were primarily for the poor or set up to support racial segregation, the lessening of segregation makes it possible for people to go to a wider range of hospitals for care. As Medicaid looks to competition and managed care to get prices and cost down, even more pressure is exerted on public hospitals, especially those whose main mission is to take care of Medicaid populations that increasingly are being shunted into managed care programs. As other facilities are faced with lowered census due to managed care pressures and the increasing use of outpatient services, they find Medicaid populations more and more attractive as paying customers.

Most organizations also have mission elements dealing with quality, cost, and access. For public institutions, access has often been at the forefront of mission, with cost lagging behind. Public hospitals have substantial investments in medical and allied health education, a factor that often contributes to such institutions having excellent reputations for high-quality services. In today's cost-conscious climate, with managed care firms seeking the best price, many public hospitals carry heavy uncompensated care loads, and teaching responsibilities will be disadvantaged. However, it should not automatically be assumed that caring for the poor and offering high-quality services are inconsistent with efficiency. Even as that may be the case, transforming the institution often can be difficult to accomplish without major changes in the organization. Thus the decision to privatize can be a means toward this end.

Not all public hospitals deal exclusively, nor even primarily, with Medicaid patients. But for those who do, it is a time for a serious re-examination of mission. If the hospital no longer serves a major need, should it be retained? Many will argue that rather than risk closing, selling, or merging and changing the mission of such hospitals, every effort should be made to keep the institution viable for the present and for the unknowable future when it might be much needed again. No argument is made here for either outcome. However, serious discussion needs to ensue over mission—what it is and should be—prior to any effort to privatize.

Ultimately, the question of access revolves around what happens to the clients/ patients who are the central concern of the hospital. If other hospitals are not only interested in serving these patients but also have the capacity and are willing to provide the service at prices below those of the public hospital, it may be time to revisit the necessity of the public hospital. On the other hand, if competing hospitals are willing to lower prices to get the patients, will they have the same incentive to keep their prices and cost low as well? Even with this limited discussion, the complexity of the issues faced are daunting, making it more important to question and probe any easy assertion as to what solution is best for an institution.

Cost Becomes a Driving Issue

For survival today, the question is not primarily access but cost. While the public hospital wants to keep its traditional clientele and attract more, it is often essential to lower cost. The difficulty in lowering cost may stem from the challenge public organizations are reputed to have in cutting back on employment. The issue of cost may also arise from a lack of sufficient patient flow. Volume and expanding business solves many cost problems. However, to stimulate volume it may be necessary to cut costs first. Some efficiencies may come from closing high-cost services, such as burn centers. But in realizing such efficiencies, the fundamental mission of access to important services may be violated. Sorting out what problems account for the higher cost is essential to an assessment of what kind of solution will be required. Will an authority system provide the increased leverage required to deal with the problems being faced? Or will it be necessary to completely sever the relationship of the hospital, turn it over to private business, and let them use the profit motive to bring cost in line with the market?

Whatever the issue that is supposed to be better addressed by one party than another, a healthy skepticism should infuse any exploration. Many people claim that efficiencies can be achieved but find the presumed opportunities fading once merger or sale is accomplished. Efficiencies can come from cutting cost, which may include closing unprofitable services. If those services are critical to the mission, then the change contemplated needs to be questioned. However, an equally rigorous questioning should be applied to every service and job slot that someone will consider essential. Sometimes, closing entire hospitals will in fact make the entire community hospital system more efficient. But when it is your hospital being closed, the act of making the overall usage of resources more efficient holds less appeal and is not something any proposed merger partner or even buyer would likely want to discuss in any depth.

Examining just how cost can best be controlled in any given situation is an essential step in determining what steps a new owner might take. One should not assume that every possible owner will cut costs in the same way. A neighboring hospital might well close some services, streamline an operation, and use their combined facilities in a more efficient manner. A new owner without neighboring hospitals might try new strategies to increase market share, thus spreading fixed cost over more patients. Many such potentially cost-saving methods can also be used to improve quality because having an ample patient flow is critical to building and sustaining quality.

Complicating Factors

Not every seemingly rational community interest solution will be selected. Other issues often sidetrack cost decisions. In some situations, the choice between a new organization from outside the area and a local hospital may well be made because the public hospital prefers to bring in a buyer who will maximize the job opportunities for current employees, a condition most likely to be the case if market share can be increased. The community cost may go up under these circumstances, but the jobs for specific groups of employees can be protected. Many owners will take a lower price for a particular hospital property under circumstances in which the seller agrees to keep more employees for longer than it might otherwise and to serve particular patient populations or to keep some loss-making services. Such assurances seem likely to be short-term, although often necessary to get a deal on transforming any hospital from one owner to another. More important is the question of which potential solution is likely to provide long-term protection to needed employees and services.

A related, primary goal of quality may well be impacted with the choice to privatize. Will quality go up or down? This is not an easy question. It may be impossible to ascertain in advance what will happen to quality if a change is made. Indeed, quality may well remain the same under any form of ownership. Quality may be improved by consolidating low-utilization services or increasing patient flow through existing services. Teaching programs, while costly, are often associated with high quality. Many ways exist to improve quality, so incorporating serious discussion of just how this will be done is a vital part of any meaningful assessment of a transformation option.

Most hospitals feel they owe a debt of loyalty to physicians and employees (of course physicians may well also be employees). Thus the goal of access extends to the question of what opportunities exist for the physicians and others who have devoted their lives and careers to taking care of the patients traditionally served by the institution.

Public Support

Public support is central to any decision about transformation. What support currently exists? Is it getting stronger or weaker? What is the likely reaction to a change? For many, the debates over limiting government will negatively impact the ability of public hospitals to get sufficient capital to compete effectively. Or will it? Chances are good that while people might express an opinion on what should be done, the number who have actually given it any serious thought will be small. Does this mean that no one will care when major ownership and control issues go on the agenda? While some institutions seem to sail through this process easily, it is potentially one of the most divisive issues that can be raised. It challenges every settled assumption about who will get what from the transaction. To say that a communications plan is essential understates the problem. What is really needed is a fairly in-depth understanding of the condition of the institution, the evolving industry, and the options available. Management styles vary considerably, so prescriptive comments about how to make this happen probably will not be of help. My own personal preference is for frequent, open, and straightforward appraisals of the strategic positioning of the institution with anyone who will listen. When the time comes for decision making, it is helpful when all the major constituencies accept the recommended directions not because they like the choice, but because they understand the options and how one particular option has been chosen.

Beyond mission, cost, quality, and access, the issue of accountability is a major issue for public institutions. The role of governments in delivering personal health services and owning and operating hospitals varies widely around the country. Thus, we know that there is no inherently superior method of providing health care. However, when one method is used, it can be very difficult to change it. Privatization of public hospitals can be heavily charged with emotion and, indeed, can have serious negative consequences for some constituencies. Consider the anguish that will come from the prospect of a hospital closing, especially for those who live nearby and count on the institution for services.

The issue of accountability thus needs to be expanded from the idea of being responsible to a board, and through them to elected officials, to one which extends the definition to a wide range of stakeholders.

CONCLUSION

Hospitals today are under great stress. Managed care in its many forms emphasizes fewer services, and when services are needed, lower-cost services. This makes hospitals a natural target for cost control. When providers are paid some form of capitation, then every service becomes a cost center, unlike earlier times when the more days of care and the more services used meant the more one was paid. Today, payment is more likely to be fixed for the diagnosis or by population. Hospitals that are unable to secure patients through capitation contracts or are unable to keep their cost low to attract cost-conscious buyers and to deliver quality services efficiently are in trouble. Under these circumstances, many hospital owners, trustees, and public officials are looking for ways to survive. For many, this means getting out of the business by selling to more efficient operators or merging with others in contiguous markets to enable the system to be downsized to fit the new market realities.

There are many ways in which public hospitals may move toward privatization. The use of public authorities is a well-established means to move the hospital into a more independent mode so that its successful operation is its primary concern. A move to convert public hospitals to not-for-profit, public interest corporations takes a bigger step toward complete privatization but remains well within the range of traditional solutions. Converting public hospitals into for-profit institutions is a step that has been taken increasingly since Medicare and Medicaid made hospitals more profitable, but it also increased the need for working capital and improved facilities.

The issues and concerns associated with this movement are many. Fortunately, debate about the transformation of the industry is becoming more vigorous. People who must face these challenges early have the opportunity to refine the issues and design improved models of health care delivery.

REFERENCES

1. Johnson EA, Brown M, Johnson RL. *The Economic Era of Health Care*. San Francisco: Jossey-Bass; 1996.

2. Brown M, ed. *Integrated Health Care Delivery: Theory, Practice, Evaluation, and Prognosis*. Gaithersburg, Md: Aspen Publishers; 1996.

3. Brown M, Lewis HL. *Hospital Management Systems*. Gaithersburg, Md: Aspen Publishers; 1976.

4. McLaughlin CP. Privatization and health care. In: Halverson PK, Kaluzny AD, McLaughlin CP, eds. *Managed Care and Public Health*. Gaithersburg, Md: Aspen Publishers; 1997.

5. Metsch JM, Haley DR, Malafronte D. Privatization of a public hospital: a quality improvement strategy. *Qual Manage Health Care*. 1997;5:19–24.

6. Gray BH. Conversion of HMOs and hospitals: what's at stake? *Health Affairs*. 1997;16:33.

7. Needleman J, Chollet DJ, Lamphere J. Hospital conversion trends. *Health Affairs*. 1997;16:187–195.

8. Camper AB, Gage LS, Eyman BDA, Stranne SK. *The Safety Net in Transition: Reforming the Legal Structure and Governance of Safety Net Health Systems*. Washington, DC: National Association of Public Hospitals and Health Systems; 1996.

9. Beauchamp D. Public health, privatization, and 'market populism': a time for reflection. *Qual Manage Health Care*. 1997;5.

10. Scott, L. Can marriage of academic and community hospitals work? *Modern Healthcare*. 1997;27:26–32.

CHAPTER 5

Privatization and Health Care

Curtis P. McLaughlin

> Whether or not the current turn toward privatization discloses a general failure
> of government, it certainly discloses a general failure of social theory.
>
> Paul Starr[1(p22)]

Starr here is referring to the fact that, during the 1950s to the 1970s, social
scientists accepted the growth of the state whether they welcomed it or abhorred
it. Therefore, most social scientists were caught by surprise by the turn toward
privatization in the 1980s and 1990s that occurred under rightist governments in
the United States and United Kingdom; labor governments in Scandinavia, New
Zealand, and Australia; socialist governments in Spain and Mexico; and throughout the former Soviet bloc.[1] Some argue that in the contest between socialism and
capitalism, capitalism has already won.[2]

A look at health care, however, shows that its privatization phenomena are
much more complex than the Cold War analogy implies. We see a variety of
changes in ownership and responsibilities for delivery and financing fueled by a
variety of motives and environmental changes. Most of the shifts are away from
government involvement in delivery, while some also move away in financing
and regulation. There are services turned over from government to private
contractors, others that are no longer provided at all by agencies, and intermediate
shifts such as hospitals moving from government ownership to not-for-profit
status and then to for-profit status. The reasons are also varied, ranging from cost
reduction to dropping the service due to political antagonism (e.g., stopping the
distribution of condoms in schools), to meeting increasing service capacity
requirements, to responding to capital markets, to rewarding efficiency and
entrepreneurship.

Starr notes that the lines between governmental and private human services
delivery in the United States have been blurring as government has maintained a

policy role but turned over the service delivery to private organizations, yet usually with continued tight government accountability and controls. He writes:

> Several other examples—private prisons, privatization of infrastructure, school vouchers, and social welfare privatization—also illustrate how privatization blurs public-private boundaries by involving private firms in the performance of functions that government cannot entirely surrender. . . .
>
> Much of the expansion in social welfare in the United States has come in the form of financial support for services delivered by private, often nonprofit, organizations. . . . But once the private organizations take on these roles, they are inevitably subject to greater public supervision. Scandal is typically the mother of control: every incident of exposed corruption produces a wave of regulation and threatens to undo the very advantages of private organization that such programs aimed to exploit. [1(p 42,44)]

PRIVATIZATION ALTERNATIVES

Because of this blurring, there is a need to develop a way of looking at and describing relationships and changes in organizational structure and controls during privatization. Exhibit 5–1 outlines a number of alternative stages along the

---

Exhibit 5–1 Schematic of Privatization Alternatives

Stage	*Organization*	*Function*		
Before privatization	Governmental	{ Regulation/oversight Financing Delivery		
After privatization		Regulation/ oversight	Financing	Delivery
	Governmental			
	Quango			
	Membership not-for-profit			
	Entrepreneurial not-for-profit			
	For-profit			

MATRIX OF POSSIBLE FUNCTIONS

privatization route. It does not include mechanisms of control as a dimension, something discussed later. A governmental agency can move functions to any of the other types of dimensions. The British National Health Service has moved away from being a deliverer of health care by turning that function over to a number of local authorities or quasi-nongovernmental organizations (quangos), which are not government agencies but have their boards appointed by the government. A health department can reduce or eliminate its public health nursing staff by contracting with local home health agencies that may be entrepreneurial, not-for-profit and/or for-profit providers.

One method of classification of not-for-profit organizations, based on Hanssman[3] and McLaughlin,[4] is shown in Figure 5–1. Most not-for-profits are some combination of the three types: donative, membership, and entrepreneurial. The Sierra Club is a good example; one can become a member with certain privileges, or donate money to specific causes, or buy books from its entrepreneurial publishing division. The donative aspect has been ignored in Exhibit 5–1, because health care delivery has long ceased to be heavily dependent on philanthropy or on direct governmental largess.

Note that this formulation of the types of changes induced by privatization does not require that the service start with the government in order to be further

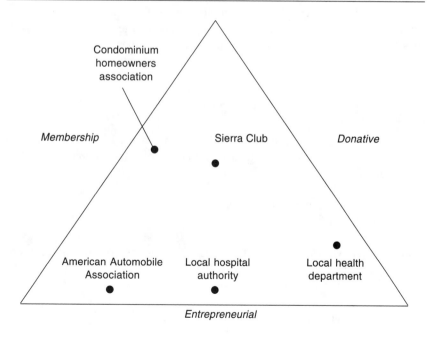

Figure 5–1 Typology of Not-for-Profit Organizations.

privatized. The recent movement of a number of Blue Cross/Blue Shield organizations to private, for-profit status could also be represented in Figure 5–1. These organizations started out on the upper left as creatures of not-for-profit membership organizations (state hospital associations and medical societies). After shedding representatives of specific interests from charters and then their boards, they moved further toward the bottom of the triangle to an interim position of being entrepreneurial not-for-profits. Recently, a number have sold out to or become for-profit companies,[5] leaving the triangle entirely.

In fact, the easiest part of the process to define is privatization as a "shift from the government to the private sector of responsibility for some or all aspects of particular activities and services."[6(p2)] However, in this chapter it is recognized that there are relative degrees of privatization, ranging from the quango to the managed care company with its stock traded on the New York Stock Exchange. It is necessary to make that distinction, because the public thinks mostly in terms of stock ownership as the model of the private sector, which is not universally the case. In addition, it is important to note the many transitions, some interim and some not, that are being made all along that spectrum in the health care sector.

For example, a local health department that is budget based, relies on its county and state allocated monies, and has no fee income is donative. It becomes much more entrepreneurial as it begins to provide and charge for direct health care services, perhaps under a family planning grant at first and then opening up a primary care clinic that accepts Medicaid patients on a fee-for-service basis. It may even become more entrepreneurial by gaining further fiscal autonomy (but also financial risk) by becoming a Medicaid managed care contractor.

ALTERNATIVE CONTROL MECHANISMS

Clarkson[7] suggests a series of control mechanisms used in the privatization process where the operation is neither sold nor discontinued completely. They include the following:

- Government financed and regulated:
  1. contracting out
  2. vouchers
  3. incentives (tax abatement and regulatory or deregulatory incentives or disincentives for demand are included here)
  4. grants and subsidies

- Not necessarily government financed but regulated:
  1. franchise agreements
  2. governmental service diminution making a private market viable

- Not necessarily government financed or regulated:
  1. volunteers
  2. self-help

All of these have been used in the United States at the federal, state, and local levels for the privatization of services, including some health care services. However, this characterization fails to include situations in which governmental institutions engage in alliances and partnerships with the private sector, or where government agencies become providers to for-profit managed care organizations.[8] This book even includes an example of a public hospital authority (a quango) buying a competing for-profit hospital.

Two other classifications that are useful in analyzing privatization phenomena are arranged by function and by structure.[8] Figure 5–2 outlines the functions that researchers have observed in public health organizations and shows how each public function potentially can be privatized. Note that privatization does not necessarily mean moving the provision of functions to for-profit entities. Figure 5–3 shows an alternative to Clarkson's model of the ways in which relationships can be structured, including a wide variety of alliances between public health and other organizations. Halverson et al.[8] note that most of the arrangements observed in the field relate to the privatization of relatively narrow areas of clinical services, such as prenatal care and obstetrical services, mainly services widely available in the private health care sector. The existence of these services in a competitive market makes their specification and evaluation much easier. One can ask for competitive bids and compare customer satisfaction and outcome measures. It is where no competitive market exists (such as an underserved rural area) that measurement and evaluation become difficult.

However, within the definition of public health used in this book, there are also issues of the shedding of publicly owned institutions such as hospitals and home health agencies. Even though these are not under the control of traditional health departments and may have had few, if any, linkages to them, this is a privatization of what has been a public health care function. One might also think of the earlier wave of "deinstitutionalization" in mental health as an example of privatization as the term is used here, since in some states the mental institutions were a single, monolithic bureaucracy, many of whose functions were transferred to local nonprofit organizations such as community mental health centers with highly variable results.

The factors behind the choices of specific structural arrangements and specific control mechanisms relate to the character of the service as a public good, the public's ability to evaluate performance, the political power of public employees involved and other interest groups, as well as existing and future constitutional and legislative mandates.

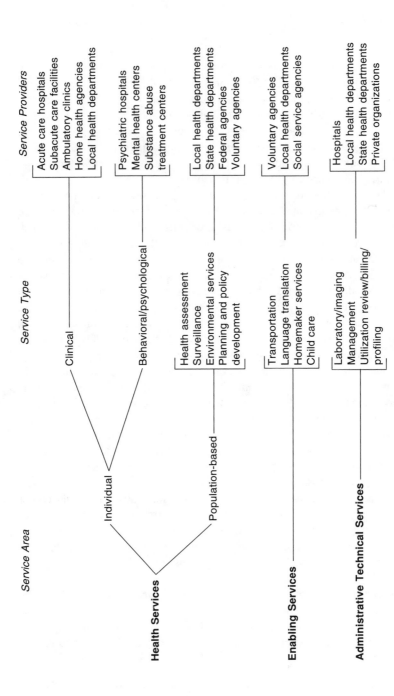

Figure 5–2 Service Areas, Types, and Providers in Public Health That Possess the Potential for Privatization. *Source:* Reprinted with permission from P.K. Halverson et al., Not-So-Strange Bedfellows: Models of Interaction between Managed Care Plans and Public Health Agencies, *Milbank Quarterly*, Vol. 75, No. 1, pp. 113–138, © 1997, Blackwell Publishers.

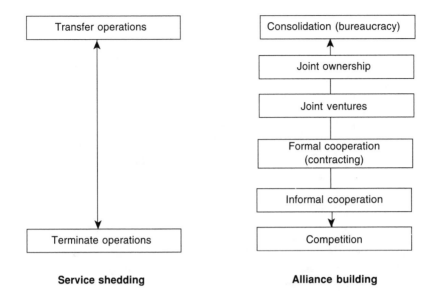

Figure 5–3 Structure-Based Models of Health Service Privatization. *Source:* Reprinted with permission from P.K. Halverson et al., Not-So-Strange Bedfellows: Models of Interaction between Managed Care Plans and Public Health Agencies, *Milbank Quarterly*, Vol. 75, No. 1, pp. 113–138, © 1997, Blackwell Publishers.

MAINTAINING ACCOUNTABILITY

As privatization of public health activities takes place, one cannot merely trust the marketplace to provide either the quantity or quality of services that are needed, especially for populations currently served through categorical and entitlement services.[9] After all, the very agencies and programs that are being privatized came into being because of market failures[4] and there have been few fundamental changes in markets and market theories since then.

Thus, there is a need for keeping formal responsibility for accountability with a combination of governmental health agencies and nonprofit private accrediting agencies. A representative set is listed below.

- Federal government: Health Care Financing Administration (HCFA), Centers for Disease Control and Prevention (CDC), and Health Resources and Services Administration
- State government: state health departments, state human service departments, and state insurance commissioners

- Local government: local health departments and local authorities (mental health, hospital, etc.)
- Private nonprofit accrediting agencies: National Committee for Quality Assurance (NCQA), Joint Commission for the Accreditation of Healthcare Organizations, and Association of Accountable Health Plans (AAHP)

These latter groups can also collaborate in developing accountability systems, such as those NCQA and HCFA have worked on for Medicaid and those CDC and AAHP have created for private managed care organizations.[10,11]

WHY PRIVATIZE?

The reasons for privatization in U.S. human services are quite different from those experienced in developing countries or developed countries with a history of nationalization of industry. The reasoning in the United States tends to be political, based on the desire to stop deficit financing, to reduce the role of government, and to experience reductions in regulation and taxation, as well as a redirection of the country's social agendas. Suleiman and Waterbury[12] suggest that in the developed countries we will see a slow cycle of privatization followed by centralization in state control in times of crisis, followed by privatization again.

Young argues that "The primary goal of privatization is to improve the efficiency of the institution and to increase the organization's productivity. Privatization shifts the authority and financial responsibility from the public governmental sector to the private sector, relieving the financial and administrative burden from government."[13(p 3)] He cites the example of New Jersey, where the requirement exists that hospitals impose a surcharge on insured patients to subsidize charity care. In urban hospitals, surcharges rose as high as 40%. This tended to run off to the suburbs what limited insured business there was in those cities. Hurley and Draper in Chapter 6 suggest that privatization can also allow governmental programs to avoid onerous government rules and regulations such as the Boren Amendment.

In health care, the trend toward privatization also stems from a number of factors in the health care marketplace and from the needs of public providers and payers. The growth of managed care organizations has forced many public agencies to serve patients under discounted-fee arrangements and capitated-reimbursement contracts negotiated with managed care organizations. These public entities have had to become as efficient as other actors in the marketplace to compete and also to maintain their perceived effectiveness in the eyes of their public overseers.[14] For example, the hand-picked mayoral advisory panel looking at the New York City Health and Hospitals Corporation recommended that the system be abolished. It asserted that it was inefficient, that it provided low-quality services, and that its 11 hospitals and its clinics, nursing homes, and home health agencies could not compete in a marketplace dominated by managed care.[15] The perceived inefficiency of the regional mental health bureaucracies was also a factor in Washington state's shift from fee-for-service to independent mental health resource managers.

The reluctance of the body politic to raise taxes has also limited the funding available for public programs. The managers of these programs have looked in turn at the restraint on the growth of health care costs achieved by the private sector using managed health care organizations and envisioned similar restraint for their programs. As public payers have shifted their clients to managed care, this has put further pressures on public sector providers to compete for those patients whom they had previously monopolized.

WHY CHOOSE TO GO FOR-PROFIT?

There are specific advantages to hospitals that do go private.[13] These include the development of a corporate planning mechanism, gaining cash to reinvest in programs and "corporate culture," terminating bankruptcy protection, being able to provide incentives to managers for taking risks, being able to develop an integrated network that reaches beyond the local jurisdiction, and being able to partner with physicians. Privatization streamlines and speeds up decision making and allows the institutions to develop a distinctive niche among the players in the area.

At the political level, these trends are also driven by the same factors that have led to privatization and outsourcing in other government sectors. Some observers suggest that the development of "market populism" and its introduction to public health is a serious threat to public health values.[16] This trend includes embracing the market as superior to the government in effectiveness in the delivery of services due to the incentives operating in a competitive environment. Beauchamp[17] argues that the unfreezing of the status quo by the Clinton administration's proposed Health Security Act and the resounding defeat of that plan have led to a commitment to a market-driven managed care process and an abandonment of government-oriented measures.

The risk to the public is that the providers of care will lose sight of their access goal and reduce their provision of uncompensated care. It is known that uncompensated care is reduced with increased competition and stress and that for-profit organizations have historically done less charity care,[18] so vigilance is required to maintain access in the face of these new structural arrangements.

One also must not lose sight of the fact that much of the growth in the costs of public health programs, such as Medicaid, has come not just from cost inflation and the application of new technology, but from the expansion of coverages and eligibility, seemingly independent of the amounts of funds actually appropriated by state and federal governments. Therefore, the drivers of the rising costs of publicly financed health care have really been much more forceful than the trends motivating corporate employee benefits managers. In some states, more than half of the births are covered by expanded Medicaid maternity benefits, and specific mandates can move eligibility standards from 61% of the poverty level to 185% of that level. Similarly, the Medicaid mental health coverages that are not federally mandated but may be supported by state statutes may shift the program focus from the small pool of chronically mentally ill patients whose disease usually manifests itself in early adulthood to a focus on the needs of children, who make up half of the Medicaid population, through a variety of interventions including Early and Periodic Screening, Diagnosis, and Treatment (EPSDT) and interagency and school referrals. Such a policy shift can easily swamp an already strained system. The same forces can also come into play when state legislatures add another category of disabled or chronically ill to the list of those categorically eligible for programmatic coverages.

Halverson et al.[8] also suggest that the information explosion may be behind the move to outsource some direct and indirect service functions. Both public and private organizations are turning to more knowledgeable and flexible independent contractors for some specialized work. Moreover, one of the strengths of managed care itself is that it is a more effective vehicle than the individual provider for learning and for improving the delivery of care by disseminating learned improvements rapidly over a wide geographic and population base.[19] This is despite the fact that private-sector health organizations have not tended to be responsible for population-based services, such as community health assessments, epidemiological surveillance, and environmental monitoring. Now it is clear that many private organizations do understand the importance of these efforts and of preventive health measures such as vaccinations. The challenge will be to get the public agencies responsible for these population-based efforts to develop alliances with private sector organizations to gather the data, interpret it, and take necessary action. This seems to be one of the first areas that should be emphasized in any public-private health alliance. Because most of such expertise currently exists in public agencies, it is very likely that they must continue to play a major role in such programs as tuberculosis (TB) screening and sexually transmitted disease (STD)-contact tracing. The case load from all providers can be aggregated in agencies to achieve economies of scale, and the clout of public health police powers is often necessary to induce client and provider cooperation. On the other hand, private organizations may still perform specific functions such as lab work and the delivery of treatments, even for those patients brought into public health clinics.

One area where change is quite likely is in the support services funded under Medicaid that assist special populations to access the health care system. It is very likely that organizations that provide other outreach services in the community such as neighborhood health centers, interagency motor pools, and homeless shelters can deliver services such as transportation, homemaker services, temporary child care, and language translation. They may well have to, since managed care organizations tend not to be equipped to provide these services and might very well consider them frills.

Among the more promising areas for privatization are the laboratory services provided by state and local health organizations. However, some public laboratories, especially at the state level, can aggregate highly specialized tests and technical skills in volumes that would be hard for private laboratories to duplicate. Therefore, the public sector must be quite careful about outsourcing only those tests for which the new provider has sufficient volume and expertise to maintain or enhance the technical quality of the service. It is also important that any new provider agrees to develop and implement methods of surveillance of test results so that public health officials are warned of problems and opportunities. Further, the provider needs to take on a range of analyses, both the high volume and the "orphan" tests to maintain access for all patients. A further requirement should be that the data be available for research, especially for epidemiological studies. The health care world has been one in which data for research were readily shared. Once those data become proprietary, it is then up to the commercial organization whether or not to release them. Public health policy makers should devote considerable effort to negotiating contracts that preserve availability of data for research and surveillance purposes.

Figure 5–3 suggests two types of service shedding: ceasing operations and moving the function or the organizational unit from public to more private ownership. The first can cause quite a bit of dislocation unless there is a mass movement of clients, as in the case of an exclusive service contract. Otherwise, the clients must fend for themselves in the marketplace and may be denied access for one reason or another. Where the organization shifts its form of ownership, the issues are more subtle. As with any change of governance, there are likely to be cycles of satisfaction and dissatisfaction as the professionals deal with mismatches in expectations and with the process of accepting new management philosophies, cultures, and technological mandates.[20] Similar mismatches of expectations are also likely to occur with clients and with public policy makers. The problems encountered with the new private operation may include quality standards for access and service, internal productivity, cash flow, recruitment and retention of key personnel, capacity development, and interorganizational relations. If the personnel are transferred, there are also likely to be problems with the blending of two cultures, especially in the areas of work methods, work norms, and acceptable client advocacy.

ALLIANCES

Alliances can allow the public and private organizations to retain their existing forms of governance and oversight, but accomplish many of the good outcomes associated with privatization: efficiency, specialization and cost sharing, improved quality, and improved access. However, issues of size, growth, autonomy, governance, control, integration, oversight, and evaluation still exist alongside the economic and political ones in the alliance situation. Both partners have to address each of these issues, even in the most informal arrangements. For example, Halverson et al.[9] cite the arrangement between a county health department and a large HMO in Washington state to share medical supplies on an as-needed basis, reducing inventory investments and increasing availability and reliability. However, such an arrangement is unlikely to succeed unless there are basic understandings that each will maintain a reasonable supply at most times, that draws on the other organization's stock will be small, and that replacements will be made promptly and be a one-for-one replacement of any items requested, in other words, that neither will take advantage of the other.

The frequently used method of specifying and using a formal alliance is the contract for services delivery.[21] The contract is a very specific, but very flexible, vehicle for specifying the terms under which a service will be delivered to or by a public health organization. For example, 44 states now have Medicaid managed care programs. In these situations, contracts are used to specify how providers will deliver services to clients of the state's Medicaid entity and/or its agent, as well as how county and city public health departments will deliver services to Medicaid enrollees. The contract is the means of establishing methods for reimbursement, for quality assurance, for access, and for performance measurement. Even then, local departments may further subcontract services such as billing and utilization review to yet another private organization.

Contracts are also involved in the privatization of whole institutions such as county hospitals. For example, in the Nash County, North Carolina example described in Chapter 17, the hospital corporation, a nonprofit entity, contracted with the county to lease and operate the county hospital for a period of 10 years. The reputed offers from for-profit corporations also involved contracts (leases) for the hospital. A variety of numbers were thrown around to describe the lease terms in this case, but it takes considerable information and financial sophistication to compare contracts to lease or buy a county hospital, because any specific proposal may differ in terms of cash payments, capital investment to be made, assumption of financial and tort liabilities, working capital requirements, and assumption of debt and uncompensated care balances. One part of that lease was to make a payment in lieu of the property taxes that the for-profit corporation would have paid. In this particular case, the political issues were not just the ownership of the hospital but the use to which the multimillion-dollar lease payment would be put, including whether it would substitute for the proceeds from a defeated school bond issue. Unfortunately, even state regulators responsible for approving such sales and leases seldom have the financial sophistication or the amount of information necessary to do a rigorous comparison of competing offers from the private sector.

A further consideration of this alliance and contract environment involved with the privatization of public health functions is that such a process really changes the management role of senior public health personnel. Usually, it moves the agency away from direct services delivery and further into the arenas of measuring costs, effectiveness, and outcomes; negotiation; relationship development and maintenance; performance evaluation; and financial analysis. Information technology is a key element of health care delivery, and this becomes even more important in the contracting mode, since actual operations are not being observed on a daily basis and records are not owned or fully maintained by the public agency responsible for the program. One has to develop methods for tracking such performance in the absence of transaction records and, in the case of capitated services, of billing records. One might be nonplussed, but should not be surprised, to find out that health maintenance organizations (HMOs) are not necessarily any better equipped than public agencies to find the cost of a specific clinical activity.

In the case of Mecklenburg County, North Carolina (see Chapter 18), a regional hospital system, formerly the county hospital system, has taken over 80% of the tasks of the county health department under a five-year contract. The county health department had 475 employees in 1995 and provided preventive clinical services, primarily to women and children at nine sites, and a full range of traditional, population-based public health services. The county wanted to cut the rate of growth in departmental expenditures. The integrated health system, Carolinas Medical Center (CMS), was a nonprofit, regional hospital authority already providing care in 12 counties in two states. Privatizing most of the county health department was not the first such transfer between the county and CMS since the latter was founded in 1949. Over the previous 15 years, CMS had acquired a county-subsidized rest home, the county nursing home (the largest in the state), and the county mental health center. CMS also provided medical control for the area's emergency medical services system, housed a number of county social services eligibility specialists, and provided health care for inmates of the county jail. To slow the growth in costs, the county pays CMS a fixed annual fee to provide the contracted services, including:

- all direct clinical services, such as maternal and child health (MCH) and family planning, care for STDs and TB, dental services for children, immunizations, and care of special needs children

- community services such as school health clinics, case management, home visits for new babies, respite care, and health education
- support services, including labs, medical records, data processing, appointment scheduling, and administration
- public health assessment and policy development, including epidemiological surveillance, community diagnosis, needs assessment and advocacy, community health planning, and public and media relations

Both facilities and employees were transferred to CMS. The residual county health department maintains the following services: vital registration, communicable disease control services, environmental health services, and oversight of the contract with CMS. The three types of direct services that were not contracted cannot be contracted under existing North Carolina state law.

The monitoring system associated with the contract calls for three types of evaluation measures to be used: (1) activity and input measures already reported annually to the state public health agency, such as client numbers, service activity, and resources made available, (2) performance measures such as immunization and screening rates, rates of appropriate prenatal care, teen pregnancy rates, and incidences of STDs and TB over a two- to five-year period, and (3) performance on high-priority community health measures identified in a 1993 survey over a 2- to 10-year period. These include rates of infant mortality, violence, substance abuse, and adolescent pregnancy, as well as incidence rates for selected cancers, heart disease, and STDs. The new system will also be subject to the state health agency's comparative report card system.[22]

While the preceding examples are concerned with privatization moving activities from local governments to private non-profits, Patterson et al.[23] report on moving state-operated MCH programs to a combination of non-profits and the private, for-profit sector (see Chapter 7). They describe the 1994 effort to redefine and restructure the MCH services provided under the Title V Maternal and Child Health Block Grant augmented with state monies. The state of Texas had been providing services directly in eight public health regions that lacked local health departments through 179 clinic sites. In other areas, these services were contracted out to 87 varied local government and nonprofit agencies with 318 sites. When the state direct service was started in the 1970s, there were no providers in these mostly rural areas, but by 1995 there were 428 rural health centers in Texas. Medicaid MCH benefits had been expanded and Medicaid managed care had been established. In 1991, the Texas Medicaid eligibility for pregnant women and infants was moved to 185% of the federal poverty level, and Congress had mandated many services for children that used to be discretionary under state law. By fiscal year 1995, 47% of all births in Texas were covered by Medicaid, many physicians had been recruited into the EPSDT program, and Texas was beginning to enroll beneficiaries into capitated managed care programs. Yet the state did not feel that it could walk away from the Title V program, because there were still more than a million children without health insurance in Texas and because the program helped support the infrastructure of the state's public health programs.

Therefore, Texas decided that it should reinvent its Title V program rather than abandon it entirely. Much of it was outdated, but there were still needs out there. It was also clear that funding at the state level would be substantially reduced soon. A committee structure was set up to study the nature and impact of the Title V program. Emphasis was given to the delivery of MCH services and the related impacts of the cuts on the public health infrastructure (or ecosystem, to use Hurley and Draper's interesting term; see Chapter 6). After developing and reviewing alternative vision statements for Title V, a new objective was defined: filling the gap, covering those low-income women and children below 185% of the federal poverty level who were not eligible for Medicaid. Existing public and private providers would be used for delivery under a "performance-based reimbursement methodology." Instead of receiving a budget allocation from the state, these providers would bill the state against a contractual dollar ceiling for approved services provided to eligible patients. Clinics operated by the Texas Department of Health and local public health agencies were downsized as patients were steered to local providers, including some recruited to the area for that purpose. Private providers were offered three-year contracts to promote stability in service availability.

This approach has also been supported by a policy of competitive bidding for new providers in those areas that were once underserved. New arrangements have occurred. For example, in 46 out of 76 counties, medical schools are now providing these services. Local health departments have also had to adjust to competitive bidding and performance-based reimbursement—a difficult task, but one that they report has improved their efficiency and their cost-finding skills. This has made them better equipped to compete in a managed care environment. Patterson et al.[23] report that between fiscal years 1995 and 1996 the same number of patients has been served, but budgets have been cut 20% and 568 positions funded by Title V and general state revenues eliminated.

What is still unknown in Texas is the impact that this shift away from categorical granting to privatization and performance-based contracting will have on the public health infrastructure, especially if, as is very likely, many other categorical programs are privatized.

TENNCARE

One of the largest experiments in Medicaid managed care has been TennCare, the capitated managed care program of the state of Tennessee. This is a five-year demonstration program based in part on the Clinton health plan. Competing state-chartered health maintenance organizations are responsible for providing a broad range of preventive inpatient and outpatient services to their enrollees with a capitation rate based on an overall state budget. Effective January 1, 1994, it had been planned to enroll 1 775 000 individuals. The plan actually covered 1.2 million and incurred a $99 million deficit during its first year.[24] During 1996, TennCare insured 1.2 million Tennesseeans, including all those eligible for Medicaid plus 420 000 additional individuals who were formerly uninsured. The latter group included those who could not afford or could not get medical insurance through commercial insurance companies. Overall, health insurance coverage in the state approached 95%. However, just about everyone involved agrees that there had been serious implementation problems associated with the program. The lead paragraph in a *Washington Post* article began, "The state of Tennessee has proved that you really can hammer a round peg through a square hole, so long as you don't mind an awful screeching sound and a fair number of splinters."[25(pA1)]

TennCare started in 1993. The fiscal year 1994 Tennessee Medicaid budget was estimated to be approaching $700 million and growing rapidly, and yet many people still lacked access to health care services, especially the working poor. Tennessee was spending a quarter of its state budget on Medicaid. Then-governor McWherter argued that "No issue is more urgent, and without a solution, the entire state government in Tennessee remains in jeopardy." In the spring of 1993, the governor asked the legislature for authorization to develop an alternative plan. The legislature agreed and then approved the plan a month later with little debate. TennCare was intended to slow the growth of state Medicaid expenditures at the same time that the covered population was increased. One reason given for the rapid legislative decision was the desire to avoid the type of deadlocking of interests that led to the defeat of the Clinton health plan. At the time, the state's providers had relatively little experience with managed care, with only 6% of the state's population in such plans.[25]

The original design called for a "gross capitation" of $1641 per person, close to the 1993 national HMO average of $1636. However, this figure was adjusted downward in the political process because the cost of charity care by hospitals would be substantially reduced and allowances were made for some copayments, a drug formulary, and the expected savings from managed care. The resulting gross capitation was set at $1214 per individual.

In response to complaints from the Tennessee Medical Society and other provider organizations, supplemental capitation for patients with serious and persistent mental illness, acquired immune deficiency syndrome (AIDS), hemophilia, and organ transplants raised the average payment to $1275. The governor also agreed to lift a tax on patient revenues earlier than planned to gain acceptance by the hospitals.[26]

Low-income individuals not covered by Medicaid gained access by paying premiums on an income-based, sliding premium scale and by copayments. The HMOs offered "no-frills" care policed by primary care physician gatekeepers, who reduced the utilization of specialists, and by insurers, who reimbursed specialists, hospitals, and pharmacies to very low levels. Articles variously refer to reimbursement of some specialists at less than 20% of normal fees, but the average was about 35%. One hospital bill for a heart transplant on a TennCare patient was reportedly negotiated down from $381000 to $186442. Primary care physicians were paid a flat capitation fee.[27]

The startup problems were horrendous. The program was created overnight, and so were 10 of the 12 HMOs. Neither providers nor patients had much experience with such arrangements. Every managed care organization lost money during the first year. The Blue Cross-Blue Shield HMO ultimately gained more than 40% of the market, but the second largest barely escaped bankruptcy through the support of a large hospital. There were serious fraud and adverse selection problems. However, many of the limitations on utilization in traditional Medicaid programs were dropped, and coverages, including inpatient psychiatric care, were continuously expanded. Over the first three years, administrative procedures improved, and so did customer satisfaction. When surveyed, 49% of former Medicaid recipients said TennCare was better for them in 1994, a proportion that rose to 68% in 1995. In both surveys, 60% of the formerly uninsured felt that they were better off. In a 1995 survey, 71% of Tennessee respondents felt that their care was good or excellent, compared with 62% of TennCare respondents. The rate of services for people under 21 quadrupled. The rate of immunizations increased, the infant death rate dropped from 9.4 per 1000 live births under Medicaid to 8.9 in the first year of TennCare, while the proportion of low-birth-weight infants stayed the same.[25]

The rate of growth of Medicaid expenses was reduced from 20% to 5%, and many uninsured were covered. However, lack of funds limited substantially the enrollment of the uninsured, non–Medicaid-eligible, especially those with pre-existing conditions. Waits for appointments have dropped and there now seem to be sufficient participating primary care physicians to provide access for the enrollees. There have been problems with the enrollment of specialists in some specialties and geographic areas.

TennCare has had a major impact on the medical community. Primary care providers are doing many procedures that were formerly done by specialists, such as sigmoidoscopy and aspirating joints, especially in large primary care practices where internal referral can take place.[27] Emergency departments have had to shed the dispensary function and move to triaging and referring out nonemergency patients, so claims dropped from 50.2 to 5.0 per 100000 enrollees between January and May 1994.[26] While nursing home care is not part of the TennCare package, prescription drugs for enrollees are, and the effect of this has been felt in this segment of the industry.[25]

The public health departments, especially those in rural areas, were not left out of the process. Most continued to supply traditional public health services to enrollees for the managed care organizations, and 50 of the 89 provided primary care, including 24-hour coverage, and acted as gatekeepers and case managers for TennCare under a contract with the state (see Chapter 15).[26]

One might legitimately conclude so far that TennCare has been an access success and a cost success, but that the quality effects are still unknown. What does seem clear is that the variance of quality of care is likely to be increased.

CONCLUSION

There are a wide variety of privatization alternatives in public health. Most of these are being used in one way or another. These are bringing about major changes in the institutions that traditionally delivered public health services and policies.

The reality of health care in the 1990s is that managed care focuses most heavily on managing costs. However, this is not just an attribute of the private, for-profit sector; it is true throughout the public health sector. The public health sector as well as corporate benefits managers are refusing to tolerate the very high inflation rates induced by the alternative of fee-for-service medicine, which fails to minimize care for profit improvement and maximizes the use of care by those who can afford it. (However, the situation in the public health sector has been exacerbated by major mandates to increase coverage and service eligibles without recognizing the major cost impacts involved.)

Either way, the public and its representatives must be vigilant in managing the tradeoffs between underutilization and overutilization. Managing this tradeoff is made difficult by the fact that costs are easy to measure and the effects of cost-saving beyond the dollars involved are very difficult to measure. The fallout of such decisions may not be known for years. In the meantime, the institutional frameworks for the delivery of care will be substantially and probably permanently altered.

When one considers the alternatives, it is clear that privatization in health care is much more complex than the privatization of banks, coal mines, and steel mills. In health care, the profit motive has always been there for the professional providers, but it is not as evident for some other stakeholders, such as hospitals and public health departments. The privatization move is not always from a government agency to an investor-owned stock company. There are many alternatives of ownership, governance, financial control, and regulation in between these two poles of a continuum, virtually all of which exist in practice. It is clear that the delivery of acute care services is rapidly being privatized, but a number of other public health functions remain under one form or another of collective governance.

REFERENCES

1. Starr P. The new life of the liberal state: privatization and the restructuring of state-society relations. In: Suleiman EN, Waterbury J, eds. *The Political Economy of Public Sector Reform and Privatization.* Boulder, Colo: Westview Press; 1990:22–54.

2. Heilbroner R. The triumph of capitalism. *N Yorker.* January 23, 1989:98–109.

3. Hanssman HB. The role of nonprofit enterprise. *Yale Law J.* 1980;89:835–901.

4. McLaughlin CP. *The Management of Nonprofit Organizations.* New York: Wiley; 1986.

5. Levinson M. Health care profit motive. *Newsweek.* April 22, 1996:56–57.

6. Bluestein FS. *Privatization of Local Government Functions or Services: Legal and Philosophical Issues.* Chapel Hill, NC: Institute of Government, University of North Carolina at Chapel Hill; 1996.

7. Clarkson KW. Privatization at the state and local level. In: MacAvoy PW, Stanbury WT, Yarrow G, Zeckhauser RJ, eds. *Privatization and State-Owned Enterprise.* Boston: Kluwer Academic Publishers; 1980:143–194.

8. Halverson PK, Mays GP, Kaluzny AD, Richards TB. Not-so-strange bedfellows: models of interaction between managed care plans and public health agencies. *Milbank Q.* 1997;75:113–138.

9. Halverson PK, Kaluzny AD, Mays GP, Richards TB. Privatizing health services: alternative models and emerging issues for public health and quality management. *Qual Manage Health Care.* 1997;5:1–18.

10. National Commission for Quality Assurance. *Medicaid HEDIS 1.0.* Washington, DC: National Commission for Quality Assurance; 1996.

11. Centers for Disease Control and Prevention. Prevention and managed care: opportunities for managed care organizations, purchasers of health care, and public health agencies. *MMWR.* 1995;44:1–12.

12. Suleiman EN, Waterbury J. Introduction: analyzing privatization in industrial and developing countries. In: Suleiman EN, Waterbury J, eds. *The Political Economy of Public Sector Reform and Privatization.* Boulder, Colo: Westview Press; 1990:1–21.

13. Young GJ. Bridging public and private sector quality assurance. *Qual Manage Health Care.* 1997;5:65–72.

14. Kralewski JE, Wingert TD, Feldman R, Rahn GJ, et al. Factors related to the provision of hospital discounts for HMO inpatients. *Health Serv Res.* 1992;27:133–153.

15. Rosenthal E. Mayor's advisors seek to dismantle hospital system. *N York Times.* August 16, 1995:A1.

16. Beauchamp D. *Health Care Reform and the Battle of the Body Politic.* Philadelphia: Temple University Press; 1996.

17. Beauchamp D. Public health, privatization, and "market populism": a time for reflection. *Qual Manage Health Care.* 1997;5:73–79.

18. Mann J, Melnick G, Bamezai A, Zwanziger J. Uncompensated care: hospitals' responses to fiscal pressures. *Health Affairs.* 1995;14:263–270.

19. McLaughlin CP, Kaluzny AD. Total quality management issues. *J Healthcare Fin.* In press.

20. McLaughlin CP, Konrad TR, Pathman DE. Maintaining the new practice networks. *Health Care Manage Rev.* In press.

21. National Association of County and City Health Officials. *1992–1993 National Profile of Local Health Departments.* Washington, DC: National Association of County and City Health Officials; 1995.

22. Keener SR, Baker JW, Mays GP. Providing public health services through an integrated delivery system. *Qual Manage Health Care.* 1997;5:27–34.

23. Patterson PJ, Simpson JS, Davis RJ, Stabeno DC, et al. Privatizing maternal and child health services in Texas: reinventing Title V programs. *Qual Manage Health Care.* 1997;5:35–43.

24. Solomon CM, Smith JL. TennCare up and running. *Health Syst Rev.* 1994;27:10–13, 16–18, 20.

25. Brown D. Tennessee's economy of care: TennCare's first three years: deluged by Medicaid, states open wider umbrellas. *Washington Post.* June 9, 1996:A1, A6.

26. Hatcher MT, Halverson PK, Kaluzny AD. Managed care and Medicaid: lessons and strategies for public health. *Health Care Manage: State Art Rev.* 1995;2:33–42.

27. Brown D. Tennessee's economy of care: the physicians adapt: when specialists aren't the norm. *Washington Post.* June 10, 1996:A1.

PART II

Applications of Managed Care and Privatization

Public health in the United States is assured through a wide range of organizational components and subsystems. The unique environments and capacities of these various components suggest that managed care initiatives will develop in different ways across the organizational landscape of public health. Part II examines applications of managed care and privatization initiatives within important subsystems of the nation's public health system. Chapter 6 describes the national experience of managed care in the Medicaid program, noting recent trends in Medicaid managed care's impact upon public health. Chapter 7 examines the efforts of Texas to privatize the delivery of Title V maternal and child health services, a major categorical program area for many state and local health departments. Chapters 8 and 9 describe recent developments in managed care for mental health services delivery and examine the effects of these developments upon the provision of publicly supported mental health and substance abuse services. Finally, Chapter 10 provides a critical assessment of private sector involvement in health care quality assurance efforts and discusses the public health implications of this often overlooked trend. These chapters clearly do not describe *all* possible applications of managed care and privatization within the public health system; nonetheless, they should offer valuable insights into the disparate ways in which managed care may affect public health structures, processes, and outcomes.

CHAPTER 6

Managed Care for Medicaid Beneficiaries: An Overview

Robert E. Hurley and Debra A. Draper

The extraordinary growth of managed care enrollment among Medicaid beneficiaries reflects the convergence of two powerful trends: the ascendancy of managed care financing and delivery systems, and the enormous appeal of shifting the delivery of public services to private contractors. As managed care has leapt from alternative to mainstream status for privately covered individuals, the same conversion is now widespread for Medicaid beneficiaries across the country. And the enrollment of persons eligible for Medicaid in managed care plans, particularly prepaid models, has the effect of privatizing Medicaid, one beneficiary at a time. The evolving role that Medicaid is playing as yet another powerful buyer embracing the instrument of prepaid managed care has had, and will continue to have, significant, far-reaching consequences on health and human services for low-income populations with and without Medicaid coverage.

While this transformation will continue to be daunting for most traditional providers of service to these groups, it is likely to be especially challenging to the public health organizations that have played integral roles in the fragile indigent-care ecosystem. Their ability to continue to deliver personal health services is being called into question. The extent to which they can and should transition from direct service to roles of monitoring, assessment, and assurance of managed care plan performance is being debated. The capacity of public health organizations to find constructive and meaningful roles and relationships with private managed care plans and their members is being widely discussed, although evidence of their ability to do so remains inconclusive. The willingness of public health agencies and officials to assume more active roles in exerting local community influence on increasingly corporatized and remotely governed delivery systems is also being examined. And the surging interest in "market populism"[1]—the belief that privatization is a kind of panacea—has ominous implications for sufficient investment in the maintenance of public sector organizations of all types.

All of these debates transcend the particular concerns and issues posed by Medicaid managed care. But it has been the growth and rapid evolution of managed care in Medicaid that has brought these issues home to many people and galvanized the attention of public health entities across the nation. This chapter reviews the rise of Medicaid managed care and its various manifestations and relate experiences of public health providers who have participated in varying degrees. The question examined is how recent developments in the policy arena related to privatization, Medicaid restructuring, and a growing preference for prepaid models are compelling public health officials to reassess the nature and extent of their participation in these initiatives. Attention is then turned to future developments in Medicaid managed care and the residual responsibilities likely to be available to public health entities. Finally, several broader questions are raised about the evolving nature of public and private relationships that might be informed by the Medicaid managed care experience.

BACKGROUND

The pace of growth of Medicaid managed care is initially reviewed with an eye to the unevenness of this growth and the policy context within which states have implemented it. The types of models adopted by states are detailed and related to the roles that local health departments have played in the past in Medicaid managed care. The sustainability of these roles is also discussed.

Growth of Medicaid Managed Care

The background on the evolution of Medicaid managed care has been extensively chronicled,[2] including the fact that enrollment in prepaid arrangements has been possible essentially since the beginning of Medicaid in 1966. Little activity occurred until the early and mid-1970s, when a limited number of well-established prepaid health plans or group practices (the term *health maintenance organization* or HMO had not yet come into common usage) enrolled relatively small numbers of Medicaid women and children with Aid to Families with Dependent Children (AFDC) eligibility. These plans included Health Insurance Plan (HIP) of New York, Group Health Cooperative in Seattle, and Group Health Association in Washington, DC. Enrollment was voluntary, and plans typically made only modest efforts to promote enrollment, reflecting concern about adequacy of payment and uncertainty about the impact that episodic eligibility would have on enrollment and service use. By 1981, enrollment in HMOs was approximately one-quarter million beneficiaries or about 2% of total Medicaid eligible persons at a time when national HMO enrollment was less than 5% and HMOs were not yet identified as a major mechanism for controlling health care cost inflation (Figure 6–1).

Most of the nation had very limited exposure to HMOs and there were not yet any preferred provider organizations, so most states did not look at managed care as even an alternative model for Medicaid financing and delivery. The one state that did, California, had obtained federal permission in the early 1970s to move MediCal beneficiaries into prepaid health plans on an aggressive, ambitious basis with the expectation that competition among plans would permit the state to obtain Medicaid covered benefits at a cost less than fee-for-service rates. Unfortunately, this effort was highly unsuccessful and scandal-ridden in terms of marketing abuses and development of phantom plans that failed to serve beneficiaries or to pay providers.[3] This fiasco achieved considerable long-lasting notoriety for the prospects for managed care for low-income persons by engendering hostility from advocates and skepticism and caution among state officials.[4]

Renewed interest in managed care surfaced in the early 1980s when the federal government granted states increased flexibility to implement programs that waived selected Medicaid program requirements. Requirements that could be waived included freedom of choice of provider, requirements of statewide program uniformity (to permit piloting of models in substate locales), deviation from

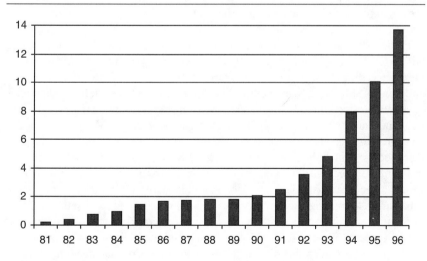

Figure 6–1 Growth of Medicaid Managed Care, Number of Enrollees in Millions. *Source:* Reprinted from Department of Health Care Financing Administration.

standard provider payment methods, and others.[3] This flexibility had the intended effect of stimulating considerable variation among states both to pursue HMO enrollment more aggressively and to devise new models of managed care, such as primary care case management or gatekeeping, to address certain persistent problems in the Medicaid program. This experimentation typically had the dual goals of cost containment and access enhancement. By the end of the 1980s, Medicaid managed care enrollment reached nearly 2 million across a widening variety of models, as described below.[2]

A subset of these waivers involved carefully devised research and demonstration programs intended to provide models that could be studied and evaluated in depth, rather than merely demonstrating cost neutrality and no adverse effects on beneficiaries as called for under the routine programmatic waivers. One of these research and development waivers was the notable Arizona Health Care Cost Containment System, which implemented an experimental Medicaid program based solely on prepaid health plans. The program—a kind of "first of the next generation" model[3] persists today, still under federal waivered status. Some other programs initiated at that time are also still operational (Santa Barbara, California, and Minneapolis-St. Paul) and they, along with Arizona, have provided the foundation for much of the research evidence regarding Medicaid managed care. These so-called Section 1115 waivers enjoyed a resurgence in the 1990s as several states have applied for permission to make sweeping changes in the structure, coverage, payment policies, and operations of the Medicaid program, in every case using managed care delivery systems as the core feature of restructuring. The most notable of these waivered programs are found in Tennessee, Oregon, and Hawaii, but several others are in development.[5]

In the 1990s managed care enrollment among Medicaid beneficiaries soared, with a fivefold increase between 1990 and 1995 and with managed care enrollment exceeding 25% of all eligible persons and close to 50% for women and children in AFDC and related eligibility categories. The growth has been stimulated by states seeking relief from huge Medicaid expenditure increases, driven in large measure by mandated eligibility expansions.[6] But non-Medicaid managed care growth has also surged during this period, and general acceptance of managed care, including greater tolerance of restrictions on freedom of choice, has climbed along with the number of managed care plans. Moreover, managed care has become a national phenomenon and is increasingly moving from large urban areas to mid-size and small cities and potentially into rural settings. Thus, the continued conforming of Medicaid to private sector changes in financing and delivery seems inevitable. Finally, growing infatuation with privatization of public services makes the sustained growth of Medicaid managed care highly probable. Throughout this period, as Medicaid managed care has grown in size and scope, it has presented intensifying challenges for public health officials.

Evolving Models of Medicaid Managed Care

First generation Medicaid managed care involved enrollment in prepaid health plans designed for commercial members. In the 1980s, Medicaid deviated considerably from this approach as several different models of care management were devised as alternatives to HMO enrollment. The nature of these models reflected interest in incremental changes, targeted arrangements to solve specific difficulties, or uncertainty about whether HMOs could and/or would participate on a meaningful scale to satisfy state goals. Previous studies have detailed the various models and efforts to try to classify them into some general prototypes.[2] The three basic models in use are briefly detailed to illustrate some of the possible roles and relationships they have posed for public health organizations.

1. Fee-for-service primary care case management. While the origins of this gatekeeper model lie in the private sector,[7] Medicaid programs have pioneered and extended this approach to care coordination and management for more than 15 years. Beneficiaries enroll with a primary care provider—a contractually obligated "medical home"—who agrees to provide or authorize all nonemergency care in return for fee-for-service payment plus, typically, a fixed per member per month case management fee.

2. At-risk primary care case management. While structuring care management duties in a similar fashion to the previous model, these programs try to promote cost-efficient delivery by putting primary care providers at some financial risk. Commonly, this involves paying them partial capitation or fee-for-service with a withhold with the opportunity for shared savings, in the same sense that a conventional independent practice association might do. No case management fee is paid in this model. These models were common during a period when HMOs were still underdeveloped, but where states felt a need to alter financial incentives of fee-for-service.

3. HMO or prepaid health plan enrollment. This model involves enrolling beneficiaries in an entity that assumes contractual responsibility to provide or arrange for virtually all covered services, in return for a capitation amount for the full scope of Medicaid benefits. Unlike the primary care case management models, where program management remains lodged in the Medicaid agency, the HMO approach involves shifting responsibility for provider network development, compensation, and utilization management to the health plan—under a detailed contract relationship.

Current enrollment figures indicate that nearly half of all beneficiaries in managed care are in HMOs, with about a third in fee-for-service case management and the remainder in the at-risk case management model, and that the fastest growing models are HMOs.[8] The preponderance of enrollees in all models are women and children, rather than people with chronic disease or disability, as most states are only now beginning to try to extend Medicaid managed care to these groups, as detailed later in this chapter. It is also noteworthy that many states have sought to accommodate beneficiary and provider needs as well as state policy and political considerations through carve-outs of special populations or services or the creation of specialized managed care arrangements. These developments are making this simple classification less meaningful than it once was.

Emergent Roles for Local Health Departments in Medicaid Managed Care

The timing and nature of points of contact between growing Medicaid managed care and local health departments (LHDs) have varied across the country due to both the models of managed care being advanced and the types and expansiveness of services offered by local health departments.[9,7] For some, there was parallel and relatively peaceful coexistence, particularly if personal health services in the LHD were limited. Medicaid managed care might have marginal effects on selected services—immunizations; early and periodic screening, diagnosis, and treatment screenings; and so on—but remained essentially an activity occurring in the acute care delivery sector. For LHDs with well-child clinics or adult services, there may still not have been contact, unless these clinics had chosen to obtain Medicaid provider status to bill for services to Medicaid eligibles. In the late 1980s and early 1990s, this became increasingly common, both as eligibility for low-income women and children was expanded and as LHDs sought to acquire new or replacement revenue streams as other sources declined. "Getting a Medicaid provider ID" became a widely promoted policy solution in this era and contributed to very real "Medicaidization"[10] of primary care and case management services within LHDs.

It was this transitioning of many LHDs into integral providers of services to Medicaid beneficiaries that ultimately led to growing concerns about the impact of managed care programs and the possible consequences of either participating or not participating in these programs. For states embarking on a primary care case management model, inclusion of current, high-volume providers was a priority, and many LHDs fit this status well. However, to participate it was necessary to meet certain staffing and availability standards (24-hour coverage, 7-days-per-week availability, and, in some locations, alternatives to hospital emergency department services as off-hour back-up). Faced with the consequences of the potential loss of a major revenue source, many LHDs made the necessary adjustments to meet these requirements.

In some instances, states showed a willingness to accommodate some compromise of these standards, even though to do so might imperil their federal waiver if it said all beneficiaries would have a fully accessible medical home. Service standards related to limits on number of enrollees, off-hour arrangements, or linkage with an identifiable individual case manager might be differentially applied to LHDs compared to individual physician practices. As large capacity providers, LHDs could absorb substantial numbers of people who did not select a primary care provider but were assigned to those providers who were participating and willing to accept new patients. Concerns were expressed by some primary care providers about double standards for LHDs and lack of true continuity, but in many locations—inner cities and underserved rural areas—individual practitioner options simply did not exist.

LHDs in many locations did add personnel and bolstered infrastructure to accommodate this new volume and the service requirements to maintain or expand revenues. In other cases, the adaptation was more reluctant and defensive, driven by concern that failure to participate would ultimately mean the loss of revenues, programs, and the ability to sustain services to people without any coverage. For LHDs that sponsored federally qualified health center (FQHC) "lookalikes," cost-based reimbursement had become an important windfall and this form of payment could be left intact in primary care case management programs, so the stakes of losing Medicaid patients and revenues were raised all the more.[11]

The New Reality: Prepaid Managed Care Everywhere

In locales where primary care case management has remained the dominant model of Medicaid managed care—such as rural areas and other markets with limited HMO penetration—LHDs have remained in a relatively stable position. But states have clearly recognized the strong appeal of contracting with prepaid health plans as a means to shift financial risk and to buy a more complete and, presumably, integrated delivery system than primary care management could ever provide.[12] At the same time they can align their buying more fully with private sector buyers who are eschewing fee-for-service systems and experiencing flattening or declining trends in premium growth.

Contracting with private plans also allows state governments to downsize their work force by offloading some administrative functions to the health plans. By relying on private contractors as agents and negotiators with providers, public agencies can be liberated from encumbrances they believe they have been saddled with by federal rules and regulations related to both providers and beneficiaries such as special payment requirements like the Boren Amendment.[3] Thus, prepaid managed care contracting becomes a means by which Medicaid agencies extricate themselves from some of the (beneficiary and provider) entitlements that have accrued in the Medicaid program.

This shifting toward HMOs in Medicaid contracting creates a very different environment for traditional Medicaid providers. Providers with sizable commercial patient volume have already seen the implications of these changes, and likely have already embarked on adjusting the way they do business in a managed care world. But providers with predominantly or exclusively Medicaid and uncompensated patients typically face a more abrupt and challenging transition. This is the case for many LHDs. They must find their way into HMO provider networks and meet credentialing criteria. They have to be able to negotiate acceptable rates. They have to comply with service and staffing standards, including hours of operation, appointment and wait time limits; conform to utilization management procedures and protocols; meet data-collection and reporting requirements; and demonstrate their ability to achieve specified performance levels in areas such as clinical quality and consumer satisfaction. Their ability to invoke privileged status as a public provider may be lost, and failure to meet standards may mean deselection. In summary, they have to perform at an acceptable and competitive level with private health care providers—perhaps for the first time.

In many locations, these demands have been attenuated in varying ways. Health plans may be compelled by Medicaid officials to contract with safety net or essential community providers.[3] In a number of states, plans are required to either pay these providers a higher rate or a supplemental payment may be made by the state to make them whole, as in the case of some FQHCs.[13] Some public health providers enjoy a virtual monopoly/sole community-provider status, so their inclusion in networks may be necessary in order for plans to meet travel time requirements of state agency contracts. Some service or reporting requirements may be adapted or relaxed or compliance delayed to allow time for public health facilities to bolster infrastructure. But managed care plans typically labor under significant pressure from state contracts and also from accreditation standards that curb their ability to make special accommodations or to deviate from standard practice in critical areas like credentialing. This pressure is likely to intensify as competition increases among plans. And the fact that many of these plans are investor owned means that they also face expectations from shareholders for reasonable returns.

Sustainability of Personal Health Services in LHDs

The cumulative effect of the conversion of Medicaid managed care to prepaid models—certainly in most urban areas of the country—and of the growing pressure on plans to meet multiple performance demands signals that LHDs interested in continuing to serve Medicaid beneficiaries will be under the gun to bolster their performance on many fronts. This development has provoked widespread debate among LHDs and other public health officials about the sustainability of personal health services, particularly in areas where substantial private sector competition and excess capacity exists. The conclusion of some health departments will be to discontinue these services. Others will struggle to maintain them because to do so will require substantial investment of resources to make them commercially viable and competitive. Still others will feel compelled to maintain them, because Medicaid revenues are crucial to support other safety-net services that cannot or will not be delivered by other providers in the community.

By the mid-1990s this issue reached nearly center stage in debates among public health officials at the local, state, and national level.[13] As one looks to future developments in Medicaid managed care, it is evident that the pace of change is unlikely to abate as Medicaid discovers that it can exercise its sizable purchasing clout through managed care companies, similarly to other powerful purchasers. Likewise, in many communities there is little willingness to make the investments needed to elevate personal health services to a point at which they can be made compatible with, if not attractive to, the provider networks of managed care organizations. But as managed care organizations work on behalf of private and public buyers to suppress the ability of providers to cross-subsidize care for uninsured persons, the availability of resources to finance uncompensated care is being diminished. Very few states (e.g., Oregon, Tennessee, and Hawaii) have been able thus far to exploit the 1115 waiver opportunity to expand the numbers of persons eligible to participate in Medicaid managed care initiatives. So, ironically, at the time when many LHDs are deciding to discontinue personal health services, the demand for such services for persons without coverage is going to grow.

CURRENT ISSUES AND DEVELOPMENTS

A closer look at current issues, developments, and controversies in Medicaid managed care can illuminate how public health may respond in terms of sustaining personal services, providing enabling and supportive services, or transitioning to new roles and relationships with managed care organizations and Medicaid agencies.

Next Frontiers in Medicaid Managed Care

As states embrace a prepaid managed care strategy, either throughout the state or only in urban areas, and extend managed care to special need beneficiaries, they are taking differing approaches to accommodating special populations, selecting contractors, determining payment rates, and developing and enforcing contracts—all of which are significant for local health departments. Virtually every state that has implemented Medicaid managed care for AFDC and AFDC-related beneficiaries (a distinction that will cease to be meaningful after welfare reform is implemented) is now involved in some fashion with extending managed care models to special need groups such as the disabled and persons with chronic disease. In nearly every instance, these programs are proving to be complex and contentious. But because these populations (30% of eligibles) consume a disproportionately high level of Medicaid expenditures (approximately 70%), the states are committed to trying to achieve savings from these beneficiary groups.[10]

As states opt for prepaid managed care, some are limiting their contractors to established, licensed HMOs that may be required to have substantial commercial membership. This strategy favors investor-owned companies who now dominate the commercial market.[14] These companies have the capital to enter new markets by responding to open procurements/solicitations, perhaps using Medicaid as a way to get a beachhead in a new market from which they may then build commercial business. They are also typically not locally based and raise serious concerns about their commitment to local community health systems as well as the sustainability of their effort if the Medicaid product line proves unprofitable.

Other states, including several of those with 1115 waivers like Tennessee, Oregon, and Illinois, allow prepaid entities that are not licensed HMOs to participate.[15] Some of these entities may be built around traditional, indigenous providers and have explicit roles for LHDs or FQHCs. These organizations may be more hospitable and accommodating to local providers, but they will also be organizationally immature and underdeveloped, and will likely invite adverse selection by drawing in disproportionate numbers of needy persons from among existing patients. Their long-term financial viability is uncertain. Concerns about selection effects and plan ownership also focus attention on rate development and rate adequacy. A growing number of states are using bidding processes rather than administered rates, which invites competitive pricing. States are interested in using market dynamics to save money through competition, and this goal has been recognized as particularly successful in Arizona (although informed observers point out this succeeded only after a decade of developing a foundation for true competitive bidding).[13]

Downward pressure on rates will only intensify the need for plans to ratchet down payments and negotiate other terms more aggressively with their network providers. This will make them less disposed to provide special accommodation to LHDs or FQHCs unless these are explicitly mandated to do so. Likewise, they will challenge more aggressively the value of supplemental services that traditional providers have rendered or perhaps refuse to pay for them. Supportive and enabling services rendered by LHDs or community health and human service providers under contracts to HMOs will be scrutinized more closely, and some plans may decide to go in-house with these. The relentless make-or-buy pressure induced by the financial constraint of capitation will be a powerful rationalizing force, producing new competitive demands on indigenous providers.

Response Opportunities for Public Health Entities

Several responses are likely to emerge among LHDs to the challenges brought on by expanded Medicaid managed care. Some LHDs with substantial case management and human service capacity may find roles for themselves in the provision of "wrap-around" services for special need populations for which HMOs are ill-prepared and inadequately staffed. These will be useful adjuncts for people for whom acute services may be of secondary importance, and they may be critical in customizing service delivery for people for whom traditional HMOs would be a rough fit. In a similar vein, past experience with low-income populations could make LHD personnel valuable in terms of outreach services to members or in enhancing cultural competence for plans with limited exposure to these populations. While this may seem a particularly natural role, many public health personnel have had little experience with commercial enterprises, and health plans may be leery or uncomfortable with enlisting their services and, instead, prefer to hire their own staff, which might be more malleable and responsive.

Some local health departments have very sophisticated delivery systems already in place in strategically located (i.e., underserved) areas and can fit effectively into health plan networks. In some urban areas, such as Philadelphia, these centers may already be organized into a unified, integrated system with substantial investment in information and other infrastructure needs.[3] They may be able to negotiate effectively from a position of strength across multiple networks. The special challenge for these entities will be to obtain adequate rates to support services to Medicaid beneficiaries while not impeding their ability to care for the uninsured, the other half of their target service population. As public providers they are constrained in their ability to add new profitable services or shed costly, unprofitable services, so payment rates are critical concerns. In addition, these public systems may face emergent competition from private systems of care that may find Medicaid patients more attractive in a period of declining revenues and excess provider capacity. The prospect of private, excess capacity raises the larger question of whether local governments may conclude direct provision is no longer needed and/or appropriate.

Another area of response, and an alternative to maintaining personal health services or shifting to enabling services, is the potential for local public health officials to alter course and move in the direction of playing assessment and assurance functions related to Medicaid managed care both for the community and for individual beneficiaries. There appears to be growing interest in this type of role, although relatively few concrete models of what it looks like are in full fruition.[12] Presumably, health departments could install themselves in proactive surveillance roles regarding local managed care plan performance by tracking the impact of Medicaid managed care on community health indicators. This might be done by collating information from managed care organizations (MCOs) with community-based surveillance systems and disclosing information to residents to raise levels of awareness and/or concern. They might also play a community ombudsman role and/or undertake systematic surveys of beneficiaries to assess experience and variation among plans.

While such a role has intuitive appeal and is not inconsistent with an aggressive assumption of public health responsibilities, there are several potential problems. Most health departments lack resources, including facilities, personnel, and skill sets to undertake such ambitious activities without a major front-end investment, and the source of this support is highly uncertain. Moreover, such agencies may lack credibility with health plans or formal standing with the state Medicaid agency, which may not have specified a role for LHDs in program monitoring and oversight. Since this would extend only to Medicaid managed care, it is unclear if the data that plans might share—such as Health Plan Employer Data Information Set (HEDIS) indicators—could be meshed with public health data to provide meaningful information on the impact of the health of the community. Finally, for those health departments that maintain personal health services and have contracts with managed care plans, serious conflict of interest questions might be raised. This suggests that embracing the assessment and assurance function might necessarily preclude the ability to sustain personal health services.

An additional tactic that might be embraced is a more generalized community education and information role. Such a role might include acting as a convener for health plans for sharing data and devising dissemination strategies. It could also include identifying issues and concerns that cut across or go beyond the interests of any single plan (or go beyond the concerns of Medicaid to all purchasers). A proactive local health department could promote organization and mobilization among plans and engage them in collaborative activities that meet the needs of the broader community in areas like immunization, school-based health services, or violence prevention. This seems like a particularly worthy role as the interests of individual professional practitioners are increasingly absorbed or subsumed by managed care organizations, and new ways are pursued to promote community spirit and investment among these competing corporate entities. LHDs, especially if they are neither encumbered with enforcement responsibilities nor aligned with a particular plan, could be instrumental in such efforts. At the same time, they will have important responsibilities to continue to articulate for the community as a whole some of the limits of privatization.

THE BROADER CONTEXT OF MEDICAID MANAGED CARE

It is useful to put these questions of how Medicaid managed care is shaping and, in some ways, redefining roles for public health agencies into a broader context related to both rapidly expanding managed care and the growing reliance on privatization of many public functions.

Working to the Contract: A Two-Edged Sword

No single issue or instrument captures both of these themes better than the contract that state Medicaid agencies enter into with MCOs. Not only is this the basic blueprint for what the state believes it is purchasing and paying for its beneficiaries from prepaid health plans, but it is also the mechanism by which public officials seek to get private contractors to do the public's work. For these reasons, enormous interest now focuses on the content and construction of these contracts that have been extremely varied among the states.[9] As these documents move toward a greater specificity and prescriptiveness, they detail the responsibilities and duties of plans, including the extent of affiliations they must develop with other organizations—such as health departments. And they may specify whether special accommodations are to be made to incorporate safety net providers into provider networks and whether certain payment arrangements are to be employed. Even more significantly, they are likely to set up performance targets for contracting plans that may relate to community health indicators and include provisions for monitoring and sanction procedures for noncompliance.

Unfortunately, many officials from other state agencies, particularly public health officials, have been slow to recognize the critical importance of these documents and the importance of having a proverbial "seat at the table" with their Medicaid colleagues when the agreements are crafted and/or negotiated with MCOs. This situation is now changing as many public health officials have recognized that the contract is a crucial point of intervention to ensure attention to public health concerns, and to the possible roles and relationships for local health departments in Medicaid managed care initiatives. This reflects growing understanding of longer term implications of managed care, of the health plan procurement and negotiation process, and of the capabilities (and limitations) of commercial managed care organizations.

Local officials are also learning that contracts cut both ways in terms of what is not included and thus not likely to be done or to be paid for. Plans may not be willing to spend capitation funds to support services not incorporated in the contracted benefit package, even if community health officials might expect them to do so. Services rendered to health plan enrollees by health departments for which health plans may have been paid, such as immunizations, cannot be billed back to the health plan unless the contract permits it. Plans may choose to go in-house with services such as home health or case managers even if LHDs have local capacity unless the contract grants preferred status to these entities. And certainly plans cannot be expected to willingly pay for services—directly or indirectly through cross-subsidies—for persons not enrolled in their plans. In a crude sense, health plans are like road contractors who can, at best, be expected to build a road strictly according to its contract specifications. They are not expected to build a better or longer road out of public-spiritedness or good citizenship. Commercial managed care organizations cannot be expected to go beyond what they been have contracted by Medicaid agencies to do. Consequently, the central role of this contract cannot be overstated.

Return on Investment Logic: A Sobering Reality

Even more pertinent to the discussion of the capacity of Medicaid managed care to meet beneficiaries' needs is whether managed care plans will make meaningful and sustained investment in prevention and pre-emption of more costly conditions. In fact, the answer to this is self-evident: they will invest in such efforts insofar as they get a reasonable rate of return from them, and/or their contracts require activities as a condition of compliance. Contracts can specify coverages, functions, and activities but struggle to operationalize the vigor and quality of performance. Prepayment has widely been held to fill in these gaps by inducing plans to invest in efforts to promote health and prevent more costly conditions from arising. However, this presumes a sufficiently sustained affiliation or enrollment so that the initiatives, literally and figuratively, will pay dividends for the plans. In other words, managed care plans are enrollment-based, not population-based, health systems as currently structured and financed.

Episodic eligibility for Medicaid and freedom to move among plans casts serious doubt on this presumption and underscores the need to find ways to preserve and promote those services that transcend what can be realistically expected from commercial MCOs. Some states and localities address this by excluding some services from capitation contracts—in effect, taxing all plans to finance some community-based services—and continue to finance providers directly for these services. Others require plans to pay for services such as immunizations from non-network public providers should their members choose to consume the services from these providers. Still other states may require plans to demonstrate community-wide investment by undertaking initiatives in violence prevention or school-based clinics to contribute to the public good on a broader basis than just to their plan members. It is likely that new, creative approaches will have to be found to confront the limits of return on investment logic and to finance activities that rebound to the entire community, including managed care plans.

Community-Based Input into Managed Care

The exuberant desire to move large numbers of Medicaid beneficiaries into managed care arrangements has led many states to undertake open solicitations for bidders to participate in a kind of "gold rush." While selection criteria used in the procurement process are becoming more sophisticated and demanding, eagerness to implement can make states inattentive to how their selections affect local delivery systems. On the other hand, health plans may intentionally underbid or overpromise to gain selection and market entry or, as is becoming more common, to get mandatory assignment of persons not making a plan selection who tend to be lower-cost members.[1] New investor-owned corporations have been formed explicitly to pursue these kinds of Medicaid-only opportunities and they rapidly build ad hoc provider networks to meet contract requirements. As profit seekers, these plans will stay in Medicaid as long as this product line is profitable and, just as surely, exit it if it is not.

Most investor-owned managed care corporations are not domestic or locally based companies, and extracting responsiveness to community needs from them may be possible only through the influence of large buyers, both public and private. But the self-interested nature of aggressive purchasing of health benefits via managed care plans does not address how consumers and communities may express individual or collective concerns about how managed care affects them. It is possible that LHDs may come to play a role in bringing to the fore community concerns about the performance and actions of managed care companies, especially if these departments can gain status and stature in the eyes of purchasers. Local health agencies that understand these changes and possess the requisite skills in community education and organization may perform a valued public service by promoting awareness and activism to give consumers and communities greater voice in matters affecting their well-being.

Community Capacity and the Indigent Care Ecosystem

Many LHDs may find it difficult, impossible, or undesirable to participate in prepaid managed care programs for Medicaid beneficiaries. Some with personal health services may phase them down and out as Medicaid revenues decline and as managed care organizations and their provider networks show interest in enrolling and serving Medicaid beneficiaries. To the extent that this leads to mainstream access to care for Medicaid-eligible persons, this is potentially a very positive development. But it may leave LHDs in an awkward position of making decisions about sustaining personal health services to persons without any insurance coverage. These persons will still need services, and without coverage they cannot gain access to the benefits and assurances of managed care.

In areas where excess or new capacity will not materialize—such as in rural, underserved locations—vacating this role for LHDs will be particularly problematic. Discontinuing services may limit access and/or increase the demands on providers to cross-subsidize uncompensated services just when commercial managed care companies may be attempting to systematically suppress cost shifting. Those providers who chose to do this may imperil their own competitive position or contribute to out-migration of private patients. This example illustrates the complex ecosystem of indigent care that has evolved through collaboration, coercion, and collusion among providers, purchasers, and policy makers. Managed care initiatives threaten this ecosystem, and LHDs will need to both educate the community about these dynamics and take actions necessary to preserve access for those persons unable to benefit from the successes of managed care.

KEY QUESTIONS AND CONCERNS

There follows a series of looming policy questions that will need to be addressed as the two-pronged advance of managed care and privatization continues.

Will the Insurance Model Ultimately Prevail as the Dominant Means To Provide Access to All?

The prevailing rationale for the ardent embrace of managed care is essentially this: for everyone in a lifeboat, the rising tide of managed care lifts all boats. The apparent success of managed care in stemming inflationary trends rebounds, in principle, to the benefits' purchasers—private and public—and to consumers for whom care remains more affordable and/or coverage more generous. But these benefits do not accrue to persons without coverage, the uninsured, whose plight is worsened by the zest for efficiency and the suppression of cross-subsidization that managed care stimulates. The case is made, and supported in some instances, that savings from managed care can be reinvested to expand eligibility for coverage in public programs. This expansion dynamic, however, simply does not apply on the private sector side, since there is no way to recapture a portion of the savings to use to expand insurance coverage to make this model fully effective for all, i.e., getting people into the lifeboats. Current policy has committed itself to a course in which the insurance model is ascendant, but universal coverage remains elusive.

Will Medicaid Managed Care Models Achieve Mainstreaming of Beneficiaries into a Single Tier of Care?

For more than 30 years, ostensible public policy has been to make Medicaid indistinguishable from other payers for care as a means to get access to mainstream providers of services. The failure in this regard is well documented, but there has been some reason to believe that contracting with managed care organizations that have substantial commercial membership could improve this track record. Evidence shows that the number of HMOs entering the Medicaid market has surged in recent years, including those with predominantly commercial membership. But it is possible that the high-water mark on this development has already been passed. In the mid-1990s, commercial HMOs began to see diminished profits, intensifying price pressure from their customers, and restiveness among investors. A clear signal being issued is that they are not willing to cross-subsidize the Medicaid product line with commercial profits. At the same time, a number of states are ratcheting down rates to health plans to gain greater savings or respond to perceptions of past overpayments. If there is a substantial exodus of commercial HMOs from this market, hopes for mainstreaming for beneficiaries will be lost, and it is unclear who and what types of capitated entities are likely to rise to replace them.

What Will Be the Predominant Shape of Future MCOs?

Will they be more or less accommodating toward the roles of local health departments? An added dimension of uncertainty arises from the continued flux in the managed care industry itself and shifting relationships among purchasers, plans, and providers. Recent experience suggests that there may be a kind of counterrevolution developing among providers who are becoming more organized and strategic in their dealing with health plans to regain, in their minds, at least, some measure of control of their destinies.[16] In some markets, this has met with purchaser support because of disappointment or disillusionment with managed care organizations, and, on a national level, there has been extensive discussion of whether the Medicare program should broaden the range of entities with which it will enter into prepaid contracts.[17] By implication, these same issues will pertain to the Medicaid program, although very significant regulatory issues will have to be addressed at the state level.[18] The question this poses in the context of this chapter is whether provider-sponsored initiatives and models are more likely to develop collaborative and cooperative relationships with local health agencies and provide them with meaningful community-based roles. On the one hand, the "localness" of many of these arrangements may be seen as a very positive feature and may promote real partnership possibilities. On the other hand, these counterrevolutionary models could actually represent reactionary, circle-the-wagons initiatives by acute care providers that could set back some of the progress toward population-based health system thinking provoked by managed care.

Will the Public Sector Achieve Greater Accountability via Private Contracting?

This chapter began by noting that policy makers have demonstrated in recent years a kind of infatuation with the idea that purchasing services from private vendors via contracts can extract more accountability and responsiveness than direct delivery. In other words, just as in prepaid health plans, public sector officials are aggressively exploring make-or-buy alternatives with a renewed interest. Success on this front requires proficiency in contract-based procurement and skill in contract monitoring and enforcement. Frankly, most states are still struggling on both of these counts, as witnessed by the recent landmark study of contracting conducted by Rosenbaum et al.[16] But the fact that contracting with managed care plans allows states to shift administrative and, to some extent, political burdens associated with vendor/provider relationships to subcontractors can be liberating, particularly when a number of these providers have succeeded in the past in gaining favorable terms from the Medicaid program. This may also be true in terms of extracting desired performance as well, as Medicaid agencies may not be able to exert effective pressure to meet certain expectations on sister state or local public agencies. They may permit or even require their subcontractors to tackle these challenges directly. Medicaid agency relationships with local health departments in primary care case management programs is a good example of this, as HMOs are expected to be more stringent in enforcement of service standards than states have chosen to be.

Will There Be a Renewal of Support for Public Health Functions and Services in the Face of Managed Care Growth?

It is too soon in the current transformation to answer this question, especially in light of what seems to be a widening backlash against managed care in many sectors and a corresponding concern that consumers need better vehicles to influence the shape of the marketplace. There is likely to be a maturing understanding of how managed care has succeeded in reducing costs and in reconfiguring delivery systems among the general public. In addition, purchasers and managed care plans are more forthrightly acknowledging the need to address consumer concerns about exercising informed choice and the dearth of meaningful comparative information. And there will be more recognition of how managed care organizations linked to individuals through their place of employment is a tenuous basis for continuity and accountability, with potential for instability at several points along this chain. It is possible—although far from certain—that public health may in fact be invited into this breach to provide the missing continuity between patients and providers and connectedness among plans, purchasers, and communities. This role is certainly not incompatible with public health roles and values, but it appears that the burden is on public health officials to make the case that they are the best candidate for this crucial work.

CONCLUSION

There is little reason to believe that the twin forces of managed care and privatization will abate in the near future. Each force presents distinctive threats and challenges to public health officials and agencies, and taken together these impacts will be especially daunting. The Medicaid experience vivifies several stark choices that public health officials will face as they explore new roles and relationships with commercial managed care enterprises. Finding accommodation with these organizations will involve many different strategies and tactics that will have to be customized and adapted to local markets. It will also necessitate cultivating new knowledge, skills, and attitudes for public health proponents who themselves will have to adapt to a world different from the one for which they have been trained. But there is also reason to be hopeful that core traditional public health values may gain new esteem as communities and their residents come to recognize some of the inherent shortcomings of managed care and the lurking dangers of unbridled privatization.

REFERENCES

1. Halverson PK, Kaluzny AD, Mays GP, Richards TB. Privatizing health services: alternative models and emerging issues for public health and quality management. *Qual Manage Health Care.* 1997;5:1–18.

2. Hurley R, Freund D, Paul J. *Managed Care in Medicaid: Lessons for Policy and Program Design.* Ann Arbor, Mich: Health Administration Press; 1993.

3. Hurley R, Kirschner L, Bone T. *The Managed Health Care Handbook.* 3rd ed. Gaithersburg, Md: Aspen Publishers; 1996.

4. Luft H. *Health Maintenance Organizations: Dimensions of Performance.* New York: Basic Books; 1981.

5. Rosenbaum S, Darnell J. *Medicaid Statewide Demonstrations: Overview of Approved and Proposed Section 1115 Proposals, Policy Brief.* Washington, DC: Kaiser Commission on the Future of Medicaid; 1994.

6. Kaiser Commission on the Future of Medicaid. *The Medicaid Cost Explosion.* Washington, DC: Kaiser Commission; 1993.

7. Moore S. Cost containment through risk sharing by primary care physicians. *N England J Med.* 1979;300:1359–1362.

8. Health Care Financing Administration. *Medicaid Managed Care Enrollment Report.* Baltimore, Md: Health Care Financing Administration; 1995.

9. Halverson PK, Mays GP, Kaluzny AD, Richards TB. Not-so-strange bedfellows: models of interaction between managed care plans and public health agencies. *Milbank Q.* 1997;75:113–138.

10. Gordon R, Baker E, Roper W, Omenn G. Prevention and the reforming U.S. health care system: changing roles and responsibilities for public health. *Annu Rev Public Health.* 1996;17:489–509.

11. Rowland D, Feder J, Salganicoff A, eds. *The Medicaid Crisis: Balancing Responsibilities, Priorities, and Dollars.* Washington, DC: American Association for the Advancement of Science; 1993.

12. Hurley R, Zinn J, Rosko M, Kuder J. *Adapting to Mandatory Medicaid Managed Care: Preparations and Perspectives among Community Health Providers.* Philadelphia: The Pew Charitable Trusts; 1997.

13. National Academy for State Health Policy. *Medicaid Managed Care: Guide for the State.* 3rd ed. Portland, Me: National Academy for State Health Policy; 1997.

14. Tannenbaum S, Hurley R. Disability and the managed care frenzy: a cautionary note. *Health Affairs.* 1995;14:213–219.

15. Interstudy. *The Interstudy Competitive Edge: Industry Report.* St. Paul, Minn: Interstudy; 1995.

16. Rosenbaum S, Shin P, Smith B, Wehr E, et al. *Negotiating the New Health Care System: An Analysis of Contracts between State Medicaid Agencies and Managed Care Organizations.* Washington, DC: The George Washington University Medical Center–Center for Health Policy Research; 1997.

17. Hurley R, Freund D. Determinants of provider selection or assignment in a mandatory case management program and their implications for utilization. *Inquiry.* 1988;25:402–410.

18. Coile R. Provider-sponsored networks: physicians organize for direct contracting. *Physician Executive.* 1996;22:5–9.

CHAPTER 7

Privatizing Maternal and Child Health Services in Texas

Patti J. Patterson, J. Scott Simpson, Robbie J. Davis,
Debra C. Stabeno, and Linda L. Bultman

Of all the traditional public health services, none is more fundamental than the provision of maternal and child health services. Historically, the maternal and child health services provided by state and local health departments have been funded through federal categorical grants established under Title V of the Social Security Act. Federal legislation in 1981 consolidated these grants into the Maternal and Child Health (MCH) Block Grant, which gave states broad powers to determine the use of these funds but also required states to share in the appropriation of funds.[1] Declining state revenues, increased managed care market penetration, and the growing accessibility of private health care providers have encouraged the state and local public health agencies in Texas to re-examine their roles in the provision of these services. The purpose of this chapter is to describe and assess the process by which the Texas Department of Health (TDH) embarked on a major initiative to "reinvent" maternal and child health services funded through the MCH block grant and related state revenues. Specific attention is given to the rationale, planning process, and implementation issues associated with this initiative.

Source: Adapted from P.J. Patterson et al., Privatizing Maternal and Child Health Services in Texas: Reinventing Title V Programs, *Quality Management in Health Care*, Vol. 5, No. 2, pp. 35–43, © 1997, Aspen Publishers, Inc.

This project has involved the efforts of hundreds of public health planners, administrators, and clinicians from across the state of Texas. Without their dedication, time commitment, and willingness to search for new and innovative approaches, this process would have been futile.

BACKGROUND

The TDH has a history of administering Title V that dates back to the implementation of the federal Social Security Act in 1939. TDH combines Title V funds with state general revenue dollars to support a variety of services, including family planning, prenatal care, preventive and primary health care for women and children, genetic screening and counseling services, case management, and payment for specialty and subspecialty services for children with special health care needs (CSHCN).[2] TDH provides these services directly in the eight public health regions in areas that lack a local health department, and indirectly through contracts with local health departments, medical schools, hospitals, community health centers, and nonprofit organizations.

During fiscal year 1995 (FY95), MCH services were provided through 87 contractors, which operated a total of 318 clinics. The TDH regional offices provided MCH services in 179 clinic sites around the state. Using funds from a variety of sources, these clinics provided prenatal care to 93410 women, family planning services to 154774 individuals, and preventive child health clinic services to 222770 children.[3] In addition, these funds supported broad-based services to entire populations. Newborn infants were screened for metabolic, endocrine, or heritable disorders, and school-aged children were screened for vision and hearing disorders and for scoliosis. These MCH funds also supported education and outreach campaigns regarding a number of health and social issues affecting women and children.

Despite the extensive and effective MCH service delivery system that developed under Texas Title V funds, evolving organizational and environmental conditions created a need for change. In the late 1980s and early 1990s, TDH expanded and broadened MCH and CSHCN services. Service priorities included increasing access to care through the development of school-based health centers and Community Oriented Primary Care projects and through expansion of case management and traditional preventive health services for women and children. Soon after this expansion, TDH recognized that its MCH funds from Title V and other sources could not keep pace with the rising costs of maintaining these programs. In order to balance the service needs of low-income women and children with the limited resources available through Title V, a thorough examination of ways in which MCH funds were being allocated and utilized in Texas was needed.

Changes were also occurring in the provider base of these services for low-income women and children. TDH instituted public health clinical services in the 1970s in places where no other providers were available. In some of these areas, private physicians, rural health clinics, migrant and community health centers, or rural hospitals had initiated clinical services for the population being served by TDH. By 1996, 428 rural health clinics had been established in Texas.[4] Thus, it became necessary to re-examine the need for TDH to continue providing maternal and child health services in each of its clinical sites.

At the same time, significant changes were occurring in health care coverage for women and children, including: expansions in the eligible population and benefits package of the Medicaid program; increases in the use of Medicaid managed care models; and movement of Medicaid clients into the private sector. In light of these service-delivery shifts, TDH recognized the importance of using Title V funds to support functions that would complement the Medicaid system. Additionally, Title V leaders at the federal level had been encouraging states to develop systems of care that focus on improving the health of entire populations of women and children, as well as the health of low-income individuals in need of clinical services.[5]

Since 1989, Medicaid services for pregnant women, infants, and young children have expanded significantly. In 1991, Texas Medicaid eligibility for pregnant women and infants was increased to 185% of the federal poverty level (FPL). In the Omnibus Budget Reconciliation Act of 1989, Congress mandated that Medicaid income eligibility increases be phased in until all children who are 18 years old or younger and at or below 100% of the FPL are covered by Medicaid by the year 2001. Congress also required that states offer to children all medically necessary services that are allowable under federal law, whether or not they are included in the state plan. This mandate has been implemented in Texas as the Comprehensive Care Program, which provides specialty services for CSHCN. Although these expansions provided significant improvements in insurance coverage for children and pregnant women, major gaps still remain for adolescents and for women who are not pregnant. For those individuals not affected by the Medicaid expansions, eligibility for Medicaid in Texas was limited to approximately 18% of the FPL.

As a result of the Medicaid expansions, a number of uninsured women and children who traditionally received care in public health clinics became Medicaid eligible. In FY95, approximately 47% of the 322669 births that occurred in Texas were paid for by Medicaid.[6] In addition, the state increased prenatal care reimbursement in the Medicaid program and actively recruited physicians and nurse practitioners to participate in the Early Periodic Screening, Diagnosis, and Treatment program. Texas also began enrolling Medicaid beneficiaries in private managed care plans that were paid capitated fees to provide all medically necessary health services. These Medicaid managed care contracts promised to affect the entire service delivery system, including public health services, and held potential for increasing access to private sector health care for these clients.

Texas' public health leaders recognized that difficult choices would need to be made regarding Title V programs and their role in Texas' changing health care system. Although Medicaid coverage had expanded significantly, more than one million Texas children still did not have health insurance.[7] Decision makers had to weigh the importance of providing education, quality assurance programs, needs assessments, and disease and injury surveillance information to the total population against the importance of providing direct health care to a relatively small portion of the people in need. Additionally, policy makers needed to consider the substantial role that Title V funds played in supporting the Texas public health infrastructure, recognizing that any changes in Title V programs were likely to have broad impact across many TDH public health programs. All of these factors weighed into the difficult decisions regarding the future uses of Title V funding in Texas. Due to the complexity of the issues and resolutions to be determined, a diverse collection of stakeholders was asked to participate in a planning process for the future of Title V programs.

REINVENTING TITLE V PROGRAMS

In November 1994, TDH initiated a strategic planning process to "reinvent" the Title V maternal and child health programs based on the needs of the target populations, diminishing resources, and the changing health care environment. A driving force in this process was the need to reduce expenditures significantly below the next fiscal year's projected level. The planning committee assembled for this process, which was named the Futures Project, embarked on an ambitious quality management process that it hoped would lead to well-informed decisions regarding where reductions should be made. The purpose of the Futures Project was to evaluate short-term and long-term strategies to address MCH and related issues. Short-term recommendations focused on changes that had to be made quickly to address available funding in the next fiscal year. Long-term recommendations provided a blueprint of priorities for spending limited Title V dollars in future years. The Futures Project was intended to review and revamp established priorities and policies for services to women and children in order to enable state, regional, and local partners to adjust their MCH programs to complement Medicaid and to strengthen the role of public health in the emerging health care system.[8]

Five committees were created to guide the planning process: a steering committee; a data workgroup; and committees for MCH and Related Services, CSHCN Services, and essential public health functions. A parallel review of genetic screening and counseling services was also included in the process. Committee membership included representatives from a cross-section of TDH programs, the eight TDH regional offices, local health departments, service contractors, professional and advocacy organizations, and service consumers. The project also included eight regional coordinators who developed and maintained linkages with other TDH staff, contractors, clients, and interested persons not serving on the project's committees.

The planning process and resulting recommendations were established to directly address issues related to the delivery of MCH services. However, the steering committee was cognizant of the fact that Title V and other MCH funding provided significant financial support for the entire public health infrastructure in the State of Texas. Changes made in MCH service delivery were likely to impact adult health programs, tuberculosis control, sexually transmitted diseases/human immunodeficiency virus programs, and all other direct services provided by the Texas Department of Health. These programs were involved in the project by including their representatives on project committees and by ensuring that their concerns were considered during planning sessions and deliberations.

A major area of focus for the Futures Project related to the direct delivery of MCH services. At the time, prenatal and well-child care, family planning, and genetics services were being provided by a variety of agencies and organizations within the state, including public and private contractors, local health departments, and TDH state employees in the regional clinic system. In contrast, most of the services for CSHCN were already being delivered by the private sector, with TDH functioning primarily in the administrative roles of eligibility determiner, payer, and service delivery monitor. The Futures Project targeted those MCH services for which private sector providers appeared to have sufficient capacity and expertise, but which continued to be directly provided by TDH. Although the project encompassed many other substantive issues, the remainder of this chapter focuses exclusively on the project's efforts to reach a solution to the question of direct service provision.

The project's mission regarding direct service provision was to critically examine and make recommendations for adapting Title V MCH programs and related activities to the changing health care environment and enhancing program efforts to improve the health status of women and children in Texas. Teams developed vision statements for the future of MCH services, reviewed the current status of programs, gathered information about alternatives for service delivery and workloads at individual clinic sites, and examined other health-related activities for the target populations. Each committee also reviewed Title V legislation, key state legislation, and literature about the role of MCH programs in addressing population-based, essential public health functions.[9]

Public input regarding major MCH issues and potential solutions was solicited and reviewed. This information was used by the committees to develop their reports and recommendations, all of which were combined into a single report for public comment. After eight public hearings across the state, all committees reconvened at a summit meeting to review public comments and develop final recommendations. TDH executives and the Texas Board of Health made revisions and approved the final product.

The Title V Futures Project recommendations addressed three major MCH service-provision components: (1) definition of the population to be served, (2) provider requirements, and (3) shifting priorities for utilization of these limited funds. The population eligible to receive preventive and primary health care with these funds was defined as women of child-bearing age and children with incomes below 185% of the FPL who were not eligible for Medicaid. Since Medicaid is the major funding source for health care for low-income women and children, MCH funding allocated for individually based, direct services should be used in a gap-filling role only. The purpose of this recommendation was to ensure that applicants who are eligible or potentially eligible for Medicaid are channeled to the Medicaid program and that limited MCH funds are spent only as a last resort for people who are not eligible for health services through other sources.

These recommendations were made operational through a performance-based reimbursement methodology: MCH contractors bill against a contractual dollar ceiling for approved services provided to eligible patients. In previous years, funding for MCH contractors was provided for individually based health services by budget categories, such as salaries, benefits, supplies, travel, and so on, assuming that staff, travel, and supplies costs would permit communities to determine their own service needs and to provide them through this funding. The performance-based system of reimbursement was instituted to increase accountability, to encourage Medicaid billing, and to increase efficiency and productivity.

Changes in the provider base for MCH services were also implemented in response to the Futures Project recommendations. Clinics operated by TDH and by many other public health providers were downsized to address the recommendation that greater emphasis should be placed on facilitating the development of accessible private systems of care, rather than on expanding the existing public sector clinic system. Public clinic days and hours of operation were reduced, and restrictions were placed on clinic service delivery capacities, particularly for acute care services. As public clinics were downsized, TDH assumed a critical new role in transitioning clients into "medical homes" by locating or recruiting new providers that would enable families to receive both preventive and acute care services from the same local provider. Although TDH continued to fulfill its role as the provider of last resort in medically underserved areas, a fundamental change occurred in the organization's mission, transforming its earlier focus on direct service provision into a broader role in ensuring that adequate services are delivered through existing systems of care in the community.

Implementing the changes to Title V service provision required movement to a competitive application process for provider contracting.[10] Although a few new TDH providers had been added when funds were available and special initiatives such as school-based health care and community-oriented primary care sites had been funded, the contractor base for Title V services had remained stable for more than 10 years. The competitive application process allowed TDH to transition the delivery of clinical MCH services from state-sponsored clinics to local providers in areas where practitioners had moved into previously underserved areas. The competitive application was phased in to allow a progression toward "medical home" providers. For the first fiscal year of the new process, the competition was limited to the existing pool of providers. For subsequent years, the application process was opened to all qualified providers. The new contracting system aimed to promote stability in the provider base by offering renewable three-year contracts rather than the traditional single-year contracts.

A final Futures Project recommendation that motivated Title V program change involved a gradual movement away from the provision of personal health services to highly targeted individuals and groups, toward a new focus in supporting population-based, community-wide efforts in essential public health services. This strategy was supported by a growing body of literature suggesting that the strengthening of essential public health services is vital for community health improvement and effective system change.[11,12] The steering committee determined that these essential services should include: providing input into development of state health policy ensuring that all women and children have health care coverage; improving health-status monitoring through surveillance and needs/resource assessment activities; establishing and reviewing quality assurance procedures and standards for Medicaid managed care programs; and providing training and technical assistance to public and private health care providers.

Consensus among the MCH, CSHCN, and essential public health functions committees prescribed that future MCH priorities and funding allocation should be based on community need as measured by local assessments of health status, health care access, and delivery systems. Extended discussions about a state needs/resource assessment centered around whether the assessment should be the role of TDH's Bureau of Women and Children (BWC), TDH, or other state agencies. The steering committee concluded that TDH should coordinate a department-level statewide needs/resource assessment and that BWC should contribute resources to plan and implement it. It was also determined that population-based services should focus on improving data-gathering capacity, establishing and maintaining a minimum data set, and retraining existing public health staff to accomplish broader population-based services.

THE PROSPECTS OF TITLE V REDESIGN: CHALLENGES AND OPPORTUNITIES

The success of the "reinvented" Title V programs in Texas must ultimately be measured against the four major objectives identified during the planning and early implementation phases of the Futures Project: (1) bringing public and private health care providers together in Texas to adapt the MCH delivery system to the changing health care environment, (2) shifting the emphasis of public health providers from the delivery of personal health services to the performance of population-based essential public health practices, (3) reducing MCH program costs and improving overall efficiency while maintaining a safety net for residents without access to community providers, and (4) communicating to providers, clients, and policy makers the concept of a "reinvented" MCH delivery system that depends upon community providers to serve as a medical home for MCH clients and upon TDH to support and assure the adequacy of the delivery system for all residents. Early observations of the new system suggest that substantial progress is being made toward these objectives, although formidable challenges remain.

Encouraging Public and Private Sector Collaboration

The first objective of the new Title V system is for public health entities, including TDH central and regional offices, local health departments, and other contractors, to work together in adapting to a changing health environment. This environment is shaped by Title V funds, which are inadequate to meet the needs of all of the uninsured women and children in the state; expanded Medicaid eligibility criteria, which are allowing greater numbers of low-income women and children to be covered under the program; and an ongoing program to enroll Medicaid beneficiaries in capitated managed care plans. In response to these changes, all public health providers must take steps to maximize use of the Medicaid program for health services to women and children. TDH must continually reassess its resource expenditures and respond proactively in a changing environment. The new system must include continuous efforts to improve communication within the MCH community across the state and to elicit committed participation in this change process.

The changing health care environment is increasing private sector competition for patients traditionally served in the public health sector. Under the Title V innovations, existing public and private contractors must now compete for available Title V funds. Additionally, a competitive bid process is now underway in TDH regions that were traditionally underserved but had experienced the entrance of new providers. This bidding process is responsible for transferring the responsibility for providing MCH clinical services from TDH regional clinics to other providers in 76 counties. In 46 of these counties, medical schools are now providing these services. In the remaining 30 counties, the new MCH service providers include hospitals, rural health clinics, private physicians, community health centers, and other entities, including a home health agency.

The issue of competition in areas where medical schools assumed responsibility for providing MCH services to the Title V population is somewhat controversial. TDH maintains a good relationship with the local hospitals and physicians in most of these areas. However, some providers feel subjected to unfair competition when medical schools are awarded service contracts. Most objections center around services to the Medicaid population, rather than services for uninsured Title V clients. TDH continues to explore management approaches for minimizing this conflict and ensuring balanced competition among a diverse collection of MCH providers.

Local health department leaders report that adapting to competitive bidding and performance-based reimbursement is a difficult process. However, they also indicate that their clinics have become more efficient and that the costs of providing services are more easily defined. Many local public health directors believe that they are now in better positions to negotiate with managed care organizations for provision of clinical and ancillary health services.

To ensure that MCH contractors adequately adapt to changes in Medicaid eligibility, TDH now requires contractors to perform a formal Medicaid eligibility screening process for all women and children seeking MCH services. Applicants who are potentially eligible for Medicaid are referred to the Department of Human Services. Contractors bill Medicaid for services to eligible clients and reserve Title V funds for services to the remainder of the low-income women and children.

Overall, the move to competitive bidding and performance-based reimbursement appears to be succeeding in improving the efficiency of MCH service delivery. Between fiscal years 1995 and 1996, state expenditures for maternal and child health services were reduced by 20%, and 568 positions funded by Title V and related general revenues were eliminated. At the time of this writing, projections indicate that the same number of patients were seen by Title V–supported clinics in 1996 as in 1995 (approximately 470954), suggesting that program costs were reduced while overall service volume was maintained.

Emphasizing Population-Based Essential Public Health Practices

The second objective of the new Title V delivery system entails a true paradigm shift in the MCH public health community. This objective maintains that TDH must increase the use of limited MCH resources for population-based, essential public health services, including: policy development, health surveillance and monitoring, quality assurance, public education, training, population-based individual services, and community development. This objective also requires that TDH decrease the use of Title V and related resources for filling gaps in direct services, except as a last resort when there are no other resources. The rationale for this objective holds that if TDH redirects resources to population-based essential public health services, the health status of the general population of women and children in Texas will improve, in contrast to direct clinical services provision, which offers health status improvement in only a small percentage of the population.

There are major reasons for moving away from individually based client services. As stated above, Medicaid is the major health care program for indigent

Texas residents, and many potentially eligible people have not applied for Medicaid. Under Title V, each state is responsible for identifying women and children who are eligible for Medicaid and for assisting them in applying. Changes in TDH's service delivery procedures would therefore help to reinforce Title V's role in promoting use of the Medicaid program.

Next, even though the majority of Title V general revenue funds have been spent on individually based, gap-filling direct services, the services do not equitably reach all potentially eligible women and children. Clinic and school-based health services targeted to women, infants, children, and adolescents are not present in every county.

Finally, Title V resources are stagnant. Both federal block grant allocations and Texas state appropriations for MCH have remained steady since 1993, while inflation in health care costs has grown at a rate of 13% to 15% per year. Given these trends, Title V direct services programs are expected to serve progressively fewer women and children, and program inequities are likely to increase.

In the long run, TDH believes that increased funding of population-based services and activities will provide greater benefits to more Texas residents than will continued support of gap-filling, direct services to a fraction of the population in need. The decision to begin redirecting funds toward population-based services is both praised and criticized in the health care community. Some observers concur with the decision to emphasize such services as policy development, health status monitoring and surveillance, newborn screening, immunizations, fluoridation, recruitment of providers, development of quality standards/assurance, provider training, and public education.

Improving Efficiency and Reducing Expenditures

The third objective of the new Title V program is to reduce expenditures, improve program efficiency, and continue some direct services for low-income families and children who are not eligible for the Medicaid program. TDH central and regional offices, local health departments, and other contractors are required to reduce expenditures, which clearly affects the extent and scope of Title V services. At the same time, TDH endeavors to continue providing or paying for some primary, preventive, and specialty health services for indigent Texas residents who do not qualify for Medicaid. TDH recognizes that Title V resources are insufficient to provide full access to uninsured low-income women and children, but the agency continues to provide individually based client services in a gap-filling role. Finally, TDH continues to serve in a case management role by assisting families in finding medical homes and in gaining access to other needed health and human service programs their needs require.

One difficulty encountered in implementing the performance-based reimbursement methodology stems from the fact that most non–Title V TDH programs continue to provide funds to communities through a categorical granting system. Most of these programs are under review to determine the feasibility of changes that would offer greater accountability for services provided. Since public health staff work comprehensively to address the needs of the entire population regardless of the funding source, decreases in resources and staff will reduce the public health infrastructure statewide.

Communicating the Concepts of Reinvention to Stakeholders

The fourth objective of the new Title V system represents one of the more complex and time-consuming aspects of the project: communicating effectively to providers, clients, local community leaders, and legislators the role of public health organizations in supporting the health of all Texans, and the need to adapt to a changing health care environment by transitioning clinical service delivery to community providers. This concept stands in stark contrast to the traditional view of public health as care for low-income persons. In many communities, the public health clinic is an icon of assistance to the poor. Despite the conceptual leap that is required, this "reinvention" process is slowly resulting in increased awareness on the part of the general public and local and state elected officials regarding the Title V block grant and the maternal and child health services provided by TDH and its contractors.

The task of communicating the concepts of a "reinvented" MCH system to key stakeholders is an ongoing one, and it is likely to follow the adoption and diffusion processes that are characteristic of many policy innovations.[13] For most of the system's key internal and external stakeholders, the initial processes of awareness and acceptance are now complete. Most TDH staff, contractors, local health departments, community organizations, and policy makers are knowledgeable about the new MCH service delivery system and are moving to adopt appropriate roles within this system. As TDH and its stakeholders make progress in fully implementing the objectives of the reinvented system, MCH clients and the public in general are beginning to understand system concepts and to accept the new ways of organizing and delivering public health services in Texas. By developing and maintaining lines of communication and coordination among service contractors, clients, policy makers, and other stakeholders, TDH continues to strive toward institutionalizing the reinvented MCH system within its own organizational structure as well as those of other agencies contributing to maternal and child health in Texas.

CONCLUSION

In Texas as in most other areas of the country, rapid and far-reaching changes are occurring within the health care system. Public health services, including maternal and child health services, must remain responsive to these changes in order to sustain and improve the health of the populations served by this system. The expansion of managed care, changes in public and private sector expenditures for health care, shifts in health manpower and resources, and proposals to reform Medicaid and welfare are likely to continue affecting community health needs and the delivery systems established to meet these needs, especially within populations at risk of underservice. Texas offers the nation one example of how public health services can be "reinvented" through privatization guided by quality management principles. Early observations suggest that this approach can be successful in responding to health system change.

REFERENCES

1. Title V Maternal and Child Health Services Block Grant of 1991, Section 501, 42 USC, §§ 701–709.

2. Texas Department of Health. *Maternal and Child Health Block Grant Application, Fiscal Year 1996.* Austin, Tex: Texas Department of Health; 1995.

3. Texas Department of Health. *Maternal and Child Health Block Grant Annual Report, Fiscal Year 1995.* Austin, Tex: Texas Department of Health; 1996.

4. Texas Department of Health, Division of Health Facility Compliance. Austin, Tex: Texas Department of Health. Unpublished data.

5. Maternal and Child Health Bureau. *State Block Grant Annual Report Guidance.* Rockville, Md: U.S. Department of Health and Human Services, Public Health Service, Health Resources and Services Administration; 1994.

6. Texas Department of Health, Bureaus of Health Care Financing and of Vital Statistics. Austin, Tex: Texas Department of Health; 1996. Unpublished data.

7. Texas Medical Association. *Insuring the Uninsured: A Plan for Texas.* Austin, Tex: Texas Medical Association; 1991.

8. Texas Department of Health. *Title V Futures Project: Final Report and Recommendations.* Austin, Tex: Texas Department of Health; 1995.

9. Washington State Core Government Functions Task Force. *Core Public Health Functions: A Progress Report from the Washington State Core Government Functions Task Force.* Olympia, Wash: Washington State Core Government Functions Task Force; 1993.

10. Texas Department of Health. *FY97 Title V Request for Applications.* Austin, Tex: Texas Department of Health; 1996.

11. Grayson HA, Guyer A. *Public MCH Program Functions Framework: Essential Public Health Services to Promote Maternal and Child Health in America.* McLean, Va: National Maternal and Child Health Clearinghouse; 1995.

12. Baker EL, Melton RJ, Strange PV, Fields ML, et al. Health reform and the health of the public. *JAMA.* 1994;272:1276–1282.

13. Kaluzny AD, McLaughlin CP, Jaeger BJ. TQM as a managerial innovation: research issues and implications. In: Kaluzny AD, McLaughlin CP, eds. *Continuous Quality Improvement in Health Care.* Gaithersburg, Md: Aspen Publishers; 1994:301–313.

CHAPTER 8

Public and Private Sector Involvement in Managed Mental Health Care

Bruce J. Fried, Matthew C. Johnsen, and Artemis H. Malekpour

Over the past decade, employers have increasingly turned to managed care financing arrangements in an effort to reduce the burgeoning costs of health insurance. These managed care arrangements involve a set of tools that include utilization review, case management, and pre-authorization, which have been useful in controlling the costs of health care without reducing the overall quality of health care. Collectively, these have been referred to as managed care arrangements. As an effort that began in the private sector, public sector insurance programs such as Medicaid and Medicare have increasingly turned to managed care funding arrangements as part of an effort to check the ever-increasing public contribution to the health care of persons who are poor or disabled. As mentioned elsewhere in this book, this trend is expected to continue until the market share of public health insurance reaches a point of saturation.

In this chapter, we focus on the transition from mental health services traditionally provided under public auspices to a variety of arrangements involving private sector organizations. The issues involved in mental health are similar to those involved in general health services: contracting, determining who shares the risk in managed care arrangements, and monitoring contracts. These issues are exacerbated in mental health, however, due in large part to the difficulties involved in placing boundaries around what in fact constitutes a mental health service and subsequent problems in costing services and evaluating contract compliance. For people with serious mental illnesses, such as schizophrenia and bipolar disorders, the trends toward managed care and privatization present even more daunting challenges. Many of these challenges are related to the historic location of mental health services for this population within public sector settings. Although managed care organizations are most often private, for-profit entities, most mental health services for this population emerged as safety net organizations within the public sector, and only in recent years have private entities begun to develop the mental health sector. While this chapter deals with mental health services in general terms, our primary focus is on services for individuals with severe mental disorders, since this population is most likely to have received publicly financed services in the past, typically through Medicaid. Because of this group's heavy dependence on services financed and provided through the public sector in the past, issues of privatization potentially affect this group in a significant manner.

This chapter reviews some of the literature that relates to these three considerations, that is, the historic public sector location of mental health services, the recent trend toward privatization of mental health services, and the recent trend toward managed mental health care. The case of mental health care makes an illustrative case for what happens when public and private interests are merged, allowing us to understand who profits and who loses in such uneasy alliances.

A HISTORICAL VIEW OF PUBLIC AND PRIVATE PARTICIPATION IN MENTAL HEALTH SERVICES

Over the last few centuries, we have witnessed dramatic changes in the provision, administration, and financing of mental health services (Exhibit 8–1). The responsibility of caring for persons with severe mental disorders initially rested with the family and community. This role was later assumed by state governments and later the federal government. Responsibility has gradually shifted back to the states, with the private sector playing an increasingly important role in recent years. Recent pressures, particularly concern with balancing the federal budget and the emergence of managed care into the mental health field, have placed an emphasis on cost containment and the avoidance of unnecessary utilization.

Public Sector Involvement in Mental Health Care

The established belief in colonial America was that the family or local community had the obligation to care for the needs of individuals with mental disorders. Persons who were mentally ill were most frequently attended in their own homes or in lodgings that local governments helped subsidize. The prevalent theory about mental illness during this period was that insanity was not a medical condition but rather a predicament of society and finances. Almshouses or poorhouses began taking in people with mental disorders, considering them wards of the community. In this respect, during this period people with mental illness were viewed no differently from the indigent population.[1] Workhouses and prisons were also used, perhaps inadvertently, as places of containment for persons with mental disorders. Such early forms of institutionalization served

Exhibit 8–1 Historical Trends in Mental Health Service Provision in the United States

Colonial America	• Family/local community responsible for care of mentally ill
	• Almshouses/poorhouses increasingly house individuals with mental disorders as wards of the community
1772	• Pennsylvania Hospital in Philadelphia serves as first general hospital with separate wing devoted entirely to care of those with mental illness
1773	• First public mental hospital established in Williamsburg, Virginia
1790s	• Introduction of new philosophy of care, "moral treatment," with sympathetic and humane treatment administered in asylum or hospital environment with emphasis on medical care
1817	• Opening of first private psychiatric hospital in Philadelphia
Mid-1800s	• Dorothea Dix leads period of reform in mental health care, resulting in development of state mental hospitals
	• Responsibility of care for mentally ill shifted to states
Early 1900s	• Emergence of "mental hygiene" movement, or idea that treatment of mental illness could be delivered in the community rather than through hospitalization
Post-WWII	• Introduction of the idea of deinstitutionalization
1946	• National Mental Health Act increases the role of federal government in mental health policy
	• Division of Mental Hygiene renamed National Institute of Mental Health
1950	• More than 300 state mental hospitals confined more than a half million of the nation's mentally ill
1955	• Advancements made in psychotropic medications, allowing the mentally ill to return to communities to receive treatment
1963	• President John F. Kennedy signs Community Mental Health Centers Construction Act
Mid-1960s	• Enactment of Medicaid and Medicare programs helps aid in the financing of mental health care for qualified individuals
1968	• Programs established for the young, aged, and substance abusers within Community Mental Health Centers
1970	• Number of inpatients in state mental health facilities reduced to about 339000

continues

Exhibit 8–1 continued

1974	• Supplemental Security Income and Social Security Disability Income programs implemented to assist in payment of mental health care using federal funds
1975	• Community Mental Health Center Amendment passed, calling for an increase in mental health services
Late 1970s	• President's Commission on Mental Health established under President Carter
1980	• Mental Health Systems Act passed as President Carter ends his term
1981	• Mental Health Systems Act essentially repealed under President Ronald Reagan
	• Signing of Omnibus Budget Reconciliation Act leads to large cut in federal funds directed toward mental health care
	• Responsibility of treatment of mentally ill shifted back to states through block grants
Mid–late 1980s	• States pursue a variety of Medicaid waiver programs, placing many Medicaid beneficiaries in managed care programs
	• Passage of the Tax Equity and Fiscal Responsibility Act of 1982 and the Social Security Amendments of 1983, establishing prospective payment for Medicare and initiating the development of DRGs
Early–mid 1990s	• President Clinton's health care reform efforts spur market-based initiatives in health care
	• Large-scale consolidation continues among providers and insurers
	• States become focal point of health care reform with increasing attention given to public-private contracting arrangements for mental health services
	• Growth and consolidation of managed behavioral health industry

more as dumping grounds for people considered insane rather than a means of treatment for the mentally ill.[2]

The 1770s witnessed the admission of some mentally ill individuals to general hospitals. The Pennsylvania Hospital was established in 1751 in Philadelphia with public and private aid. A section of the hospital was set aside to serve the "insane," that is, people "unhappily disordered in their senses," who wandered about "to the terror of their neighbors, there being no place in which they might be confined and subjected to proper management for their recovery."[3] The first public mental hospital was established in Williamsburg, Virginia, in 1773, appropriately named the "Publick Hospital."[2] In the last decade of the 18th century, the term "moral treatment" was introduced to describe a new philosophy of care for persons with mental illness. The sympathetic and humane treatment of patients with mental disorders would now be provided in an asylum or hospital environment, with an emphasis on medical care.[1] In 1817, the Pennsylvania Friend's Asylum opened in Philadelphia, serving as the first private psychiatric hospital.[2]

A period of reform in the mid-19th century, led by Dorothea Dix, resulted in the establishment of a number of state hospitals to house and treat persons who were indigent, who had mental disorders, and who required separation from families or communities. The emergence of state hospitals signaled a shift in responsibility from local communities and families to the states. By the mid-20th century, more than 300 state mental hospitals had been established,[1] with New York and Massachusetts leading the way. The goal during this period was to not only contain but also treat persons with mental illness using both public and private facilities.[2]

During this same period, however, states were increasingly burdened with the cost of caring for persons with mental illness, and as patients tended to remain in these facilities for extended periods of time, overcrowding began to occur. Coupled with the difficulty in staffing, the quality of state mental hospitals suffered, and the ideal of treating this population was gradually supplanted by the reality of merely providing custodial care.[1] State hospitals became long-term facilities, in many cases housing patients for their entire adult lifetime. By the 1950s, more than half a million people in the United States were confined to mental hospitals.[4]

The early 20th century saw the development of new attitudes toward people with mental illness and novel approaches to dealing with the problem of mental illness in society. The early 1900s saw the emergence of the "mental hygiene" movement, or the idea that mental illness could be treated at an early stage in the community, eliminating the need for hospitalization.[1] Outpatient and aftercare programs were created with the goal of delivering follow-up treatment to individuals subsequent to their release from mental facilities. Not long thereafter, newly diagnosed individuals were also cared for on an outpatient basis.[2] Boston Psychopathic Hospital was one of a number of new facilities designed to diligently treat the mentally ill in settings close to the patients' homes and families. There was also an increase in the number of university-operated psychiatric wards located in general hospitals.[2] Notwithstanding these initiatives, state psychiatric hospitals remained pivotal to the care and housing of individuals with severe mental disorders.

The experience of World War II changed the country's perception of mental disorders. Mental illness accounted for 40% of all individuals deemed unfit to be inducted into military service, and many individuals discharged from the military were diagnosed with some form of mental illness. State mental hospitals continued to suffer from physician understaffing, and living conditions were frequently deplorable. Military physicians, despite their lack of training in the field, became increasingly exposed to mental illness through their wartime experiences.[2] At the same time, experts within the mental health field began to believe that persons with mental illness would receive greater benefit if treatment were administered outside the hospital setting.[1] Advancements made in antipsychotic medications allowed patients with severe mental illness to return to communities to receive their care. There was large-scale support for community-based care and treatment in the "least restrictive environment." All of these factors contributed to the onset of deinstitutionalization.[4]

The origins of the movement toward deinstitutionalization can be traced to 1946 with the establishment of the National Mental Health Act, which gave the federal government a more pronounced voice in mental health policy. The Division of Mental Hygiene, initially established in 1930, was renamed the National Institute of Mental Health and given increased funding and responsibilities. Robert Felix, the first director of the National Institute of Mental Health, contributed not only to the identification, treatment, and prevention of mental illness, but also to the idea that individuals with mental illness could be effectively treated in community settings as he promoted the development of outpatient clinics.

The federal government assumed an increasingly important role in financing mental health services as a result of President Kennedy's signing of the Community Mental Health Centers Construction Act in 1963.[5] Under this legislation, federal funds were made available to build a community-based system of mental health services. With the construction of community mental health centers (CMHCs), the number of state mental hospitals was expected to be cut in half.[4] One goal of CMHCs was to quickly detect the onset of symptoms and utilize preventive measures that would reduce the symptomatology associated with mental illness and the need for hospitalization and lengthy hospital stays. It was also hoped that CMHCs would stimulate use of community resources to support persons with mental illness in the community and that coordinated and continuous treatment plans would be developed.[5]

The CMHC program mandated comprehensive services, affiliation agreements between organizations, catchmented responsibilities, and citizen boards. Ideally, CMHCs would serve all members of the community, and the community mental health service system would be held accountable for the delivery of care to all persons from their area who needed service. The existence of CMHCs was intended to facilitate communication within the mental health system and provide comprehensive care. Key program components included 24-hour emergency treatment, inpatient and outpatient services, partial hospitalization, education and consultation within the community, services related to diagnosis and pre- and post-treatment, and rehabilitation. Research and evaluation were also considered integral to the mission of CMHCs. Making the community accountable for the care provided to its citizens who were mentally ill, it was believed, would ultimately save money.[2]

The reality of CMHCs was that those for whom the legislation was initially designed—individuals with severe and persistent mental disorders—were largely excluded from receiving services. The treatment of patients through the use of psychotherapy benefited individuals suffering from neuroses, rather than people with severe mental disorders.[5] The utilization of mental health services greatly increased in the latter half of the 20th century, largely due to the increased availability of services for patients not considered severely mentally ill.[6] Programs for children and adolescents, older persons, and persons who abuse substances were established within CMHCs beginning in 1968, as Congressional legislation turned its focus on these populations, believing the needs of the severely mentally ill had sufficiently been met.[5]

As a result of deinstitutionalization and the development of CMHCs, the number of individuals housed in state mental health facilities dramatically decreased between 1955 and 1970, from more than 550000 to about 339000. By 1980, state hospital admissions for the mentally ill had dropped even further, to 130000.[4]

Despite a lack of Presidential support during the Nixon and Ford administrations, with Congressional support, mental health services continued to prosper. In the 1960s and 1970s, with the introduction of Medicare and Medicaid—which provided financing for physical and mental health services—deinstitutionalization and, in effect, transinstitutionalization persisted, moving patients from state mental hospitals to community programs or nursing facilities.[6] It became increasingly apparent that CMHCs, created specifically to provide treatment for persons who were severely mentally ill once they left state mental health facilities, were not, in fact, assuming this responsibility for care. While federal entitlement programs allowed persons who were mentally ill to receive acute inpatient treatment in general hospitals, these hospitals often lacked the expertise or facilities to provide needed psychiatric services.[5] The "revolving door syndrome" became a common phenomenon for persons who were severely mentally ill. Patients would be discharged from state hospitals only to be lost to a virtually nonexistent community support system. Repeated readmissions to state hospitals were quite common.

The Community Mental Health Center Amendment of 1975 attempted to address the issue of inadequate service to persons with mental disorders through mandated programs.[2] The inception of federally financed Supplemental Security Income and Social Security Disability Income helped provide mental health services to persons without private health insurance or who were unable to pay "out-of-pocket" for necessary services.[4]

The President's Commission on Mental Health was created under the leadership of President Carter to assess the mental health needs of the nation and recommend appropriate measures. In 1980, the Mental Health Systems Act was passed as Carter was leaving office. Its purpose was to support the continuing efforts made by CMHCs to identify the needs of special populations.[1] With the election of Ronald Reagan, however, the act was essentially repealed. Under Reagan, federal funding of mental health care was drastically reduced with the signing of the Omnibus Budget Reconciliation Act of 1981. Under this legislation, states received block grants to be used to provide health, mental health, substance abuse, and other human services. This signaled a major shift in responsibility from the federal government to state governments. Community mental health centers ceased to be extensions of federal government mental health policy, and instead became little more than agencies with which state and county governments contracted to provide mental health and substance abuse services. Under the terms of this act, states were permitted to obtain waivers that required Medicaid beneficiaries to enroll in managed care plans and to develop alternative forms of managed care (Section 1915(b) and Section 1115 waivers, as discussed later). States were also permitted, under defined circumstances, to develop statewide managed care systems that did not meet federal statutory requirements.[7] The responsibility for providing care to persons with mental illness thus shifted back to the states, which were already fiscally challenged.[5] Clearly, this set of changes increased pressure on state governments and set the stage for the development of programs to control costs.

The Emergence of Managed Mental Health Care

Before 1980, payments for mental health services were made based primarily on a fee-for-service basis. Whether through private or public insurance arrangements, health professionals were paid on a fee-for-service basis, and, for the most part, hospitals were paid under cost-based reimbursement. Under these circumstances, treatment plans could be individualized to meet each patient's needs, and psychiatrists had considerable autonomy in determining care their patients would receive. Often the biggest obstacle mental health professionals faced was insufficient numbers of psychiatric beds.[8]

To control costs in the general health care sector, a direct means of cost control was undertaken through passage of the Tax Equity and Fiscal Responsibility Act of 1982 and the Social Security Amendments of 1983. As a result of these federal initiatives, a prospective payment system was mandated for Medicare through diagnosis-related groups (DRGs). The change from cost-based reimbursement to prospective reimbursement had a profound effect across the health care sector, including services provided within the mental health sector.

In the 1980s, as employment-based benefits for behavioral health care (mental health and substance abuse) expanded in the private, predominantly fee-for-service insurance market, for-profit specialty psychiatric and chemical dependency inpatient facilities grew, and costs of employee health plans skyrocketed. The costs to employers of mental health and substance abuse services increased correspondingly. The Health Insurance Experiment carried out in the 1970s, for example, found that fee-for-service populations had mental health expenditure levels almost three times greater than populations enrolled in the prepaid health plan.[9]

What emerged from these experiments—in the private sector and more recently in the public sector—was a set of organizational and funding mechanisms known collectively as managed care. As defined by the Institute of Medicine, managed care is "a set of techniques used by or on behalf of purchasers of health care benefits to manage health care costs by influencing patient care decision making through case-by-case assessments of the appropriateness of care prior to its provision."[10(p57)] In practice, however, the goal of managed care has been to cut costs by eliminating care considered unnecessary and utilizing more economical methods of treatment in place of more expensive services. Thus, treatment administered in outpatient settings is preferred to inpatient care,[11] and treatment provided by less expensive clinicians is preferable to care provided by high-priced professionals. Proponents of managed care systems believe that through a more reasonable system of allocating services, the quality of care delivered can be augmented while, simultaneously, expenditures can be reduced.[12]

A major attraction of managed care for mental illness and substance abuse services is its potential to reduce the direct and indirect costs of these disorders—to purchasers of health care who pay unnecessarily high premiums, to employers who lose productivity, to families who lose the contributions and support of their affected members, to society that bears the costs of crime, criminal justice, carnage of drunk drivers, and to the millions of Americans who directly suffer from mental illnesses and substance abuse every year.[13]

Managed care is, in fact, a broad concept that includes a variety of mechanisms for monitoring and delivering health care and thus it has a variety of forms. At one end of the continuum, managed care includes loosely coupled preferred provider organizations (PPOs), which are composed of individual physicians, physician groups, and hospitals that accept discounted fee-for-service payment in exchange for the promise of a designated volume of patient referrals. PPOs utilize a network of providers contracted by the insurance company to provide care at discounted rates.[10] Patients enrolled under this type of plan are allowed to choose their physicians, as well as the hospital in which inpatient services should be rendered, from a list of participants. Primary care physicians and specialists are both used under this arrangement. This option allows PPO members to personally select their providers of care, albeit from a predetermined roster. Both health maintenance organizations (HMOs) and PPOs often place restrictions on treatment options in an effort to contain costs.[14] This may be done explicitly through utilization review and preauthorization by the managed care entity, and/or implicitly, through financial incentives presented to health care providers.

Point-of-service (POS) plans allow and partially reimburse prepaid members who receive treatment outside the plan. Enrollees are still responsible for some of the cost incurred, but the POS option provides an increased level of flexibility and consumer choice. To increase their attractiveness to enrollees, some group and staff model HMOs are beginning to offer PPOs and POS plans as alternatives to their members.

At the other end of the managed care spectrum are more tightly coupled group and staff model HMOs in which members receive benefits within an established range for a prearranged payment over a specified time period.[11] Staff model HMOs employ directly a group of salaried physicians and other health professionals to provide care to enrolled patients. Often, HMOs employ the services of nonphysician providers in efforts to reduce the cost of care. In the mental health field, psychiatrists and even psychologists are being replaced by less expensive mental health professionals. Group rather than individual therapy may be favored, and there is great emphasis placed on short-term treatment methods.[10] HMOs deliver their services using one of three general models, although hybrids and diversified offerings are now common among HMOs. The staff model HMO essentially employs physicians to work in the HMO facility, providing them with a salary. Group models utilize one or more groups of physicians by contracting their services at predetermined rates. The network model allows physicians to negotiate with HMOs for a capitated fee for each member for whom the physician provides care. Physicians retained through this model, also known as an individual practice association, are allowed to render services within their private offices,[14] usually on a discounted fee-for-service basis. Under this model, physicians may act as gatekeepers to coordinate services required by patients.

Managed care principles may also be applied to traditional indemnity insurance models, utilizing such review mechanisms as prior authorization, utilization management, and case management. Among the most common approaches is utilization management (UM). In the mental health field, UM incorporates various methods to monitor, assess, and steer services provided to persons with mental disorders. Frequently, an insurance company contracts with a UM firm whose case managers are assigned to work with the mental health professional in devising a quality and cost-effective treatment plan for the patient. Case managers may precertify hospital admissions and treatment strategies, scrutinize reviews of time spent in facilities, and in general, seek to discourage costly care. Utilization management approaches to the delivery of health care are frequently used in conjunction with other managed care strategies.[11]

The key element shared by virtually all managed care approaches is the prospective or concurrent review of care provided to individual patients, with the power to deny provision of care thought to be unnecessary, inappropriate, or not cost-effective. Although advocates of managed care programs often maintain that their efforts will lead to improvements in the quality of care—through the elimination of unnecessary procedures or the substitution of less-restrictive for more-restrictive care—it is clear that the heart of managed care systems lies in the goal of reducing health care costs.[15,16] As discussed later in this chapter, it is not clear that there is overutilization of services by individuals with severe mental disorders. In fact, a case could be made for the idea that persons with serious mental illness may actually underutilize services and that the restrictions of managed care may lead to poor patient outcomes and increased cost for the health care system.

While health care costs increased throughout the 1980s, many companies found that mental health and substance abuse claims against corporate health insurance programs were rising more rapidly than other health care costs. Between 1983 and 1988, the medical price index rose at approximately 11% per year. Mental health and substance abuse service costs to private employers increased almost twice as rapidly, at a rate of nearly 20% annually.[17,13] Because of rising expenditures associated with mental health services and the perceived unmanageability of these services, many U.S. corporations felt a need for specialized mental health care expertise. Many independent companies and insurers began offering separate "carve-out" behavioral health care insurance products to employers. A new managed behavioral health care industry emerged to administer mental health benefits and employee assistance plans for large corporations.[17] These programs feature management teams devoted exclusively to mental health and chemical dependency; case management personnel who are specialty credentialed under the supervision of board-certified psychiatrists; use of specifically developed mental health and chemical dependency level-of-care assignment and case management criteria that address medical necessity, medical appropriateness, and levels of care determination; and specialty behavioral group, staff model, and PPO networks with a continuum of care, access to a full range of disciplines, and negotiated discounts. The most common role for managed behavioral health care companies is to conduct utilization review and case management on behalf of a payer. They may also operate employee assistance programs and set up provider networks. Most recently, these firms are moving into risk-based contracting, which essentially means that the behavioral health care company assumes some of the claims risk for a population and is responsible for providing and managing services. The employer or insurer "contracts out" to a private vendor for mental health and substance abuse services.[18]

Other key features of managed behavioral health companies include continuous quality improvement programs, specialized behavioral information systems, outcome management systems, clinical practice guidelines, and provider network management systems. The market response to these vendors has been strong and positive, resulting in rapid growth of a managed behavioral health care carve-out industry. The results for industry have been impressive. In the case of IBM, for example, the 1990 carve-out of mental health benefits to a managed mental health care vendor was followed by a drop in mental health expenditures from $97.9 million in 1992 to $59.2 million in 1993.[19,20]

There are several arguments supporting the carve-out concept for mental health managed care. The first is that a specialized organization may be required to manage an area as specialized as mental health; carve-outs are essentially a distinct health plan for a specialty area with separate budgets, provider networks, and incentive arrangements.[18] The second argument supporting carve-out arrangements is that resources are specifically set aside, or protected, for providing mental health services. This argument suggests that carve-out arrangements actually protect those needing mental health services because there is a pot of mental health money that is in fact separate and distinct. Theoretically, this should discourage competition for good mental health risks, since money is reserved and available for the service needs of potential bad risks.[18]

MANAGED MENTAL HEALTH CARE IN THE PUBLIC SECTOR

Managed care is now the dominant mechanism used by private health insurers to coordinate and manage mental health and substance abuse services. By 1994, 108 million Americans had mental health and substance abuse services delivered through managed behavioral health care firms.[13] This represents 58% of all persons with private health insurance, though less than 20% of people covered by publicly funded health insurance such as Medicaid and Medicare. The growth market for managed care, then, is clearly in the public sector. The growth and ongoing consolidation of the managed behavioral health care industry is now allowing these organizations to enter markets for which they would have been ill-prepared in the past because of the sizable start-up costs associated with state Medicaid contracts.[19] The growth of the managed behavioral health industry comes at the same time as increased concerns of government officials and the public with escalating costs of Medicaid and Medicare.

States have been experimenting with various forms of managed care for Medicaid beneficiaries both to gain control over rising costs and to assure improved access to primary care.[21,22,13] These experiments have been conducted under two federal Social Security waiver authorities, Section 1915(b) and Section 1115. Currently, 1915(b) "freedom-of-choice" waivers allow 45 states to limit a beneficiary's choice of provider to HMOs and other primary care case management systems, 14 of which include mental health or addiction treatment populations. More recently, states have shifted to 1115 waivers that afford more flexibility in waiving eligibility rules for non-Medicaid/uninsured individuals (e.g., the working poor). Most 1115 waivers shift some or all of Medicaid-covered mental health and substance abuse services into managed care systems. Should Congress put the Medicaid program in a federal block grant to the states, these waivers will be obviated. However, many states will use a block grant to accomplish the same ends.

In addition, decisions must be made about who runs any mental health carve-out established by the state.[23] Many carve-outs are planned or set up through contracts with private, for-profit managed behavioral health care firms, as is the case in Massachusetts and Tennessee. In some cases, such as in Minnesota, HMOs subcontract for separate provision of mental health services. In a few cases, such as North Carolina and California, carve-outs are accomplished through reorganization of the public mental health system and nonprofit agencies to create publicly administered managed care programs.

The assumption implicit in managed care proposals is that a comprehensive array of services, coupled with the flexibility to provide such services on the basis of individual medical and psychological necessity, will produce outcomes and control costs more effectively than traditional fee-for-service financing.[24] To date, however, little rigorous evidence supports the relative effectiveness of the various managed care options in the public sector.[21,22,13,25] Moreover, private sector results may not be generalizable to the public sector. Public systems generally target people who are poor, who have severe and persistent mental illness and substance abuse disorders, and who often have other problems that complicate their care. For many public-sector patients, providers must also coordinate with housing, social services, primary health care, criminal justice, education, and vocational services. The public sector is also the agent of last resort for the uninsured—now estimated at 41 million people—and other people with no other way of accessing services.

Private managed care companies have, as yet, little experience providing services to people with disabling mental illness, or with the specialized services they need. Although one attraction of private managed care companies to behavioral health care may involve cost cutting and cost avoidance, it is not at all clear that significant savings can be achieved in Medicaid mental health care for persons with severe and persistent mental illnesses. Most of the demonstrated savings to date have been in managed care arrangements for nondisabled adults and children, who generally require fewer services. A variety of joint ventures between private and public agencies are being developed to marry the respective strengths of each system to provide service in cost-effective ways.

States may structure their managed care programs in a variety of ways.[23] Those adopting a fully integrated approach link all mental health care and substance abuse services for adults and children under a single plan that includes physical health care. In programs adopting a full carve-out strategy, no mental health or substance abuse services are provided within the basic health care plan; both basic and intensive services are provided through a separate behavioral health care system. Programs adopting a partial carve-out strategy employ a hybrid of the first two options: basic mental health services are covered as part of the standard health plan, but adults and children with more disabling disorders who need more intensive services are carved out into a separate managed mental health care plan. Excluding high-risk individuals is another option. In this approach, basic mental health services are included within the physical health benefit and run by a managed care entity, such as an HMO. Other mental health care is provided through traditional fee-for-service and state grant-funded programs under auspices separate from the managed care program.

The Privatization of Public Mental Health Programs

The most consistent research finding on the impact of managed mental health care on costs within the corporate sector is that it is most effective when three key components of managed care are present: provider networks, assumption of financial risk by the provider or managed care firm, and utilization management. Under these circumstances, costs are reduced, access increased, and clinical outcomes remain comparable to fee-for-service arrangements. Under less comprehensive managed care arrangements, results are mixed and inconsistent.[13]

There is substantially less evidence, however, on the impact of managed mental health care in the public sector. There are, of course, substantial differences between employee groups and people served under public auspices. Public systems typically target persons who are poor, who have disabilities (including severe and persistent mental illnesses and substance abuse disorders), and who often have concomitant co-morbidities and problems of living that complicate their care.[13] While cost savings and positive clinical outcomes may have been realized in the corporate setting, it is not at all clear that managed mental health care strategies are effective or appropriate for poor people with chronic severe mental illness.

The Massachusetts carve-out plan succeeded in cutting Medicaid costs by 22% in its first year while increasing access to care by 4.6%. However, rehospitalization rates for children and adolescents increased in the year following implementation of the managed care system, and there were significant concerns about the quality of care for children with emotional problems. In studies conducted in Hawaii and Rochester, New York, generally positive outcomes were found. However, generalizations are difficult to make because of the time limitedness of these studies. The Substance Abuse and Mental Health Services Administration is currently sponsoring the Managed Care for Vulnerable Populations study. This is a multisite study in which managed care arrangements are compared with fee-for-service Medicaid arrangements at each of 15 study sites. An array of utilization, cost, and outcome variables are being examined in this study. The results of this effort should provide a clearer and more detailed picture of what managed care arrangements work for which target populations.

Privatization in relation to mental health care thus allows organizations within the private sector to bid for state contracts to provide mental health services. These may include for-profit and not-for-profit private organizations as well as publicly funded organizations. In this environment, the question arises as to the appropriate role of state government as purchaser of services. Does it assume the somewhat limited role of simply ensuring adherence to quality standards? Two general strategies have been adopted by state governments and are distinguished by whether they retain their role as an insurer, i.e., whether they continue to bear the risk and carry out insurance functions such as paying claims, or transfer this risk to another party.[7]

Where states continue to bear the risk while contracting with providers to provide mental health services (the first strategy), state governments can utilize financial incentives and care coordination strategies to achieve quality and cost objectives. These include primary care case management and mental health case management programs. Under a case management approach, the existing fee-for-service system may be retained, but providers would be paid an additional case management fee to coordinate care. Another approach is for the state itself to function as the managed care plan.[7] This requires the state to develop specific expertise in managed care techniques, and, as such, has had only limited application.

A more common approach in recent years is for states to transfer risk and the insurance function to a number of plans. State governments commonly accomplish this by implementing full-risk, capitated managed care programs where plans are paid a fixed fee per beneficiary per month. Among the challenges for state governments is that they must learn how to purchase managed care plan services, how to select and contract with managed care organizations (MCOs), how to set rates, and how to monitor access and quality. This approach has the advantage of providing greater financial certainty to state governments by transferring financial risk to another entity. States may also have the ability to negotiate rates that are less than projected fee-for-service costs. The major disadvantage, of course, is that incentives may be created to reduce access and quality. A second disadvantage is that privatizing this financing structure may shift the provision of care away from a significantly developed public mental health service delivery system, and may not provide sufficient support to ensure the survival of public sector mental health care. Some would see this as a highly negative, unanticipated consequence of this type of funding arrangement.

Recent Trends toward Managed Mental Health Care

Managed care is increasingly being implemented at state and county levels to contain the cost of mental health care. Managed care companies are bidding for state contracts in order to provide services for people in the public sector who rely on entitlement programs.[11] Case management is often used by state agencies to allocate resources and determine treatment plans. Similar to the trends in privatization, the distinction between the private and public sectors in the practice of managed mental health care may become less pronounced as the two systems learn from each other's strategies. Private sector entities are becoming more aggressive in the management of cases, while public sector agencies are assuming a greater role in risk sharing.[10]

With the inception of managed care, and recognizing the limitations of re-sources, psychiatrists and other mental health professionals are becoming increasingly wary of rendering treatment deemed medically necessary.[26] Accreditation standards have been established by the National Committee for Quality Assurance to ensure that quality mental health care is delivered in a timely manner to the satisfaction of consumers.[27] A key issue facing managed care is whether to integrate mental health services into a general medical plan. Advocates of this proposal believe that integrated provider organizations will be more likely to address mental health problems in order to avoid utilization of high-cost services at a later date. The disadvantage to integration is that decision makers of treatment plans may be neither aware of nor interested in mental health issues. Thus, people in need of mental health services may be overlooked.[11] It is important that standards be developed to ensure that "gatekeepers" who determine access to care have substantial understanding and expertise in the delivery of mental health services. It is the goal of those responsible for establishing accreditation standards that emphasis be placed on the management of mental health outcomes rather than mental health providers in efforts to contain costs.[27] Through managed mental health care, accountability can be monitored to ensure that quality care is delivered in an efficient and effective manner.[11]

UNANSWERED QUESTIONS ABOUT PRIVATIZATION OF MENTAL HEALTH SERVICES

Among the difficulties in understanding the impact of privatization is the vast array of public-private arrangements in mental health. In some situations, state mental health authorities, or state Medicaid agencies, contract directly with managed care organizations to manage the mental health benefits for the Medicaid population. In other situations, the state may contract with a managed care organization, which in turn contracts with a "public" agency, such as a community mental health center, to provide mental health services. Thus, the line between public and private is not as distinct as it once was.

Within this environment, defining the appropriate role for public entities such as state departments of mental health, local mental health authorities, community mental health centers, and state Medicaid funding agencies will be a challenge. In some instances, for example, community mental health centers may evolve into one of several behavioral health service providers competing for mental health contracts. In other cases, such as the 1915(b) children's Medicaid waiver in North Carolina (Carolina Alternatives), the public area mental health programs become both the managed care entity and the provider agency. They may or may not directly bear financial risk. It is clear, in any event, that most states are willing to experiment with the private sector in managing and/or providing mental health services for the Medicaid population. Whether these organizations have the expertise to deal effectively with the challenges associated with providing mental health services within a capitated managed care framework remains to be seen.

State departments of mental health may very well move away from the direct provision of mental health services and into the assumption of planning, enforcement, and licensing roles. For some states, this will involve a new set of roles associated with capitation rate setting, contract development, and monitoring.

A related issue involves the role of the state hospital in future mental health systems. In most states, the state mental health authority operates state psychiatric hospitals, while the state Medicaid agency typically controls Medicaid spending for inpatient psychiatric treatment. There is often little coordination between these funding streams, and little history of collaborative treatment. Maintaining these types of arrangements may also encourage cost shifting within a mental health services system. For managed care systems to operate in an optimal manner, the incentives across the system need to be aligned, and the role of the state hospital within the larger reshaped mental health system needs to be explicitly considered.

The mechanics of capitation and costing of services present particular problems in mental health services. There is as yet little consistency in how mental health services are packaged, particularly with a chronic and severely disabled group. There are significant problems not only in costing programs and service packages, but simply in articulating what services are included in a program. Part of this is due to the uncertainty associated with severe and persistent mental illness, particularly with respect to the need for hospitalization and crisis intervention, difficulties with drug compliance, and variations among patients in their need for intensive "wrap-around" services. Placing this group of patients under capitation is truly a risky endeavor. It is unclear how any organization—public or private—can effectively manage such a labile patient group under a capitated arrangement.

Rural communities face persistent problems in providing care to individuals with severe mental disorders. Because economies of scale are rarely realized in rural communities, specialized mental health services are often lacking. Individuals are more likely to be seen by generalists without specialized expertise in treatment of severe mental disorders. Where specialized services and programs are available, geographic distances may limit access. With the development of various managed care initiatives, there is concern that access to appropriate mental health services will be even more restricted than under a fee-for-service approach. A central tenet of managed care is that services tend to be overutilized as a result of incentives facing providers and consumers. A key question is whether such overutilization is a salient issue in rural communities, particularly in reference to a chronically ill population. Will managed care, with its emphasis on utilization controls, have a deleterious effect on mental health services in rural communities?

Another set of questions relates to the idea of systems of care. Since the 1960s, the public sector has been largely responsible for the development and nurturance of community support systems. These support networks typically include both formal organizations (social services departments, vocational rehabilitation organizations, health and mental health provider organizations), as well as informal linkages on the community level. In some instances, these support networks are fragile and underdeveloped, while other communities have well-established consortia to deal with mental health and other issues. These networks serve a number of functions, including coordination and communication about particular patients or clients, and sharing of information about services and community needs. They may also be an outlet for consumer voice. An important question is the effect that a change to a managed care funding arrangement would have on the viability of these networks. Proponents of managed care point out that one of the advantages of managed care is the fact that it is managed—thus allowing easier access to needed services, presumably, than a system that is not managed. What is not clear in this argument, however, is the extent to which the managed care also involves managed systems of care. Does managed care imply managed systems? Or does the managed care approach really imply a managed core of providers— that is, a smaller network of organizations that are critical players within the MCO network? This would appear to be an area in which carefully planned research today could assist planners, CMHCs, and public and private entities to better address the challenges of tomorrow.

Related to this issue is the problem of patient-related communication. The nature of severe mental illness requires strong communication links among a variety of individuals and organizations involved in the individual's care: case managers, physicians, group home supervisors, therapists, pharmacists, and so forth. To what extent will managed care facilitate or inhibit this type of necessary grassroots communication? Will the financial power of a managed care entity contribute to or deter effective patient-related communication?

While there are many aspects of privatization that are not clear, it is certain that organizations will assume new roles in this environment. Some of these roles will require organizations and managers to learn new skills and will certainly affect interrelationships among organizations. It is axiomatic that there is much each sector—public and private—can learn from the other. For persons with serious mental disabilities, a challenging group for any sector, the strengthening of interchange among private and public sectors will certainly be a key to achieving the goals of cost-effectiveness, access, and quality in the provision of mental health services.

REFERENCES

1. Fellin P. *Mental Health and Mental Illness: Policies, Programs, and Service*. Itasca, Ill: FE Peacock; 1996.

2. Talbott JA. Fifty years of psychiatric services: changes in treatment of chronically mentally ill patients. In: Oldham JM, Ribci M, eds. *Review of Psychiatry*. Washington, DC: American Psychiatric Press; 1994:93–120.

3. Rothman DJ. *The Discovery of the Asylum: Social Order and Disorder in the New Republic*. Boston: Little, Brown & Co; 1971.

4. Wisor RL Jr. Community care, competition, and coercion: a legal perspective on privatized mental health care. *Am J Law Med*. 1993;19:145–175.

5. Grob GN. The paradox of deinstitutionalization. *Society*. 1995;32:51–59.

6. Mechanic D. Establishing mental health priorities. *Milbank Q*. 1994;72:501–514.

7. Devers KJ. The challenges of implementing market-based reforms for public clients. In: Wilkerson JD, Devers KJ, Given RS, eds. *Competitive Managed Care: The Emerging Health Care System*. San Francisco: Jossey-Bass; 1997.

8. Jellinek MS, Nurcombe B. Two wrongs don't make a right: managed care, mental health, and the marketplace. *JAMA*. 1993;270:1737–1739.

9. Newhouse JP, Insurance Experiment Group. *Free for All? Lessons from the RAND Health Insurance Experiment*. Cambridge, Mass: Harvard University Press; 1994.

10. Wells KB, Astrachan BM, Tischler GL, Unutzer J. Issues and approaches in evaluating managed mental health care. *Milbank Q*. 1995;73:57–75.

11. Mechanic D. Key policy considerations for mental health in the managed care era. In: Manderscheid RW, Sonnenschein MA, eds. *Mental Health, United States, 1996*. Rockville, Md: U.S. Department of Health and Human Services; 1996:1–16.

12. Boyle PJ, Callahan D. Managed care in mental health: the ethical issues. *Health Aff*. 1995;14:7–22.

13. Goplerud E. *Managed Care for Mental Health and Substance Abuse Services*. Rockville, Md: SAMHSA Managed Care Initiative; 1995.

14. English JT, McCarrick RG. The economics of psychiatry. In: Kaplan HI, Sadock BJ, eds. *Comprehensive Textbook of Psychiatry*. 5th ed. Baltimore, Md: Williams & Wilkins; 1989:2074–2083.

15. Institute of Medicine. *Controlling Costs and Changing Patient Care? The Role of Utilization Management*. Washington, DC: National Academy Press; 1989.

16. Appelbaum P. Legal liability and managed care. *Am Psychologist*. 1993;48:251–257.

17. Freeman MA, Trabin T. Managed behavioral healthcare: history, models, key issues, and future course. Presented at Center for Mental Health Services; October 5, 1994; Rockville, Md.

18. Frank RG, McGuire TG, Newhouse JP. Risk contracts in managed mental health care. *Health Affairs.* 1995;14:50–64.

19. Essock SM, Goldman HH. States' embrace of managed mental health care. *Health Affairs.* 1995; 14:34–44.

20. Battagliola M. Breaking with tradition. *Business Health.* June 1994:53–56.

21. Callahan JJ, Shepard DS, Beinecke RH, Larson M, et al. Mental health/substance abuse treatment in managed care: the Massachusetts Medicaid experience. *Health Affairs.* 1995;14:173–184.

22. Christianson JB, Manning W, Lurie N, Stoner T, et al. Utah's prepaid mental health plan: the first year. *Health Affairs.* 1995;14:160–172.

23. Koyanagi C. *Managing Managed Care for Publicly Financed Mental Health Services.* Washington, DC: Judge David L. Bazelon Center for Mental Health Law; 1995.

24. Hoge M, Davidson L, Griffith E, Sledge W, et al. Defining managed care in public-sector psychiatry. *Hosp Community Psychiatry.* 1994;45:1085–1089.

25. Mechanic D, Schlesinger M, McAlpine D. Management of mental health and substance abuse services: state of the art and early results. *Milbank Q.* 1995;73:19–55.

26. Cann RE, Gould B, Hill ED, Stock HF, et al. Managed care, mental health, and the marketplace. *JAMA.* 1994;271:587–578.

27. Rovner J. Accreditation standards proposed for managed-mental-health care in USA. *Lancet.* 1996;347:1108–1109.

CHAPTER 9

Managed Care and the Delivery of Public Mental Health and Substance Abuse Services

Mady Chalk

Managed care is rapidly becoming central to the delivery of medical, mental health, and substance abuse services in both the private and public sectors. Yet very little is known about the impact of managed care programs on access, utilization and cost of services, and treatment outcomes. In the fields of mental health and substance abuse treatment, these uncertainties are compounded by rapid changes in knowledge about and classification of disorders, standards of care, diagnosis and treatment interventions, and accepted roles of professionals in the treatment process. Efforts to monitor and assess the quality of mental health and substance abuse treatment services provided through managed care programs are confounded by the heterogeneity of programs and the populations seeking treatment for these disorders. The objective of this chapter is to examine the critical challenges to quality management that emerge from efforts to privatize the delivery of public mental health and substance abuse services through managed care programs. Attention is given to the distinguishing characteristics of mental illness and substance abuse treatment that give rise to these challenges, and to the policy questions that need to be considered in addressing these challenges.

MANAGED CARE FOR MENTAL HEALTH AND SUBSTANCE ABUSE TREATMENT

Managed care programs come in a variety of shapes and sizes, but may be loosely defined by their use of administrative and financial mechanisms designed

Source: Adapted from M. Chalk, Privatizing Public Mental Health and Substance Abuse Services: Issues, Opportunities, and Challenges, *Quality Management in Health Care,* Vol. 5, No. 2, pp. 55–64, © 1997, Aspen Publishers, Inc.

The views expressed in this chapter do not necessarily reflect those of the Substance Abuse and Mental Health Service Agency or the U.S. Department of Health and Human Services.

to control access to care, the types and modalities of care delivered, and the amount and costs of care. To date, most managed care programs have placed primary emphasis on cost containment and resource allocation, although the objectives of managed care also include monitoring and improving treatment processes and outcomes. A theme reflected in many conceptual and empirical studies of managed care maintains that "whether applied to mental, [substance abuse], or physical health, all forms of managed care represent attempts to limit the use of services."[1]

Each form of managed care, whether in the private or public sectors, uses specific procedures to control access, quality, and treatment costs. These procedures include utilization and peer review, precertification, gatekeeping, practice profiling, concurrent review, prospective (rather than retrospective) payment, case management, and clinical guidelines and protocols. In addition to these specific mechanisms, general principles of benefit design are used both by managed care plans and the public and private sector purchasers of medical, mental health, and substance abuse treatment services to exert control over service utilization and costs. These design principles include decisions on the type and number of services to be covered, coinsurance and copayment amounts, yearly and lifetime maximum coverage limits, and penalties for unapproved or out-of-plan utilization. Managed care plans may redefine benefits if such changes promise to reduce overall costs of care.

In the present competitive market for mental health and substance abuse treatment services, small managed care plans are rapidly consolidating into larger corporations to take advantage of such benefits as larger risk pools, greater access to capital, and more extensive networks of affiliated health care providers. The frequent mergers and acquisitions in this rapidly growing industry are evident in the frequency with which market share and earnings rankings shift among competing firms. Currently, the 10 largest managed behavioral health care firms generate about 90% of the total revenue collected by the industry.

Most state mental health and substance abuse administrators are exploring the feasibility of some form of managed care for publicly funded behavioral health services. States and counties are moving large numbers of people with publicly financed health insurance into mandatory managed care programs in an effort to control costs and reduce inefficiencies. As of June 1994, 7.8 million Medicaid beneficiaries were enrolled in some form of managed care, a number double that for 1993.[2] At the same time, policies are under consideration at state and local levels that would allow private managed care plans to deliver mental health and substance abuse services funded by other public sources, such as the federal substance abuse prevention and treatment block grant, the federal community mental health block grant, and state and county revenues.

Change is being handled piecemeal. Some states and counties are contracting with managed care plans for the care of tightly circumscribed populations, such as

Aid to Families with Dependent Children (AFDC) recipients, persons with multiple mental illnesses, or children with disabilities. Others are enrolling broadly defined population groups into these plans, such as Medicaid beneficiaries and the medically indigent. Some jurisdictions allow health plans to assume full financial risk for all services required by the public beneficiaries they enroll, while others "carve out" certain services to be directly provided in the public sector or through separately managed contracts.[3]

Public purchasers of managed care services confront critical policy issues with little guidance. Most decisions are being made without the benefit of information about the characteristics, costs, and outcomes of alternative managed care options, especially for the low-income, severely disabled consumers commonly served in public sector systems. Purchasers face the sobering reality that the knowledge base for such critical tasks as estimating capitation rates and calculating risk adjustments is very weak, especially for the disabled and other vulnerable populations. Similarly, the scientific base for clinical care protocols and utilization management policies in these populations is thin. Knowledge about the effects of regulations, accreditation systems, quality assurance procedures, and performance measurement is anecdotal where it exists at all.

Despite these uncertainties, managed care programs in all of their different forms are being implemented across the nation for individuals with mental health and substance abuse treatment needs. Health care analysts observe that "without owning health care facilities or, for the most part, employing providers, the companies providing managed behavioral health care have brought about a dramatic shift in patterns of use. . . . In a growing number of instances, the behavioral health care companies are forming integrated delivery systems, thus linking the functions of direct provision of care and plan management."[1(p132)] This environment has raised a number of questions about quality management that have yet to be addressed in the policy and research literatures.

KEY ISSUES, OPPORTUNITIES, AND CHALLENGES FOR QUALITY MANAGEMENT

There are some distinct characteristics of mental illnesses and substance abuse problems that have important implications for the organizational and operational characteristics of managed care plans, and the quality management approaches that are needed when these plans assume responsibility for the care of public beneficiaries. Discussion of the history of differences in insurance coverage and treatment of mental and substance abuse disorders is beyond the scope of this discussion but is useful to keep in mind. A number of issues have emerged in the private sector that have an impact on privatization initiatives in the public sector.

Social Costs of Mental Health and Substance Abuse Problems

Mental illnesses and problems with alcohol and other drugs involve social costs that are borne by families, the community—including large and small employers—and the criminal justice and educational systems. Analysts estimate that at least one-third of all criminal justice costs relate to alcohol and other drug abuse.[4] The nation's direct health care costs and indirect costs (e.g., productivity losses) of alcohol and other drug abuse totaled more than $314 billion in 1990.[5] A series of analyses conducted by the Center on Addiction and Substance Abuse found that the costs for treating physical illnesses directly attributable to alcohol and other drug use (not including heavy additional costs of tobacco use) was more than $51 billion in 1993. Federal expenditures to treat substance abuse-related physical illnesses (e.g., trauma, adverse birth outcomes, endocarditis, human immunodeficiency virus and acquired immune deficiency syndrome, renal and hepatic failure, and ulcers) through Medicaid, Medicare, block grants, and military and veterans health programs totalled over $18.5 billion in 1993.[6] Further, a substantial proportion of people with mental illnesses have co-occurring substance abuse disorders for which they are being treated, the costs of which have not been adequately assessed.

The social costs of mental illnesses and substance abuse problems suggest that decisions about treatment must include more than specifically medical issues.[4] It is not clear to most clinicians, however, how to include these related problems in assigning patients to levels of care, settings, or modalities of treatment. Nor is it clear to what extent managed care firms include these related problems in their notions of what treatment is. A major issue that needs to be considered in evaluating the outcomes of substance abuse treatment is what effective forms of treatment are expected to do.[7] This issue is not simply a philosophical question but one that forms the basis for major decisions about the nature of treatment, including the appropriate goals, patient placement, staffing patterns, and treatment durations. In turn, these treatment expectations provide a basis for evaluating the effectiveness and "worth" of interventions.

The emphasis both in treatment and in patient outcomes research has been shifting in the last 10 years toward assessment of functioning, or the ability of patients to perform daily activities. To patients, effective treatment means not only relief from direct symptoms of mental illnesses or alcohol and other drug problems but improvement in social and occupational functioning. Beyond that, employers paying for treatment want their affected employees returned to an effective level of work performance following treatment. Families, neighbors, and police want to curtail the community disruptions and crime often associated with exacerbated episodes of these disorders. Thus, these social problems, rather than mental illnesses or substance abuse disorders themselves, appear to be the major sources of concern to society. A key quality management issue for privatization initiatives in behavioral managed care, then, involves the extent to which social costs and socially defined problems will be adequately considered by private managed care plans when decisions are made regarding benefit design, utilization management policies, and approved treatment modalities for their enrolled public beneficiaries.

The Chronicity of Mental Health and Substance Abuse Problems

Most direct costs associated with severe mental illnesses and chronic alcohol or drug abuse disorders are related to their chronicity. No matter how effectively managed, the costs and use of treatment services may extend for significant periods of time and require the use of multiple health and social services. For public beneficiaries, Medicaid has traditionally served as the funding source for acute mental health services, detoxification, and some substance abuse rehabilitation services that emphasize inpatient hospitalization. In many states, particularly those where Medicaid beneficiaries are served through capitated contracts with managed care plans, mental health and substance abuse agencies share the costs of treatment services for long-term treatment episodes only. Some states are now narrowing their scope of responsibility in this area through redefinition of Medicaid benefits and eligible populations. As a result, clients enrolled in Medicaid managed care plans may be not severe enough to qualify for state block grant–funded mental health or substance abuse services but have exhausted their managed Medicaid benefit and, thereby, "fall through the cracks" for significant periods of time. In addition, having a long-term client's needs met by several different agencies, each responsible for the allocation of limited resources, may heighten the potential for cost shifting among different parts of the public sector.

The Stigmatization of Mental Health and Substance Abuse Problems

Mental illnesses and substance abuse disorders remain more stigmatized than most other conditions, regardless of the gains that have been made in the last 15 years in treatment of these problems. Use of illegal substances increases the stigmatization not only of individuals seeking treatment but of those who treat such individuals. And finally, stigmatization not only affects the resources managed care firms may be interested in devoting to treating these problems but increases concerns about confidentiality, especially when an external organization reviews the appropriateness and duration of treatment.[8] It is of great concern to advocates and treatment providers that because of stigmatization, arrangements that reduce the privacy of the care-seeking process will discourage some people from using services.[4]

POLICY IMPLICATIONS FOR QUALITY MANAGEMENT

A number of important policy issues are raised by the current trend toward privatization of public mental health and substance abuse treatment systems through managed care programs:

- Consideration must be given to alternative methods of organizing and structuring these programs to produce desired improvements in efficiency and cost containment while also addressing both personal and societal needs in mental health and substance abuse treatment services.
- Strategies are needed within these programs to balance the proprietary and self-preserving values of private corporations with public sector treatment philosophies grounded in addressing the full range of social, psychological, and physical problems confronting the patient.
- Management approaches are required that will facilitate the development and maintenance of strong interorganizational relationships between public and private sector organizations, so that operational and cultural differences do not result in fragmented and inaccessible systems of care.
- Reliable methods of performance measurement need to be combined with private sector incentive systems to ensure that managed care plans remain accountable and responsive to policy goals and objectives in the public sector.
- Avenues for consumer participation and control need to be secured within privatization initiatives to ensure that the vulnerable populations served by public sector programs continue to have a voice and a stake in their treatment.

Each of these policy implications is discussed below.

The Organization and Structure of Privatization Initiatives

Privatization has been defined as the use of private means to further public ends and, more simply, as the purchase by public authorities of services from private agencies. Although the introduction of competition in purchasing services is intended to increase the numbers of potential providers, reduce costs, and provide a wider range of services, the capacity of states to monitor managed care systems and ensure that they are accountable presents considerable difficulties. Privatization has led to a shift in the role of the public sector in assuring the provision of treatment services and, within the public sector, to a significant change in the roles of and relationships between state Medicaid and mental health and substance abuse agencies. These changes have altered the relationship of state agencies to treatment providers and consumers from monitoring or providing direct treatment services to funding and managing systems of care. The changes also have begun to shift the power relationships between and among state agencies. The configuration of state government has a direct impact on how state authorities can affect policy and program decisions. The shifts that have begun to occur and will continue, particularly if administration and financing of Medicaid is moved to the states, may reduce the impact of state mental health and substance abuse agencies on policy related to the vulnerable populations for which they are responsible.

In the design of any managed care delivery system, decisions must be made about organizational structure and levels of integration; design of the behavioral health care delivery component; populations to be covered; eligibility criteria; pooling of funding sources; and accountability mechanisms. The decisions that need to be made in developing public sector managed care systems speak directly to the meaning of partnership.

Carve-in designs integrate behavioral health care with primary medical care. In these designs, general practitioners and health maintenance organizations (HMOs) often serve as gatekeepers. A great deal of concern has been raised, given the history of discomfort of HMOs and general practitioners with diagnosing and treating patients with severe mental illnesses and/or substance abuse disorders, about their ability to provide for the needs of these populations. Often, in these arrangements, HMOs subcontract with another vendor to provide behavioral health care services, increasing the layers of administration, reducing the dollars available for direct service provision, and, in addition, reducing the purchaser's (in this case a state's) ability to influence the behavioral health care delivery system.

Carve-out designs allow the state to contract directly with behavioral health plans and maintain greater control over the mental health and substance abuse services provided to public beneficiaries. This design, however, usually makes integration with primary care more difficult and may even increase fragmentation. Managed care carve-outs in the public sector often are designed for particular populations, opening the possibility of increasing fragmentation among treatment providers and systems. Further, inefficiencies are often created when enrollees of carve-out health plans require services managed by other state agencies, such as health services, social services, criminal justice, or education. In these cases, the health plans may either duplicate the efforts of state agencies by directly providing the needed service, or they may incur additional administrative and transaction costs by establishing contractual service agreements with these state agencies. Even among public agencies, coordination may be difficult to achieve, as these agencies often have different priorities regarding the accessibility, continuity, and costs of treatment.

The organizational and structural characteristics of privatization initiatives may also have important implications for the accrual of treatment costs and benefits. Evidence suggests that the costs of treating mental health and substance abuse problems may be offset at least in part by reductions in the number of medical services that are required by those individuals who are treated.[9] This offset effect is of particular concern in the public sector, where shrinking budgets have resulted in considerable pressure on state governments to reduce health care costs. In carve-out designs, however, offset effects are rarely observed, because the benefits of mental health and substance abuse treatment often do not accrue to the public agencies and private health plans that manage these services, but rather to other public systems, such as criminal justice, education, and welfare. The inability to provide adequate evidence of cost offset may further reduce the willingness of taxpayers to support benefits for mental health and substance abuse treatment services.

Organizational Values and Mission in Privatization Initiatives

Immediately behind the question of structural and organizational design in privatization initiatives are a wide range of policy issues related to the organizational missions and values of private health plans and their compatibility with public sector priorities in mental health and substance abuse treatment. Critical policy questions include whether private sector companies can really understand and appreciate the values and clientele of public sector agencies; whether private sector interest in public clients is genuine or motivated primarily by large capitation budgets; and whether private sector companies can truly incorporate public sector values and cultural diversity.

Encompassing the range of services required by the public client into integrated delivery systems will have a direct impact on costs over the short and long range. Available evidence strongly suggests that the costs of public sector treatment can be reduced by diverting hospital admissions to outpatient care and by negotiating substantial price reductions with hospitals for limited numbers of admissions. Surprisingly, however, few states currently require managed care plans serving public beneficiaries to apply savings from one treatment setting to the provision of other needed services such as vocational rehabilitation, health care, parenting, and educational services. If the primary aim of managed behavioral health plans is to wring costs out of the service delivery system, how are the social sequelae of mental illnesses and alcohol and other drug disorders to be addressed?

Until very recently, most states have not attended to the need to include provisions in contracts that prevent managed care organizations from incurring windfall profits from underservice and restrictions on access to specific treatment modalities. For example, in a recent interview the vice president of a managed behavioral health care organization operating in the public and private sectors was asked to describe the characteristics of a client for whom residential substance abuse treatment had been deemed a medical necessity. The honest but compelling response was that he could not describe such a client because, although his firm's benefit plan included a residential benefit, it had never been deemed "medically necessary" for a client to use such treatment.

In states that have been through several years of implementation of public sector managed behavioral health care, only now will researchers begin to learn something about whether managed care firms are willing to stay the course. In Massachusetts, some evidence suggests that the large savings that are possible through introduction of managed care in the public sector have already been wrung out of the system, and that the next phase of implementation may be more costly and result in greatly reduced revenues for the managed care firms involved in administering the program.[10]

Interorganizational Coordination, Integration, and Culture

In discussions with providers, consumers, and public sector purchasers alike questions have been raised about the extent to which integration of public and private systems of care will highlight the differences in the populations served by the two systems. The public mental health and substance abuse treatment systems have been devoted to providing services of last resort. For private managed care firms, these clients often challenge the operational definition of "medical necessity" used as a device for allocation of resources. Providers who have been accustomed to serving private clients with limited insurance benefits for treatment of mental and alcohol and other drug problems may be considerably challenged by the severity of illness and persistent need for care that most public clients present. It is apparent that unless providers accustomed to serving public clients are included in managed care networks that contract with the public sector, expertise is likely to be lost and will be difficult to replace.

The future of the publicly funded treatment system as we know it (which is composed primarily of community-based treatment programs rather than individual, office-based clinicians) is in jeopardy. It is clear to those who interact on a regular basis with states and treatment providers that treatment agencies with entrepreneurial managers will fare better under privatized, integrated systems. Treatment providers will need to assess their strengths and weaknesses and establish the parameters of their service provision. Some may seek to diversify and expand their service delivery capacity to extend services to populations they have not formerly treated; others will fare better if they specialize and carve out a niche for a specific population. Treatment agencies that choose to stand alone, particularly small agencies, are very likely to fail.

Operationalization of some privatized systems has encountered considerable difficulty from lack of sufficient consideration of the state of the infrastructure at the point of implementation, as well as the need for a realistic timetable for development. Private sector vendors in states new to managed care will need to assist public sector treatment providers in making the transition to managed care and to a more competitive service delivery system, and it is to their best financial interests to do so. Developmentally, many public sector treatment programs have a great deal to learn about forming provider networks, financial risk assessment and management, management uses of data, information systems, capitation, case mix, utilization management, and use of research findings that may improve outcomes. In some instances, substance abuse and mental health state agencies in concert with private sector vendors are providing training and placing information resources at the disposal of public sector treatment programs. In many more instances, providers are scrambling to learn what they need to learn to function in a competitive, privately managed treatment system.

Both state purchasers and private vendors need to pay attention to and anticipate the effects of managed care on other systems and agencies, and the potential to shift costs and responsibilities to other sectors. In the recent past, costs have been shifted from the criminal justice and education systems to the mental health and substance abuse treatment systems. This situation may begin to work in reverse in the current environment. For example, as public sector managed behavioral health care organizations decrease access to residential treatment—which provides not only treatment but 24-hour supervision as well and is often the treatment of choice of judges responsible for sentencing drug abusers—juvenile and other criminal justice populations with substance abuse and mental disorders may remain for longer periods of time in detention centers, jails, and prisons. In the past 10 years, criminal justice systems increasingly have contracted with public sector providers to offer treatment services within jails and prisons. However, as public sector managed care emerges, substance abusers and individuals with severe mental illnesses more often will need to be treated for longer periods of time or exclusively within the criminal justice setting, adding to the already high costs of incarceration.[11]

Performance Assessment, Private Sector Incentives, and Public Accountability

Performance standards are empirical indicators selected to represent the degree of accomplishment of certain desired goals. They provide objective evidence of program activities and their results, but only if they are based on information that is valid, reliable, and complete.[12] Performance standards also are an effective way to communicate expectations. Standards, therefore, need to deal not only with structure and operations, but with expected financial and clinical outcomes.

Although managed care arrangements are being implemented in many states, adequate performance standards are scarce. This omission has led to confusion with regard to expectations and accomplishments, dissipation of savings, and lawsuits regarding lack of due diligence in vendor selection. As specialized mental health and substance abuse managed care organizations have developed, they have faced some of the same conflicting goals that have always characterized the mental health and substance abuse treatment systems. Analysts in the field of mental health and substance abuse treatment observe, "it is particularly difficult to manage and maintain a focus on the promotion of client-centered goals when their achievement conflicts with organizational requirements. The development of standards and oversight offers a means of assuring that one set of goals are not sacrificed by the drive to achieve the other."[12(p2)] Given the special vulnerability of patient populations compromised by mental illnesses and alcohol and other drug problems, "means are needed to assure a balance between security and confidentiality, access, individualization, . . . and expedient processing, and to deal with individual need and constrained resources while, at the same time providing more than the usual level of patient voice."[12(p3)]

These issues are magnified as managed care organizations limit patients' freedom of choice of providers and access to various modalities of treatment through financial incentives and direct rationing. These limitations pose substantial risks to vulnerable populations "who may be impaired by disorders that make them less able than most to complain about poor treatment, undertreatment or overtreatment, or outright abuse and neglect, and are less able to effectively utilize grievance and appeals systems."[12(p3)] Accountability of managed care systems, therefore, must go beyond financial performance and include indicators of access and clinical and operational adequacy, including credentialing.

The contracting document, including the incentive system it contains, may be the most important tool for enhancing accountability and partnership between public and private sector managed care organizations. In the former system of categorically funded treatment programs, inputs were used to monitor the system; under managed care, outputs such as intermediate and long-term treatment outcomes, duration of treatment, and readmissions are beginning to be used in monitoring treatment programs.

With regard to the accountability of managed care organizations themselves, a great deal of work remains for privatization initiatives. Although there are a number of efforts underway to develop performance measures for public sector managed care, at the present time, no valid accreditation or quality-of-care guidelines exist that can be of help to public purchasers in differentiating between competing managed behavioral health care plans. In fact, "the uncontrolled proliferation of report cards and performance standards, both for managed care and managed behavioral healthcare, threatens to become a torrent that could drown both the systems themselves and the consumers who are the intended beneficiaries of the standard-setting initiatives."[12(p4)]

Efforts currently underway to measure health plan performance in the public sector have presented some difficulties: most have attempted to apply performance measures developed for private sector managed care to public sector managed care. Accreditation guidelines have been developed for primary care networks, but purchasers, consumers, family members, service providers, and government officials involved with behavioral health care view these with caution. Focused on acute care and based in medical models of treatment, these guidelines have been viewed as inappropriate to organization and financing of treatment for severe and persistent mental illnesses and chronic substance abuse disorders. Those instances in which performance measures have been developed specific to managed care for mental and substance abuse disorders reflect the differing priorities and interests of their sponsors. Unity is hard to find, although self-interest is not. It also should not be forgotten that multiple, specific standards impose significant compliance costs on managed care organizations that are typically passed on to patients and taxpayers (through Medicaid or private insurance) in the form of higher administrative fees or capitation rates. This issue affects mental health and substance abuse managed care organizations more than medical plans. Behavioral health plans are often less labor- and capital-intensive than medical managed care entities, and since they treat only a small proportion of the publicly and privately insured populations, they need large enrollee populations to achieve economies of scale and reduce actuarial risk. Data collection and reporting efforts, therefore, are costly to perform across large populations and with few resources.

The existing knowledge regarding incentive structures in managed behavioral health care is very shallow. There is little services research that offers information about how alternative payment systems used in the variety of managed care plans affect care processes and outcomes. At the federal level, the awareness of this paucity of information has resulted in a number of expert panel meetings, convened to assist federal agencies in defining the issues that need to be focused upon with research into managed behavioral health care and setting priorities for that research. Health services researchers point out that "the highest priority for research must be to establish the consequences for quality of care when external management reduces inpatient care or overall service use."[4] In order to evaluate quality of care, a broader set of outcome and process measures than have been used in past research must be developed and, more importantly, used and measured consistently across a number of studies.

Consumer Involvement and Control

Measuring patient satisfaction and implementing grievance and appeals processes are well established in private sector managed care. Corporations, as purchasers of managed care services, have insisted upon these methods of ensuring consumer "voice." These methods are likely to be insufficient in public sector implementation of managed care due to the vulnerability of the populations being treated. For consumers in public sector managed care systems, there are a number of key protections that purchasers, managed care organizations, providers, and consumer advocates should consider: creating systems that are open to consumers, including making medical necessity or other patient placement criteria available to consumers, and soliciting input of consumers during the process of development of these criteria; ensuring necessary access to out-of-plan services so that consumers have reasonable access to appropriate treatment even if these services cannot be provided within the plan; providing clear and understandable written materials that describe the organization and operation of the managed care plan in all of its detail; instituting protections against disenrollment and undertreatment, given the financial incentives in competitive markets to disenroll or neglect expensive, difficult-to-treat clients; and evaluating the qualifications, training, and experience of gatekeepers to ensure that they are capable of addressing the needs of individuals with mental health and substance abuse problems.[13]

CONCLUSION

Introduction of managed care into the public sector has raised a number of issues for consumers and providers, none more important than the issue of defining the goals for mental health and substance abuse treatment in this society. The question of whether treatment systems for substance abuse and mental disorders should be charged with meeting public health and safety concerns, or alternately, whether these systems should be charged with reducing or eliminating primary symptoms of drug abuse or mental illness only has yet to be directly confronted. If treatment systems, including those organized and financed under managed care arrangements, are to do more than reduce symptoms (as most consumers in the public sector have come to expect and most providers to attempt) then funding and guidelines need to be developed that reflect these broader goals.

Privatization of public sector treatment services under managed care arrangements is likely to have complex effects on access, utilization, cost, and outcomes of treatment. The rapidity with which privatization is occurring requires that researchers move rapidly, but thoughtfully and efficiently, to evaluate the impact of these effects. A necessary prerequisite to these efforts is a comprehensive examination of the alternative treatment goals and values among public and private purchasers, providers, and consumers. These goals and values must form the foundation upon which effective quality management approaches are built to guide the development and maintenance of viable privatization initiatives in mental health and substance abuse treatment.

REFERENCES

1. Iglehart J. Managed care in mental health. *N England J Med*. 1996;334:131–135.
2. Health Care Financing Administration. *Medicaid Managed Care Enrollment Report: Summary Statistics as of June 30, 1994*. Washington, DC: U.S. Department of Health and Human Services; 1994.
3. Goplerud E. *Managed Care for Mental Health and Substance Abuse Services*. Rockville, Md: Substance Abuse and Mental Health Service Administration; 1995.
4. Mechanic D, Schlesinger M, McAlpine DD. Management of mental health and substance abuse services: state of the art and early results. *Milbank Q*. 1995;73:19–55.
5. Rice DP, Kelman S, Miller LS, Dunmeyer L. *The Economic Costs of Alcohol and Drug Abuse and Mental Illness: 1985*. Rockville, Md: Substance Abuse and Mental Health Service Administration; 1993.
6. Merrill J, et al. Substance abuse and federal entitlement programs. New York: Center on Addiction and Substance Abuse, Columbia University; 1995. Unpublished paper.
7. McClellan T, Weisner C. Achieving the public health potential of substance abuse treatment: implications for patient referral, treatment matching, and outcome evaluation. Presented at the National Institute for Drug Abuse Symposium on Health Services Research in Drug Abuse; August, 1994; Rockville, Md.
8. Borenstein D. Managed care: a means of rationing psychiatric treatment. *Hosp Community Psychiatry*. 1990;41:1095–1098.
9. Pallack MS, Cummings NA, Dorken H, Henke CJ. Managed mental health, Medicaid, and medical cost offset. *New Directions Mental Health Serv*. 1993;59:27–40.
10. Norton EC, Lindrootn RC, Dickey B. Cost shifting in managed care. *Association for Health Services Research 1996 Annual Meeting: Abstracts*. Washington, DC: Association for Health Services Research; 1996. Abstract.
11. Morrissey J. Shifting boundaries, reducing costs: managed behavioral health care and the criminal justice system. New York: The National GAINS Center for People with Co-occuring Disorders in the Justice System, Policy and Research Associates; 1996. Unpublished paper.
12. Gelber S, Duggar B. *Performance Standards: Measurement Tools for Managed Mental Health and Substance Abuse Programs*. Rockville, Md: Substance Abuse and Mental Health Services Administration; 1996.
13. Moss S, Kushner J. *Purchasing Managed Care Services for Alcohol and Other Drug Treatment*. Technical Assistance Publication Series, Financing Subseries. Vol. III. Rockville, Md: Center for Substance Abuse Treatment; 1995.

CHAPTER 10

The Privatization of Quality Assurance in Health Care

Gary J. Young

After years of debate over the relative merits of private sector versus public sector models for financing and delivering health care services in the United States, the U.S. health care system currently reflects a decidedly strong preference for the private sector. Health care reform proposals that call for a stronger public role in the financing and delivery of health care services have proven to be politically unacceptable. Meanwhile, competition and managed care are having a dramatic impact on the structure and functioning of health care markets in many parts of the country. Investor-owned hospital corporations are gaining market share throughout the country by aggressively acquiring voluntary nonprofit hospitals.[1,2] And at the state and local levels, public hospitals are being closed or converted to private institutions.[3]

However, this "privatization" of the U.S. health care industry has raised concerns about the quality of health care. Americans are anxious about whether cost-control pressures and corporate cultural values will cause providers to place the bottom line above the best interests of their patients. These concerns have led to demands for greater external oversight of health care quality.[4] While for the better part of this century the public sector has assumed the primary role for the external oversight of health care quality, it may cease to have this responsibility in the future. Just as the private sector has emerged as the predominant force for greater efficiency in the delivery of health care services, so too is the private sector gaining importance as a source of quality oversight strategies. Indeed, the United States may be witnessing a subtle but important shift in the respective roles and functions of the public and private sectors for ensuring quality of care. This

Source: Adapted from G.J. Young, Bridging Public and Private Sector Quality Assurance, *Quality Management in Health Care*, Vol. 5, No. 2, pp. 65–72, © 1997, Aspen Publishers, Inc.

chapter discusses these developments, associated policy issues, and implications for the future role of the public sector in ensuring quality of care.

PUBLIC OVERSIGHT OF QUALITY

The United States has a long history of public oversight of health care quality. This oversight role began at the state level in the form of occupational licensure statutes for medical personnel.[5] Since the late 1800s, states have used physician licensure as a means to regulate entry into the medical profession.[5] Most states today also have licensing programs for other types of health care occupational groups, such as nurses, dentists, chiropractors, and psychologists.[6] To administer licensing programs, states typically have a licensing board for each regulated occupational group. These boards establish licensing criteria related to educational credentials, written examinations, and training requirements.[5] These boards are also empowered to take disciplinary action against licensed practitioners under certain circumstances.

Public oversight of the quality of health care facilities did not become widespread among the states until after World War II. The Hill-Burton Hospital Construction Act, enacted by Congress in 1946, provided the major impetus for hospital licensure at the state level. This legislation provided federal funds to states for hospital construction but conditioned eligibility for the funds on a state's adoption of a hospital licensing statute.[5] Over time, states have expanded their licensure programs to cover other types of health care facilities, including nursing homes, home health agencies, and ambulatory surgery centers. These licensing programs, which are usually administered by state health departments or agencies, entail periodic inspections of facilities to determine their compliance with licensure requirements that typically focus on a facility's physical layout and operational characteristics.[5]

The passage of the Medicare and Medicaid legislation in 1965 resulted in public oversight of health care facilities at the federal level. Congress mandated that all health care facilities participating in these public health insurance programs be certified as meeting a set of requirements intended to ensure a minimum level of health and safety for program beneficiaries. Detailed certification requirements currently exist for a variety of health care facilities, including hospitals, nursing homes, home health agencies, hospices, and rehabilitative agencies.[5] Additionally, in 1972 Congress established a program for the ongoing oversight of the care provided to Medicare beneficiaries. The initial legislation created peer standards review organizations (PSROs) that were responsible for conducting systematic retrospective reviews of patient medical records to assess whether the care received was appropriate, necessary, and of adequate quality. Subsequent legislation in 1982 replaced PSROs with peer review organizations (PROs), but the primary objectives of the program have remained the same.

Public oversight of health care quality has been explicitly justified as a response to a weak private market for health care quality.[7] Consumers are said to lack the information and expertise needed to assess quality of care and, therefore, cannot comparatively shop for a health care provider as they do for, say, laundry detergent. Consequently, government intervention is required to ensure minimally acceptable levels of care for all consumers. Commentators, however, have criticized licensure and other oversight programs as being both ineffective and anticompetitive.[5] Licensing programs are said to do little more than create market entry barriers that insulate those who have already gained entry into an occupation or industry from competition. While these criticisms are based at least as much on ideology as they are on data, public oversight of health care quality appears to be far more extensive in the United States than it is in European countries, even though the latter maintain public sector approaches to the financing and delivery of health care services.[8]

THE ROLE OF THE PRIVATE SECTOR IN PUBLIC QUALITY ASSURANCE PROGRAMS

In many public sector efforts to oversee quality of care, the government, at both the federal and state levels, has delegated significant implementation responsibilities to members of the private sector. For example, in a significant number of states, medical licensure boards are largely comprised of physicians in private practice who are nominated to the board by the state's medical society.[7] Some states use contractors to assess the compliance of certain types of facilities with licensure requirements. The federal government manages the Medicare PRO program in cooperation with 54 contractors across the country that perform the medical record reviews upon which judgments of appropriateness, necessity, and quality are based.[9]

Another example of this public sector–private sector interrelationship for overseeing health care quality is Medicare's certification program for hospitals. Since the inception of Medicare, the federal government has relied substantially on the private accreditation activities of the Joint Commission on Accreditation of Healthcare Organizations (Joint Commission) for purposes of certifying hospitals to participate in Medicare. The Joint Commission, an Illinois nonprofit corporation, was formed in 1951 by several organized groups of providers for the purpose of conducting voluntary accreditation of hospitals. It is the country's oldest private accreditor of health care facilities, having evolved from an earlier hospital accreditation program that was sponsored by the American College of Surgeons.

Federal law requires the Department of Health and Human Services (DHHS), the federal agency responsible for Medicare and Medicaid, to recognize Joint Commission accreditation as evidence that a hospital is also in compliance with Medicare's hospital certification requirements. Hospitals that obtain Medicare certification on the basis of Joint Commission accreditation are said to have deemed-certification status. As an alternative to Joint Commission accreditation, hospitals may submit to a government inspection typically carried out by a state health department at the behest of DHHS. More than 75% of Medicare-participating hospitals are certified on the basis of Joint Commission accreditation.[5,10]

EXPANSION OF THE PRIVATE SECTOR ROLE IN EXTERNAL QUALITY ASSURANCE

Although both federal and state governments have relied on the private sector in carrying out quality oversight programs in the past, several developments point to an expanding role for the private sector in defining and monitoring quality of care. First, private accreditation programs have been gaining prominence within the country's external quality assurance framework. The Joint Commission, which once offered hospital accreditation exclusively, now provides accreditation services to many other types of health care facilities as well as health care networks.[11] In addition, since the formation of the Joint Commission in the early 1950s, a number of other private accrediting bodies have been formed to oversee the quality of care provided in health care facilities. The National Committee on Quality Assurance (NCQA) has emerged as the predominant private accreditor of health maintenance organizations (HMOs) and has gained national recognition as a powerful voice on quality assurance issues. Other accrediting bodies include the National League of Nursing's Community Health Accreditation Program (CHAP), the Accreditation Association of Ambulatory Health Care (AAAHC), the Commission on the Accreditation of Rehabilitation Facilities (CARF), and the Accreditation Council on Services for People with Disabilities.

The growth in the number and diversity of accreditation programs has enhanced the visibility and status of private accreditation as a "seal of approval" for health care facilities.[12,5] It also is creating a competitive environment for accreditation services.[12,11,13] There are now many examples where two or more accrediting bodies are competing to offer accreditation services to the same type of health care facility. Both the Joint Commission and CHAP compete for business from nursing homes. The Joint Commission also competes with AAAHC to provide accreditation services for free-standing ambulatory clinics. Several accrediting bodies currently vie for business within the managed care industry.[12] In time, many health care facilities may be able to choose between two or more accreditation programs based on which seal of approval they think will be most valuable to them in attracting the business of purchasers and health care plans.[12]

DHHS also has an emerging policy to expand the number of private accrediting programs that can offer deemed-certification status to health care facilities for purposes of Medicare participation. While DHHS has had legislative authority to take this action since Medicare was passed into law, until recently, deemed-certification status was limited primarily to Joint Commission accreditation of hospitals. In the early 1990s, DHHS extended deemed-certification status to home health agencies if they are accredited by either CHAP or the Joint Commission.[5] DHHS is now in the process of extending deemed-certification status to ambulatory surgery centers that are accredited by either the Joint Commission or AAAHC.[14] DHHS appears to be interested not only in expanding the number of accrediting bodies that can offer deemed-certification status, but also, where possible, in promoting competition for such accreditation services.

A second development is the movement to make available to consumers—insurance companies, self-insured employers, and individuals—comparative information about the quality of health care providers. This movement builds on scientific developments within the field of health services research that have improved methods for evaluating quality based on providers' treatment outcomes (as opposed to their structural characteristics or the processes by which care is delivered).[15] Using these methods, several efforts have been undertaken to disseminate profiles of providers' various treatment outcomes, such as, in the case of hospitals, mortality and infection rates.[16] These profiles are commonly referred to as report cards.

The dissemination of outcome data is intended to strengthen the private market for health care quality. In theory, these data help consumers overcome the information barriers they have historically faced in selecting health care providers on the basis of quality differences.[15] Consumers are expected to use outcome data to select the providers that will deliver the highest quality care for a given price. Providers with poor outcomes will face a decline in their volume of business and thus will be motivated to make changes to improve the quality of their care.

The public sector has played an important leadership role in providing consumers with comparative information on quality. A seminal event occurred in 1986 when the federal government published hospital-specific mortality data for specific procedures and conditions. Several states have also begun publishing outcome data for health care providers.[16] In disseminating outcome data, the public sector has departed from its traditional role of ensuring that health care professionals meet minimum levels of competence and health care facilities meet minimum standards of quality. In theory, the dissemination of outcome data provides consumers with more than a means to identify incompetent providers; it provides a way to discriminate among providers on the basis of more fine-grained quality differences.

Private industry is responding to the growing demand for comparative information about the quality of health care providers. Several of the leading private accrediting bodies have modified their confidentiality policies to increase the amount of information they disclose to the public about the facilities they accredit. For example, the Joint Commission now releases to the public detailed performance data on many of its health care facilities indicating the facility's level of compliance with various quality standards.[17] The NCQA has been a major player in the development of the Health Plan Employer Data and Information Set, which is a report card on health plans consisting of over 30 quality measures.[18] Research and consulting firms are also working with business coalitions and other large purchasers to develop performance measurement systems and report cards for assessing quality of care.[19]

A third development is the formation of voluntary, community-based efforts to oversee quality of care. These community-based efforts consist of coalitions of local purchasers and providers who collaboratively establish a program for measuring and monitoring both cost and quality within the community. Perhaps the most well-known effort is the Cleveland Health Quality Choice (CHQC) Initiative. The CHQC initiative represents a voluntary partnership of local businesses, hospitals, and physicians. As part of the initiative, clinical outcomes and patient satisfaction measures are collected as indicators of the quality in the 29 hospitals in the area and shared with coalition members in the form of two reports of comparative data each year.[20] Other community-based programs to oversee quality have been implemented in the Boston, Minneapolis-St. Paul, and Rochester, New York, metropolitan areas.[21-23]

These community-based efforts constitute a distinct model for using outcome data to strengthen private markets for quality. In contrast to more broad-based outcome dissemination efforts at the federal or state level, these programs create an organizational structure for collecting, monitoring, and disseminating outcome data within a specified community. The structure provides a mechanism for promoting continuous quality improvement through benchmarking and best-practice development. Thus, community-based programs represent a shift in the locus of quality control—from the public sector to the private sector, and from the federal or state level to the local level.

PRIVATIZATION OF EXTERNAL QUALITY ASSURANCE: THEORETICAL ISSUES

The growing leadership role of the private sector in external quality assurance offers a variety of potential benefits and, at the same time, raises a number of concerns. Potential benefits include those traditionally associated with the provision of goods and services in private markets.[24] Thus, privatization may promote efficiency in quality oversight activities. For example, in the Medicare certification context, multiple accrediting bodies offering deemed-certification status within the same markets can potentially promote price competition with respect to accreditation services. The rising cost of accreditation services has been a major concern to providers.[25,26] Community-based efforts can also help promote efficiency by pushing accountability and control of oversight activities down to the local level, where purchasers and providers can weigh the added value of the oversight activity against its costs.

Another potential benefit relates to the effectiveness of quality assurance activities. A stronger private sector role in quality assurance activities can inject flexibility into the way quality is defined and monitored. Public sector regulatory programs have been notoriously slow to address quality issues associated with the emergence of new types of health care facilities and new organizational arrangements for delivering health care services. Several years ago, the Government Accounting Office completed a study in which it found that with few exceptions, states had failed to expand licensing and other regulatory programs to address quality issues raised by free-standing health care centers.[27] Because public regulatory programs must often comply with time-consuming public notice and comment rule-making procedures, their ability to respond to the types of quality issues surfacing in a dynamic health care market is limited. The private sector does not face these constraints and, thus, theoretically can respond to quality issues in a more timely manner.

Private sector initiatives in quality assurance also reflect democratic notions of plurality and free choice. Community-based quality assurance efforts can be conducted to reflect local customs and norms in ways that federal or even state regulatory programs cannot. For example, some communities may wish to attach greater emphasis to certain quality indicators about which their community is most concerned, perhaps because of the presence of vulnerable populations or a prior history of poor outcomes. A community-based quality assurance effort in Minnesota rejected traditional outcome measures (e.g., mortality) in favor of population-oriented indicators of wellness.[22] In addition, the participation of multiple accrediting bodies in Medicare certification activities can promote diverse philosophies toward health care delivery generally and quality assurance specifically. Professor Clark C. Havighurst, a leading expert on private accreditation, has been a strong advocate for a multiplicity of accreditors in health care to facilitate consumer choice.[28]

Privatizing quality assurance can be viewed from a less optimistic perspective, however. A stronger private sector role in the oversight of health care quality may lead to a diminished public presence in this arena. Of course, private sector activities may serve to supplement rather than substitute for public sector regulation. However, as state and federal budgets become increasingly strained, public officials will likely be tempted to rely more heavily on the private sector to oversee quality. Future health care reform initiatives may curtail or eliminate public sector regulatory programs or eliminate them altogether. Significantly,

President Clinton's Health Security Act focused on consumer report cards as the primary quality assurance tool without considering any potential role for public sector licensing and certification programs.[7,19]

The prospect of a declining public role in overseeing quality of care raises at least two major concerns. One concern is that the private sector will not be able or willing to adequately meet consumer needs for quality assurance. As Jost has noted, quality assurance programs produce information that is by and large a public good; once the information is produced, others can access it with little or no cost to themselves.[4] The public good characteristics of quality assurance information suggest that the private sector will not supply all the information needed. The implication is that there will be a lack of competing accreditation programs for some health care facilities. Consumers will also lack adequate outcome data for assessing the quality of certain health care services. Moreover, a private sector model for quality assurance assumes a competitive health care market in which providers have the motivation and capacity to differentiate their quality status—whether it be based on accreditation, superior technical outcomes, or some other quality indicator. Such markets do not exist everywhere in the United States, however. In rural areas of the country, one or two providers often dominate a market. Historically, rural hospitals have been much less likely than their urban counterparts to pursue Joint Commission accreditation.[29]

Certain consumer groups may be particularly disadvantaged under a private model for quality assurance. Under such a private model, consumers have more responsibility for their own welfare than they do under a public regulatory program. Consumers are responsible for searching for information about the quality of providers and interpreting the information in the context of the choices available to them for a health care provider. Commentators have asserted that for most consumers, comparing the quality of providers based on outcome data or accreditation status is a complex cognitive task.[4,19] These observers suggest that consumers will not be able to make effective use of much of the quality information that is disseminated to them. Whether or not this assertion is true for the majority of consumers remains an empirical question, but certainly a private sector system alone may not provide adequate safeguards for consumers whose cultural or educational background has not prepared them for using complex data.

A second concern relates to the accountability of private sector organizations for their quality assurance activities. Historically, private sector participation in public quality assurance programs has been in accordance with specified roles and responsibilities for which the private participants were accountable to the public agency managing the program. Thus contractors in Medicare's PRO conduct their activities pursuant to a very detailed scope of work. State contractors performing licensing inspections are similarly constrained. Even the Joint Commission, which because of its status as a franchise in relation to the Medicare certification program has operated with considerably more discretion than government contractors, has come under increasingly tighter controls by DHHS.[30] However, in the absence of a public sector presence in the country's system for external quality assurance, the private sector will have much wider discretion concerning quality assurance activities.

The problem with this scenario is that private sector quality assurance programs are fraught with potential conflicts of interest. The sponsorship and governance of many accrediting bodies are heavily made up of representatives of the providers the accrediting bodies oversee. Private accrediting bodies also depend financially on the fees they collect from accredited providers. In addition, companies that develop report cards for business coalitions may depend on the cooperation of those providers they report on to provide them with data. The need for this cooperation may compromise the independence of those companies in performing their work. There are also concerns that most purchasers participating in the types of community-based initiatives previously discussed will be more concerned with costs than quality.[4] To the extent that this is true, many community-based initiatives may ultimately devolve into cost-containment efforts that only give lip service to quality assurance.

THE FUTURE ROLE OF THE PUBLIC SECTOR IN EXTERNAL QUALITY ASSURANCE

The foregoing suggests a continued, albeit modified, role for the public sector in overseeing the quality of health care. The critical challenge will be to identify ways that bridge public sector and private sector quality assurance activities. One way is for the public sector to focus on identifying geographic and service markets where there appears to be an inadequate development of quality-assurance programs. As a country, the United States has for some time operated on the presumption that private markets for health care quality are inadequate. Given the private sector developments previously discussed, this presumption may eventually be abandoned in favor of another: private markets for health care quality are adequate unless there is concrete evidence to the contrary. Where evidence of market failure exists, the government could intervene to ensure adequate quality of care. For example, the government could use its substantial clout as a larger purchaser of health care services to help organize private markets for health care quality. This might entail initiating the formation of community-based quality assurance programs; building strategic alliances with private accrediting bodies to promote accreditation for certain types of facilities or services; and providing technical assistance to develop dissemination mechanisms for quality assurance information. Government efforts could also be used to strengthen licensure and other regulatory programs.

Another role for the public sector is in research. The government can continue to support research on outcome measurement and assessment, focusing on how consumers of different cultural and educational backgrounds interpret and use outcome data. Research in this area can lead to standardized data-reporting formats that facilitate the ability of consumers to use the data to make choices concerning their health care providers. The government could mandate that certain formats be used just as the Securities and Exchange Commission mandates standard reporting formats for disclosing information pertinent to securities transactions.

In addition, the role of the public sector could extend to ensuring that private sector entities involved in external quality assurance are accountable to the public for their activities. DHHS functions as a superaccreditor in its selection of accrediting bodies for Medicare's deemed-certification process. Although DHHS has promulgated criteria for reviewing accrediting bodies for purposes of deemed-certification status, these criteria do not explicitly address governance arrangements and other areas of organization and management that might compromise the independence of the accrediting body in performing quality assurance functions.[31] DHHS might consider criteria addressing the nature and level of consumer representation on the boards of private accrediting bodies. The government could adopt similar criteria for community-based programs involved in quality assurance. Finally, accountability might also be sought through the judicial system to ensure adequate civil liability exposure for private sector entities that negligently perform quality assurance activities.[32]

CONCLUSION

The private sector is assuming an increasingly larger role in the external oversight of health care quality. Some commentators have raised concerns that traditional public oversight activities will be curtailed or eliminated, leaving significant gaps in the country's external quality assurance systems. This chapter considered private sector developments in quality assurance relative to their potential benefits and problems. The public sector can continue to fulfill its important role in quality assurance by capitalizing on the benefits associated with private sector efforts while using its resources to intervene in those circumstances under which the private sector has not been successful.

REFERENCES

1. Lutz S. A record year for hospital deals. *Modern Healthcare.* December 18–25, 1995:43–52.
2. Lutz S. Not-for-profits up for grabs by the giants. *Modern Healthcare.* May 30, 1994:24–28.
3. Kassirer JP. Our ailing public hospitals: cure them or close them. *N England J Med.* 1995;33:1348–1349.

4. Jost TS. The necessary and proper role of regulation to assure the quality of health care. *Houston Law Rev.* 1988;25 special issue:525–598.

5. Jennison B, Young G, Brown S. *Licensing, Accreditation, and Certification.* Boston: Little, Brown & Co; 1993.

6. Graddy E. Interest groups or the public interest—why do we regulate health occupations? *J Health Politics Policy Law.* 1991;16:25–49.

7. Jost TS. Oversight of the quality of medical care: regulation, management, or the market? *Arizona Law Rev.* 1995;37:825–868.

8. Jost TS. Recent developments in medical quality assurance and audit: an international comparative study. In: Dingwall R, Fenn P, eds. *Quality Regulation and Health Care.* London: Routledge; 1992.

9. Lohr K, Walker A. The utilization and quality control peer review organization program. In: Lohr K, ed. *Medicare: A Strategy for Quality Assurance.* Washington, DC: National Academy of Sciences Press; 1990:343–437.

10. Jencks SF. The government's role in hospital accountability for quality of care. *J Qual Improvement.* 1994;20:364–369.

11. JCAHO moves in on accrediting turf held by NCQA. *Business Health.* 1994;12:14.

12. Dimmitt BS. Managed care organizations are increasingly seeking a stamp of approval from an independent organization. Does it matter which group does the job? Do employees care? Should they? *Business Health.* 1996;13:38–43.

13. Appleby C. Accreditation groups vie to offer eminent seal of approval in home care. *Healthwork News.* March 25, 1991:33–41.

14. GI *Federal Register* 67,041.

15. Pauly M. The public policy implications of using outcome statistics. *Brooklyn Law Rev.* 1992;58:35–54.

16. U.S. General Accounting Office. *Health Care Reform: "Report Cards" Are Useful but Significant Issues Need To Be Addressed.* Washington, DC: General Accounting Office/HEHS-94-219; 1994.

17. *AHA News.* 1994;30:4.

18. Stephenson GM, Findlay S. HEDIS: almost ready for prime time. *Business Health.* 1995;39:41–50.

19. Penzer JR. Grading the report card: lessons from cognitive psychology, marketing, and the law of information disclosure for quality assessment in health care reform. *Yale J Regulation.* 1995; 12:207–256.

20. Casey PJ. Cleveland communities collaborate in effort to evaluate hospital efficiency and quality. *QRC Advisor.* 1995;11:1, 6–7.

21. Jordan HS, Straus JH, Bailit MH. Reporting and using health plan performance information in Massachusetts. *J Qual Improvement.* 1995;21:167–177.

22. Terry P, Fowles J, Isham G, Wetzel S. Beyond report cards: a health profile for Health Partners Health Plan and the Business Health Care Action Group. *HMO Practice.* 1994;8:171–175.

23. Rochester, New York consortium ends outcomes data experiment. *Modern Healthcare.* 1992;2:30.

24. Savas E. *How To Shrink Government: Privatizing the Public Sector.* Chatham, NJ: Chatham House Publishers; 1982.

25. Burda D. AHA criticizes JCAHO. *Modern Healthcare.* 1989;19:5.

26. Green J. AHA sends signal to JCAHO. *AHA News.* Dec. 24, 1994:2.

27. Packer J. States go easy on freestanding facilities—GAO. *Modern Healthcare.* 1991;21:16.

28. Havighurst C. The place of private accrediting among the instruments of government. *Law Contemp Problems.* 1994;27:3–14.

29. McGeary M. Medicare Conditions of Participation and accreditation for hospitals. In: Lohr K, ed. *Medicare: A Strategy for Quality Assurance.* 2nd vol. Washington, DC: National Academy of Sciences Press; 1990:292–342.

30. Jost TS. Medicare and the Joint Commission on Accreditation of Healthcare Organizations: a healthy relationship? *Law Contemp Problems.* 1994;57:15–46.

31. 42 CFR ch 4, § 488.8.

32. Schuck T. Tort liability to those injured by negligent accreditation decisions. *Law Contemp Problems.* 1994;57:185–198.

PART III

Case Studies in Public Health and Managed Care

Managed care and privatization initiatives are highly sensitive to the attributes of the health care organizations affected and the environments in which they operate. To fully appreciate the complexities of these initiatives and their public health implications, it is necessary to observe in detail the processes by which they are developed and implemented in specific organizations and communities. Part III comprises case studies of managed care and privatization initiatives underway in selected organizations and communities across the United States. As a preface to these case studies, Chapter 11 presents a typology of interactions between managed care organizations and public health agencies that may assist readers in evaluating and comparing individual cases. Chapters 12 to 20 then describe the experiences of individual organizations and communities. Each case study concludes with a series of discussion questions intended to assist readers in identifying its salient characteristics.

CHAPTER 11

Managed Care, Public Health, and Privatization: A Typology of Interorganizational Arrangements

Glen P. Mays, Paul K. Halverson, and Arnold D. Kaluzny

Political and marketplace considerations are leading public health agencies and managed care plans to interact on a number of different levels and for a variety of reasons. The diverse relationships currently taking shape between managed care plans and public health agencies can be classified and described along three broad dimensions. The strategic attributes indicate the motivations, goals, and objectives that lie behind these alliances, from the perspectives of both managed care plans and public health agencies. The functional attributes reveal the range of activities and operations that are carried out through these alliances, as well as the individuals, groups, and populations served by these collective activities. Finally, the structural attributes of these relationships disclose the mechanisms through which health plans and public health agencies interact, and offer an indication of the strength and durability of the associations between these organizations. This chapter uses these three dimensions to identify a typology of models through which managed care plans and public health agencies interact. This typology may then be employed to analyze and compare the multiplicity of relationships taking shape between these types of organizations. The case studies in the following chapters, as well as examples in this chapter, illustrate the various models in the typology.

MODELS OF INTERACTION BETWEEN MANAGED CARE AND PUBLIC HEALTH

It is important to note that the strategic, functional, and structural attributes that characterize relationships between managed care plans and public health agencies

Source: Adapted with permission from P.K. Halverson et al., Not-So-Strange Bedfellows: Models of Interaction between Managed Care Plans and Public Health Agencies, *Milbank Quarterly*, Vol. 75, No. 1, pp. 113–138, © 1997, Blackwell Publishers.

are not mutually exclusive. Rather, these attributes are complementary and mutually reinforcing. A single observed relationship between a managed care plan and a public health agency can be described and classified simultaneously according to its strategic objectives, its functional accomplishments, and its structural characteristics. Moreover, these three attributes have numerous interrelationships and codependencies. Strategic objectives have substantial influence on both the functional and structural characteristics of relationships between health plans and public health agencies.

It is also important to recognize the operational definitions of public health agencies and managed care plans that we use in examining these organizations and in distilling their models of interaction. Our observations of public health agencies in this chapter are limited to the "official" governmental public health agencies that are operative in the local geopolitical subdivisions of a state. These agencies are most often governmental units of cities, townships, or counties, but they may also exist as multicounty authorities. Our observations of managed care plans in this chapter are limited to those organizations that operate a health maintenance organization (HMO). Many of the managed care plans we examine offer other managed care "products," such as preferred provider organizations and point-of-service plans. We restrict our analysis to managed care plans offering HMO products because we have failed to identify cases of public health agencies interacting with plans that do not offer this type of product.

Finally, it should be noted that this review focuses primarily on linkages between managed care plans and public health agencies at the local level, under the premise that the majority of individual and community-based public health services are delivered at this level. Nevertheless, the role of state health departments in managing, evaluating, and contributing to these alliances should not be overlooked. This role includes critical policy and program-level activities that enable and support alliance development at the local level, such as Medicaid contract management and enforcement; performance evaluation and monitoring; certification and inspection in conjunction with state departments of insurance; and funding for collaborative service delivery programs. State health department efforts provide a context and foundation for all of the alliance models examined in this study. Indeed, the models of strategic, functional, and structural alliances described here are likely to be sensitive to the context and environment in which they emerge. The range of models we observe and describe are, at least in part, reflective of the diversity of environments in which they are found.

Strategic Models of Interaction

At the most basic level, collaborative relationships between managed care plans and public health agencies can be classified according to the strategic intent and purpose of the relationship. Three basic models of strategic purpose that have been observed among interorganizational alliances in business and industry also appear highly applicable to relationships between managed care and public health (Table 11–1).[1] The most transitory of these alliances, the opportunistic model, allows health plans and public health agencies to exchange knowledge and expertise that will assist each organization in pursuing its own independent interests and objectives. Under this model, organizations collaborate only long enough to acquire the desired knowledge that will enable them to embark upon a new activity or area of service. These alliances take shape when a managed care plan seeks to begin enrolling Medicaid beneficiaries or other population groups that are typically served by public health agencies, or when a public health agency seeks to develop its own managed care program for serving some or all of its clients. These two circumstances may occur at the same time, resulting in an opportunistic relationship that ultimately allows two competing Medicaid managed care plans to develop, one of which is operated by the public health agency.

A second type of strategic relationship between managed care and public health involves the joint production of some product or service that is needed by both types of organizations. Under this shared services model, health plans and public health agencies agree to share the costs of establishing and maintaining such initiatives as childhood immunization databases, communicable disease registries, public health media messages, and community health surveillance projects. A key aspect of this model is that health plans and public health agencies typically have different motivations for engaging in these cooperative initiatives, and consequently they derive different types and levels of benefit from the projects. A health plan's objective may be to acquire data for its own group of enrollees or to market its services to potential enrollees, while a health department's objective may include identifying health threats in the community at large and distributing health information on a community-wide basis. Through the shared service model, organizations may achieve multiple, divergent objectives through common efforts.

The stakeholder model represents a third type of strategic relationship between public health and managed care that occurs when each organization assumes a key role in the operation or the "production process" of the partnering organization. Thus, the managed care plan assumes a role that is central to the public health mission of the health department, while the department likewise assumes a role that is central to the health care management objectives of the health plan. Typically, the relationship between the two organizations entails delivery of health services to a defined population that is of concern to both the health plan and the public health agency. This defined population may consist of a health plan's enrollee group, a health department's service population, or the intersection or union of these two populations. Organizations engaging in this type of strategic relationship undertake collaborative action to achieve mutual objectives

Table 11–1 Basic Strategic Models of Interaction between Managed Care Plans and Public Health Agencies

Model description	Strategic goals of managed care plans	Strategic goals of public health agencies
Opportunistic model		
Interaction is established to obtain knowledge and expertise in a new field or activity that will assist participating organizations in pursuing their own interests.	Acquire skills in managing the care of vulnerable population groups; using epidemiologic techniques for disease identification; and designing and managing health promotion and disease prevention interventions.	Acquire skills in projecting and managing costs of service delivery; conducting cost-effectiveness analyses for services needed by clients; negotiating service contracts; performing case management and utilization review.
Shared services model		
Interaction is established to jointly produce a service needed by both organizations in pursuing their own interests.	Share the costs associated with data collection efforts such as immunization registries and community health surveillance. Health plans use these data to improve the management of enrollees' care and to project costs associated with covering new enrollees.	Share the costs of data collection efforts and ensure the completeness of data by securing the participation of all major health care providers. Health agencies use data for identifying health risks in the community and targeting community-wide interventions.
Stakeholder model		
Interaction is established with organizations that are central to the core mission or "production process" of an organization, to realize improvements in the quality and efficiency of the goods or services produced.	Secure the participation of public health agencies as key service providers to health plan enrollees. Support the health promotion and disease prevention efforts of public health agencies that directly impact the health of current and/or potential health plan enrollees.	Secure the involvement of health plans in maximizing the quality and accessibility of health services provided to clients of public health agencies. Use health plans to achieve optimal delivery of services to clients.

in the defined population, such as improving health status; expanding accessibility of health services; encouraging appropriate utilization of services; and containing the costs of providing services.

The strategic nature of alliances established between public health agencies and managed care plans ultimately hinges upon the strategic objectives and intent of the participating organizations. In many areas, the strategic objectives of public health agencies may differ substantially from those of managed care plans. In general, local public health agencies maintain a focus on maintaining and improving health at the community level, with an emphasis on directly providing those services and activities that are not adequately performed by other organizations in the community.[2] Public health agencies, therefore, often emphasize the provision of personal health services to individuals without private health insurance, and the performance of nonclinical, population-based activities such as environmental monitoring, community health assessment, and community-wide planning and policy development. In contrast, managed care plans often maintain a strategic focus on managing the medical needs of their enrolled subscribers, and remaining responsive to the demands of employers and other organizations that purchase their services. For-profit plans have the additional imperative of providing returns on investment for shareholders, while nonprofit plans may have additional objectives related to community service, medical education, and research.

Where the strategic objectives of public health agencies and managed care plans do not overlap substantially, opportunistic alliances and shared service alliances may be the predominant forms of collaboration. Stakeholder alliances may occur when the strategic objectives of public health agencies and managed care plans are sufficiently aligned, as when a plan serves Medicaid beneficiaries or other vulnerable populations that are also served by the public health agency, or when a nonprofit plan's mission of community service parallels that of the public health agency. Multivariate analysis of relationships in 63 public health jurisdictions provides support for this contention, indicating that nonprofit plans are significantly more likely to develop alliances with public health agencies than are for-profit plans, and also indicating that alliances are more likely to develop in jurisdictions characterized by high levels of managed care penetration and consolidation.[3] This latter finding suggests that the strategic interests of managed care plans and public health agencies may be more aligned in "mature" managed care markets, where plans have responsibility for serving large shares of the total community population.

Functional Models of Interaction

Collaboration between managed care plans and public health agencies occurs in a wide range of functional areas that are related to, but not necessarily determined by, the overall strategic purpose of the collaboration. The collaborative efforts we observed can be summarized with six broad functional attributes: health planning and policy development; outreach and education; data collection and community health assessment; provision of enabling services; provision of clinical services; and case management services. Within each of these areas, collaboration may target a wide range of population groups. Coordinated efforts may be restricted to a particular subgroup of a health plan's membership, or they may extend to a community's total population. The population group that is targeted by the collaborative effort is intrinsically related to both the strategic and the functional characteristics of the relationship. For example, service alliances in the functional area of outreach and education may target broad segments of the community, since a health plan may use such a joint venture as a marketing opportunity, while a health department may use the venture for community-wide health education. Alternatively, opportunistic alliances in the functional area of clinical services provision may be restricted to the subpopulation of health plan members who are eligible for Medicaid, since each organization seeks to gain expertise while focusing as narrowly as possible on its own population of interest.

A common functional area of collaboration among managed care plans and public health agencies involves collective efforts in health planning and policy development. Through a wide range of both formal and informal structures, public health agencies and health plans may act collectively to identify major health threats in the community; plan jointly sponsored community interventions; or develop coordinated efforts to inform federal, state, and local officials about health policy issues affecting the community. In several of the communities included in our study, for example, public health agencies have gained membership in local associations of managed care plans and have begun to use these forums as opportunities for planning and initiating such joint activities as community health assessment projects and proposals for modifying state Medicaid contracts.

Collaborative efforts in outreach and education are also common. Many of these efforts seek to impact health status and care-seeking behavior by targeting population segments within the general population. However, some initiatives may seek to impact clinical practice by targeting physicians and other service providers. Jointly sponsored community health fairs exist as a common example of this model, wherein managed care plans and public health agencies collectively provide screening services, health education and counseling, and even health-related products such as bicycle helmets or smoke detectors to community members. In other communities, public health agencies and managed care plans jointly sponsor initiatives for educating community physicians regarding appropriate practices for tuberculosis diagnosis and treatment, child lead poisoning screening, or childhood immunization.[4]

Additionally, coordinated data collection and community health assessment activities are undertaken to share the costs of acquiring and maintaining information on disease incidence and prevalence, service utilization and outcomes, and health-related behaviors and risk factors. Examples of these activities include: agreements between public health agencies and managed care plans that allow the exchange of treatment records for managed care enrollees who are treated in health department clinics; an agreement for the joint operation of a computerized immunization registry; and a jointly funded effort to survey the community population for health risks and behaviors.

Three other functional areas of collaboration between managed care plans and public health agencies relate to the delivery and management of personal health services. Collaboration may entail the provision of enabling services such as transportation, child care, and language translation services needed by individuals to obtain full access to the local health care system. These services are more commonly areas of expertise for public health agencies than for managed care plans. Provision of clinical services may also be entailed in these collaborative arrangements, including preventive and primary health services in home-based or office-based settings. Both health plans and public health agencies may have clinical areas of expertise that are shared through cooperative arrangements. Finally, collaboration may involve the provision of case management services to ensure continuity, appropriateness, and cost-effectiveness in the utilization of health services. Traditionally, managed care plans hold the bulk of experience in this functional area, but health departments may claim this authority within the public sector or for selected diseases such as tuberculosis and sexually transmitted diseases.[5] A local health department in Tennessee, for example, provides case management services to the Medicaid enrollees of several different managed care plans operating in the jurisdiction, and also provides specified clinical and enabling services through the public health clinics it operates. In contrast, an agreement between a health department and HMO in Maryland allows the HMO to provide both case management and clinical services for health department clients who are at risk for breast or cervical cancer.

Each of the six functional areas identified above are of critical importance, both to managed care plans in their mission of maximizing efficiency and quality in health care delivery and to local public health agencies in their community-wide health promotion and disease prevention objectives. Nonetheless, managed care plans and public health agencies are likely to have different levels of knowledge and expertise in these functional areas. Interaction and collaboration in these areas are therefore truly rational responses.

Local health departments clearly have other functional responsibilities beyond the six areas identified here, as do managed care plans. For public health functions such as vector control, water quality, and food safety inspection, it may prove inefficient, ineffective, or unfeasible to perform these functional activities through interorganizational alliances with managed care plans. Certain functions may require a local governmental presence and preclude private sector involvement, such as regulation, evaluation, and oversight. Other functions require certain types of resources and expertise that managed care plans have no incentive to acquire or provide. Interaction between managed care plans and public health agencies is necessarily limited to those functional areas where interests are shared.[6]

Structural Models of Interaction

Diverse interorganizational structures are used to achieve the various strategic and functional objectives of alliances between managed care plans and public health agencies. These strategic and functional objectives have much bearing on the structural characteristics of the alliance. Structural characteristics are also likely to be influenced by the nature of the participating organizations and their leaders, as well as external factors in the political, economic, and social environment.[6,7]

The interorganizational structures used to support collaboration between managed care and public health can be ordered along a continuum that reflects the level of organizational integration achieved between the two types of organizations (Figure 11–1). This same approach is used to describe the structural characteristics of interorganizational alliances in business and industry.[8] At one extreme of the continuum, complete independence exists among managed care plans and public health agencies, and few if any efforts are underway to collaborate or interact in any manner. At the other extreme of the continuum, complete integration is achieved between a managed care plan and public health agency such that the functions of the two entities are consolidated into a single organizational structure. The structural models of interaction that fall within and include these extremes offer a range of potential benefits and costs to the participating organizations.

Complete Independence of Managed Care and Public Health

The absence of interaction between managed care plans and public health agencies serves as a baseline model for this analysis of interorganizational structures, since this model appears to remain the most prevalent. A survey of local health department directors in 63 diverse cities and counties across the United States finds that less than half of the departments located in jurisdictions served by managed care plans maintain any formal or informal relationship with a plan.[9] Interviews with the administrators of managed care plans and public health agencies in several of these jurisdictions suggest a number of factors that may inhibit the development of managed care–public health relationships, includ-

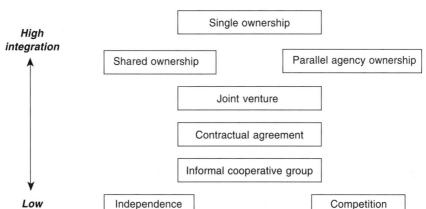

Figure 11–1 Structural Models of Interaction between Managed Care Plans and Public Health Agencies.

ing an internal focus of health department and/or managed care leadership; lack of congruence between the service area of the managed care plan and that of the health agency; differences in the populations served by managed care plans and public health agencies; differences in the organizational missions and values of managed care plans and public health agencies; and lack of visibility as an effective and efficient provider of health services in the community on the part of the public health agency and/or the managed care plan. Factors such as these may lead public health agencies and managed care plans to fail to recognize the potential value of interaction.

An important distinction exists within this baseline model that relates to the selective nature of health plan interaction. Available evidence suggests that most local health departments do not establish relationships with any of the health plans serving their jurisdictions. Other departments, however, establish relationships with some health plans within the local community, but not with others. The factors that lead health departments and managed care plans to engage in this selective interaction may be very different from those that result in a complete lack of interaction between the two types of organizations. Motivations that would lead an organization to interact with some, but not all, of its potential partners may include: the desire to limit the administrative (transaction) costs of interfacing with all organizations; the need to work only with those organizations that have a certain patient volume, service capacity, area of expertise, or accreditation; the desire to work only with organizations having similar values, missions, or cultures; and the desire to restrict interaction to those organizations demonstrating a favorable cost structure or a willingness to operate under specific financing arrangements, such as capitation.

Informal Cooperative Groups

Informal cooperative groups allow managed care plans and public health agencies to interact in a loosely structured environment with comparatively little organizational investment and risk.[8] Membership in these groups includes representatives from local managed care plans and the local health department, and may also extend to area hospitals, physicians, and other health care providers. Member organizations use these groups to share information, technology, and resources, and to engage in joint planning and policy development activities. These groups may also be used by members as forums for negotiating more formalized and integrated structures of interaction.

Some cooperative groups may conduct regular meetings and use other communication mechanisms, such as newsletters. These activities are particularly common among groups performing joint planning and policy development functions. In one Oregon county, for example, a cooperative group composed of the leaders of major managed care plans, hospitals, and the local health department meets monthly to conduct community-wide planning and policy development (see Chapter 14). To continually improve upon its process, the group's members attend national and regional conferences together on topics relevant to community health improvement. Other groups may interact through established informal patterns of communication and resource exchange that are initiated on an ad hoc basis. A public health agency and health maintenance organization in Washington state use this model to share medical supplies on an as-needed basis, in addition to other, more formalized mechanisms of interaction (see Chapter 13).

Informal cooperative groups allow managed care plans and public health agencies to accrue some of the benefits of collaborative action without sacrificing much individual autonomy and control. These structures typically do not entail large investments of resources, and therefore may be limited in their impact upon community health. The absence of contracts and binding agreements may create a reluctance among participating organizations to commit substantial resources to joint efforts, as well as a tendency for these organizations to shy away from difficult, complex, or long-term projects. At the same time, cooperative groups are typically based upon strong and long-standing personal relationships between organizations and their leaders. The familiarity and trust that underscore these relationships may not be present among the managed care plans and public health agencies serving many communities, making more formalized relationships the preferred structures for interaction. A survey of 63 local health departments provides evidence of this phenomenon, finding that more than three-quarters of existing relationships with managed care plans are formalized by contract.[9]

Contractual Agreements

As the most common structural model of interaction between managed care plans and public health agencies, contractual agreements are used for a wide range of strategic objectives and functional purposes. Two basic forms of contractual agreements are evident. In the first form, managed care plans negotiate a subcontract with public health agencies to provide services to enrollees of the health plan. Health plans then reimburse public health agencies either on a fee-for-service or capitated basis for services delivered to enrollees. Under some agreements, public health agencies may provide only specified services, such as family planning, sexually transmitted disease treatment, or home health services. In other agreements, the health department may function as an independent practice association by providing all primary care and case management services, and by subcontracting with other organizations for inpatient and specialty care. A local health department in Memphis, Tennessee, for example, holds contracts with four different managed care plans to provide and manage the care of their enrollees who are beneficiaries of the statewide TennCare Medicaid program in exchange for a fixed fee per enrollee (see Chapter 15).

The majority of subcontracting activities occurring between managed care plans and public health agencies appear to focus exclusively on Medicaid beneficiaries who are enrolled in the health plans. While interorganizational arrangements for serving the commercial (employed) enrollees of managed care plans are less common, they do exist. A contract between a large managed care plan and a county health department in Arizona enables the health department to provide tuberculosis treatment and control services to commercial as well as Medicaid enrollees. Similarly, a local health department in rural Wisconsin provides home health services to commercial and Medicare enrollees of several managed care plans that operate out of the surrounding urban areas. As many traditional sources of funding for public health services become less certain under state and federal reform efforts, growing numbers of public health agencies may explore opportunities for revenue support by serving commercially insured populations.

A second form of contractual agreement between managed care plans and public health agencies involves contracting with health plans for providing services to health department clients. In this scenario, the health plan assumes the role of service provider and receives capitated reimbursement from the public health agency in exchange for serving the agency's clients. Unlike many of the contracts that public health agencies may have with other types of providers, contractual agreements with managed care plans often entail intensive case management and utilization review activities that potentially may result in more efficient and effective care being delivered to health department clients. A county health department in Maryland, for example, contracts with an HMO for providing breast cancer and cervical cancer prevention services to low-income uninsured women over the age of 40.

Joint Ventures

In some communities, health plans and public health agencies move beyond purely contractual relationships to establish jointly operated programs and services. Under joint ventures, the managed care plan and public health agency participate collaboratively in the financing, administration, and delivery of services. These collaborative arrangements may be formalized through multiple contracts and agreements between the participating organizations or through the formation of a new corporate entity jointly owned by the partnering organizations. The health plans and public health agencies that engage in these efforts share in the control and governance of the new program or service, while also sharing the financial risk and clinical accountability that are associated with the activity. The shared control and responsibility entailed in these endeavors are the characteristics that distinguish this model most clearly from exchange-based relationships operating under the contractual agreement model.[8]

This model is used successfully by an HMO, a nonprofit hospital, and a county health department in Washington state to jointly fund and operate a community health clinic for serving uninsured and underinsured individuals as well as Medicaid beneficiaries (see case study in Chapter 13). The clinic is staffed by health professionals from each organization, and is supported with funding from each organization. Clearly, these more integrated alliances may offer the opportunity not only to pool resources but to gain access to additional resources using collective expertise and capacity.

Health Plan Operation by Parallel Agency

In the three remaining structural models of interaction, managed care plans and public health agencies are integrated to some degree within a common organizational structure. The first and least integrated of these models occurs when a managed care plan is established within an agency of local government that is organizationally parallel to the local public health agency. Although not directly owned and operated by the health agency, the health plan is controlled by the same governmental entity that controls the health agency. This organizational structure typically allows for very close working relationships between the two organizations, and may entail merger or integration of common operations and responsibilities to avoid duplication. The public health agency may assume responsibility for directly providing specified preventive and public health services to the enrolled population of the health plan, and/or may monitor and evaluate the adequacy of public health services offered by health plan providers.

This model is successfully operating in a California jurisdiction, where the locally operative public health department and a competitive managed care plan are both arms of the county government. The health plan serves all county employees, along with MediCal (Medicaid) beneficiaries, the county's medically indigent population, and the employees of several commercial businesses. Under this arrangement, the health plan assumes responsibility for providing most medical services, while the public health department retains the responsibility for providing certain public health services such as human immunodeficiency virus (HIV) counseling and testing, communicable-disease contact tracing, and operating school health clinics. Other public health services continue to be provided both by the health plan and health department to ensure maximum community coverage, including immunizations, family planning, and sexually transmitted disease treatment. The health department also negotiates memoranda of understanding with the county health plan and other health plans serving MediCal and medically indigent populations to set standards for public health services that are provided directly by the health plans rather than by the public health department.

Shared Operation of Health Plan

Vertical integration of managed care and public health may also occur through partnerships between public health agencies and other health care providers. These partnerships are typically established between health agencies and hospitals, which share the ownership and/or administration of a jointly established managed care plan. The shared arrangement brings the acute care capacity of the hospital and the primary and preventive care capacity of the health department into a single organizational structure that can assume financial risk and clinical accountability for a continuum of health needs within a population. This arrangement also allows the participating organizations to share the financial risks associated with operating the health plan, rather than assuming all of the risk alone. Shared ownership may also assist in meeting the capital requirements necessary to obtain state and/or federal licensure as an HMO, or to achieve accreditation from organizations such as the National Commission on Quality Assurance.

This structural model is used by a consortium of organizations in Portland, Oregon, to create a competitive managed care plan that serves Medicaid beneficiaries in a three-county area (see case study in Chapter 14). Participating organizations include two county health departments, a local academic medical center, and a coalition of community health centers throughout the state. Through the shared arrangement, one of the health departments provides primary and preventive health services and case management for health plan enrollees, while the hospital manages all inpatient and specialty care. Community health centers and the remaining county health department serve as additional primary care providers. Despite their ownership of a competing health plan, the health departments maintain contact to provide specified public health services such as communicable-disease and family planning services to the enrollees of other managed care plans. The health departments also continue to provide many clinical public health services to the community at large, regardless of enrollment status or ability to obtain reimbursement.

Sole Ownership/Operation of Health Plan

The most integrated structural model of managed care–public health interaction occurs when a managed care plan and public health agency are wholly contained within a single corporate entity. In all previous structural models discussed, the managed care plans and public health agencies maintain separate corporate identities alongside their collaborative alliances. The sole ownership model departs from this trend by establishing a true vertically integrated delivery system. Where this model exists, the managed care plan is organizationally integrated not only with the public health agency, but also with units providing hospital care and ambulatory care. Individuals enrolled in the plan can pass seamlessly from the preventive and public health services offered through the public health unit to the primary and acute care services offered in other settings within the system. At the same time, the public health unit continues to provide both clinical and environmental public health services to members of the community at large who are not enrolled in the health plan. Likewise, the hospital and ambulatory care units within the system do not limit their services to enrolled members. A single organization assumes financial and clinical responsibility for the full range of health services needed by enrolled members and for the public health services needed by members of the general community. This same organization is also responsible for providing both reimbursable and charity care in the inpatient and ambulatory settings.

This structural model is used by a local public health and hospital corporation in Denver, Colorado, which includes within its organization a public health agency, a managed care plan, an acute care hospital, and a network of community health centers (see Chapter 12). The managed care plan within this system serves both county employees and Medicaid beneficiaries. The hospital and health center components of this system assume responsibility for delivering most personal health services, allowing the public health agency to focus on community-wide endeavors such as education and assessment initiatives, policy development activities, and programs for high-risk population groups such as patients with HIV. The managers of this system indicate that cost savings generated through the managed care component enable the organization to provide greater levels of service in nonrevenue areas such as inpatient and ambulatory charity care and community-wide public health initiatives.

It should be noted that the consolidated ownership model also entails certain risks. In this model, there are few organizational structures that delineate the boundaries between the public health and medical care components. Therefore, in periods of resource scarcity or financial difficulty, few safeguards exist for ensuring that public health services receive an appropriate allotment of total organizational resources. In periods of crisis, an organization's medical care obligations may appear more immediate and visible than its obligations for performing traditional public health activities such as disease prevention and health promotion services or nonclinical services such as health assessment, environmental monitoring, and policy development. The 1995 financial crisis and subsequent federal bailout of the Los Angeles County public health system illustrates the need for caution in implementing consolidated systems that integrate public health, managed care, and hospital components.

CONCLUSION

The typology of interactions presented in this chapter uses concepts from organization theory to reduce and simplify the multiplicity of relationships found between managed care plans and public health agencies. While not exhaustive, this typology nevertheless provides a framework for examining salient characteristics of these relationships, and for noting trends and patterns in these characteristics across organizations, communities, and markets.

The case studies that follow this chapter provide opportunities for applying this typology to current developments in local health care markets (see Table 11–2).

Table 11–2 Models of Interaction and Privatization Examined in the Case Studies

Model	Location	Chapter
Consolidation under single ownership and administration	Denver, Colorado	12
Shared ownership and operation	Portland, Oregon	14
Joint ventures	Olympia, Washington	13
Contracting	Memphis, Tennessee	15
	Mecklenburg County, North Carolina	18
	Milwaukee, Wisconsin	16
	King County, Washington	20
Informal cooperation	Portland, Oregon	14
	Olympia, Washington	13
	Milwaukee, Wisconsin	16
Public-private competition	Portland, Oregon	14
	King County, Washington	20
Public agency conversion	Jersey City, New Jersey	19
	Rocky Mount, North Carolina	17

The case study of Denver Health and Hospitals (Chapter 12) illustrates the approach of consolidating public health, managed care, and hospital components within a single organizational structure. The model of shared ownership and operation is examined in the case of a managed care plan that is jointly operated by public and private health care organizations in Portland, Oregon (Chapter 14). Joint ventures between public health agencies and managed care plans are examined in the case study of Olympia, Washington (Chapter 13). Alternative contracting arrangements between public and private health care organizations are described in the case studies of Memphis, Tennessee (Chapter 15); Mecklenburg County, North Carolina (Chapter 18); Milwaukee, Wisconsin (Chapter 16); and King County, Washington (Chapter 20). Examples of informal cooperation between managed care plans and public health agencies are also profiled in the case studies of Portland, Olympia, and Milwaukee. Alternative views of competition between public and private health care organizations are presented in the Portland and King County case studies. Finally, the dynamics of hospital conversions from public to private ownership are explored in the cases of Jersey City, New Jersey (Chapter 19) and Rocky Mount, North Carolina (Chapter 17).

REFERENCES

1. Kanter RM. Collaborative advantage: the art of alliances. *Harvard Business Rev.* 1994;72:96–108.

2. Institute of Medicine. *The Future of Public Health.* Washington, DC: National Academy Press; 1988.

3. Halverson PK, Mays GP, Miller CA. The determinants of interaction between managed care plans and public health agencies: implications for quality, accessibility, and efficiency in health care delivery. *Association for Health Services Research 13th Annual Meeting Abstracts.* Washington, DC: Association for Health Services Research; 1996. Abstract.

4. Halverson PK, Mays GP, Miller CA, Kaluzny AD, et al. Managed care and the public health challenge of TB. *Public Health Rep.* 1997;112:19–25.

5. Centers for Disease Control and Prevention. Essential components of a tuberculosis prevention and control program. *MMWR.* 1995;44:1–16.

6. Zuckerman HS, Kaluzny AD, Ricketts TC. Strategic alliances: a worldwide phenomenon comes to health care. In: Kaluzny AD, Zuckerman HS, Ricketts TC, eds. *Partners for the Dance: Forming Strategic Alliances in Health Care.* Ann Arbor, Mich: Health Administration Press; 1995:1–18.

7. Halverson PK, Kaluzny AD, Young GJ. Strategic alliances in health care: opportunities for the Veterans Affairs Health Care System. *Hosp and Health Services Admin.* In press.

8. Lorange P, Roos J. *Strategic Alliances: Formation, Implementation, and Evolution.* Cambridge, Mass: Blackwell Publishers; 1993.

9. Halverson PK, Mays GP, Miller CA, Richards TB. Organizational linkages in public health: interactions between local health departments and other health care providers; 1997. Under review.

CHAPTER 12

Case Study: Integrated Public and Private Health Care Systems in Denver, CO

Glen P. Mays

Both the public health system and the private health care market that serve Denver, Colorado, are large, consolidated, and economically healthy. A newly created independent health care authority operates a quasi-governmental health system that integrates public health functions with hospital and community health services under a contract with the city and county of Denver. This system offers perhaps the most complete example of a public sector integrated delivery system serving individuals with public and private health care insurance as well as those without health care coverage. In the private health care market, several large health maintenance organizations (HMOs) and hospital-based integrated delivery systems operate comprehensive systems of care with strong components that address community health issues. This case study examines the dynamics and interactions among the extensive public and private health care systems serving Denver.

OVERVIEW OF THE COMMUNITY

Metropolitan Denver lies on the high plains of central Colorado just east of the Rocky Mountains. The five-county metropolitan area contains a population of 2.1 million residents, although slightly less than 500000 of these residents live within

The author wishes to thank individuals at the following organizations for their invaluable contributions of time and information: Denver Health and Hospitals; Denver Children's Hospital; University Hospital; St. Joseph Hospital; Provenant St. Anthony Hospital; Porter Adventist HealthCare; HealthOne System; Kaiser Foundation Health Plan of Colorado; CIGNA Health Care of Colorado; FHP of Colorado; Qual-Med Plans for Health; HMO Colorado; Blue Cross and Blue Shield of Colorado; MetraHealth of Colorado; and PruCare of Colorado.

the city and county of Denver. The area continues to experience rapid population growth that began in the early 1990s with an expanding local economy of computer and telecommunications firms. This recent growth stands in stark contrast to the population decline and high unemployment that characterized the area after its oil industry faltered during the 1980s.

Denver's population contains a diverse group of ethnicities and cultures (Table 12–1). Residents of Hispanic origin comprise 23% of the county's total population, and almost 12% of the population speak Spanish at home. African Americans comprise 12% of the county population. The county exceeds many similar urban areas in the educational attainment and affluence of its population. Almost 80% of Denver residents are high school graduates, and 30% hold bachelor's degrees. The median family income is only slightly below the national average, and fewer than 18% of residents live below the federal poverty threshold.

The cost of living in Denver marginally exceeds that of the nation as a whole. The cost of living index for the second quarter of 1996 was 103.1% of the national average. Health care costs in Denver were 21% higher than the average, housing costs 15% higher, and utilities were 25% lower than average.

Denver's population appears to be both younger and healthier than that of comparable urban areas (Table 12–2). Less than 14% of the county's population has reached age 65. Infant mortality stands at 8.1 for whites and 10.4 for nonwhites (per 1000 live births). Leading causes of death include heart disease (124.6 per 100000 population), cancer (128.5 per 100000), and cerebrovascular diseases (28.3 per 100000).

The city and county of Denver contain a relative abundance of health service providers. Like many urban areas, access to health services remains a concern in low-income and minority neighborhoods where private providers are scarce, health insurance coverage is low, and language and cultural differences pose barriers to care. An estimated 12.5% of the state-wide population did not have

---

Table 12–1 Demographic Characteristics: Denver, Colorado

Population (1996)	496470
Percent of metropolitan-area population	23.4
Median age in years (1996)	34.3
Percent 65 years and older (1991)	13.8
Percent non-Caucasian (1991)	30.3
Percent speaking Spanish at home (1991)	11.9
Percent completing high school degree (1991)	79.2
Percent below federal poverty level (1989)	17.1
Median household income (1989)	$25106
Average percent unemployed (1996, metropolitan area)	3.8

Source: Reprinted from *County and City Data Book*, 1994, Bureau of the Census, U.S. Department of Commerce.

Table 12–2 Health Status Indicators in Denver, Colorado, 1995

Infant mortality rate per 1000 live births	8.2
Percent of births to mothers age 10–17	7.1
Percent of infants with low birth weight	10.5
Percent of births with prenatal care later than first trimester	27.7
Deaths per 100000 population, age-adjusted	597.6
Cancer, all types	128.5
Lung cancer	31.7
Female breast cancer	21.7
Heart disease	124.6
Other cardiovascular diseases	168.2
Cerebrovascular diseases	28.3
Chronic obstructive pulmonary diseases	27.4
Motor vehicle accidents	15.3
Suicide	20.6
Work-related injury	2.6
Percent of deaths due to pneumonia and influenza	3.6
Human immunodeficiency virus/acquired immune deficiency syndrome (HIV/AIDS)	4.3
Diabetes mellitus	1.9
Injury by firearms	2.3
Alcohol-induced deaths	2.3

Courtesy of Colorado Department of Public Health and Environment, Denver, Colorado, 1997.

health care coverage in 1994.[1] A total of 3204 active nonfederal physicians practiced in the city and county of Denver during 1994, yielding a comparatively high ratio of 64.5 physicians per 100000 people (Table 12–3).[2] A relatively low proportion of these physicians practice in primary care disciplines, with only a small percentage practicing in the specialties of family medicine, general medicine, pediatrics, and obstetrics/gynecology.

Eleven community hospitals contained within four multihospital systems serve the city and county of Denver and the surrounding metropolitan area, with a total inpatient capacity of 2821 beds, or 568 beds per 100000 people (Table 12–3). Consolidation continues to occur rapidly in the local hospital market, as evidenced by a recent hospital closure (1995) and several nonprofit hospital acquisitions by the for-profit corporation Columbia/HCA. Two public hospitals—the local Denver Health and Hospitals authority and the state-affiliated University Hospital—provide the bulk of charity care in the area.

A network of 10 community health centers operates as part of the Denver Health and Hospitals authority.[3] These federally qualified health centers (FQHCs) provide primary care services to uninsured and underinsured populations, as well as Medicaid and Medicare beneficiaries. Some of the centers also receive federal funding to provide specialized HIV services under the Ryan-White program, as well as substance abuse services under the federal block grant program. A

Table 12–3 Health Resources in Denver, Colorado

Indicator		Source
Number of nonfederal physicians (number per 100000 people) (1992)	3204 (65)	American Medical Association[2]
Family practice	177 (4)	
General practice	46 (1)	
Internal medicine	587 (12)	
Obstetrics/gynecology	174 (4)	
Pediatrics	271 (5)	
Number of community hospital beds (1995)	2821	American Hospital Association[1]
Beds per 100000 population	568	
Number of community hospitals (1995)	11	American Hospital Association[1]
Number of HMOs (1995)	10	American Association of Health Plans[4]
Number of federally qualified health centers (1994)	2	U.S. Bureau of Primary Health Care[3]
Local public health expenditures (1992)	$11000000	National Assocation of County and City Health Officials (unpublished data, 1995)
Percent from federal sources	0%	
Percent from state sources (including federal pass-throughs)	25%	
Percent from local sources	55%	
Total federal funding for community health centers (1995)	$8967128	U.S. Department of Commerce[5]
Total federal funding for migrant health centers (1995)	$1319875	U.S. Department of Commerce[5]
Total federal block grant funds for preventive health services	$1983935	U.S. Department of Commerce[5]
Total federal block grant funds for maternal and child health services	$7570130	U.S. Department of Commerce[5]
Total federal block grant funds for substance abuse services	$4532108	U.S. Department of Commerce[5]
Total federal funding for homeless health services (1995)	$1128227	U.S. Department of Commerce[5]

Source: Reprinted from Colorado Department of Public Health and Environment, 1997.

federally funded homeless health clinic also operates in Denver's downtown area, under the management of a private nonprofit corporation.

Managed care has become a dominant form of local health services delivery and financing for commercially insured individuals as well as Medicaid and Medicare beneficiaries in Denver. Almost 50% of commercially insured residents in the Denver metropolitan area receive health services through HMOs and another 24% are enrolled in preferred provider organizations (National Research

Corporation. 1994. Unpublished data). A total of 10 HMOs report operating in the city and county of Denver in 1995.[4] Two of these HMOs enroll Medicaid beneficiaries, five hold Tax Equity and Fiscal Responsibility Act risk contracts for serving Medicare beneficiaries on a capitated basis, and one plan serves Medicare beneficiaries under cost-based reimbursement. Three of Denver's private multi-hospital systems also operate HMO products that primarily serve employee groups. Additionally, the Denver Health and Hospitals authority operates an HMO that serves both municipal employees and Medicaid beneficiaries. A statewide 1915(b) Medicaid waiver program requires recipients of the Aid to Families with Dependent Children (AFDC) program and the Supplemental Security Income (SSI) program to enroll either in a primary care case management plan or in a capitated HMO.

The local public health department for the city and county of Denver resides within the consolidated Denver Health and Hospitals authority (DHH). This authority also encompasses a general acute care hospital, a network of community health centers, and a managed care plan serving county employees and Medicaid beneficiaries. DHH functioned as a municipal government agency under the authority of the Denver mayor and city council until January 1997, when state legislation and municipal contracts took effect that established the entity as a health care authority independent of both state and municipal control. The new authority structure allows the DHH system to escape cumbersome municipal regulations regarding contracting, purchasing, and personnel actions.

MANAGED CARE IN THE PUBLIC HEALTH SYSTEM

As Denver's definitive public health and public medical care system, DHH began its foray into managed care during the 1980s after the private market for managed care had already begun its rapid growth. The city and county of Denver hoped to contain the costs associated with providing health care coverage to municipal employees by launching a county-sponsored health plan. For this purpose, DHH entered into a joint venture with a successful for-profit HMO that maintained a large enrollment in the Denver market as well as other metropolitan areas in the mountain states and Pacific West. The jointly operated plan served municipal employees in exchange for a capitated fee from the municipal government. Under the arrangement, DHH assumed responsibility for the provision of hospital inpatient and outpatient services, while the HMO managed primary care services through its network of private physicians and clinics. The HMO also managed administrative services such as utilization review, pre-approval, and physician profiling. Through this venture, DHH developed the capacities and skills required for operating a managed care plan.

Eventually, DHH terminated its agreement with the HMO and took over full ownership of the joint venture. DHH administrators suggest that, by assuming the full financial risk of the employee health plan, the system could leverage funds that the municipality spends on employee health care coverage in order to expand service in other, non–revenue-generating areas. DHH's chief executive reports that revenue generated through the CityCare Plan allows the system to provide greater levels of uncompensated care through its hospital and community clinics, and enhanced levels of public health services that are not supported by federal and state funding. Approximately 20% of the county's work force is currently enrolled in the plan, and county premiums amount to $5 million, or approximately 3% of the system's total revenue.

In 1994, the DHH system began to apply its newly acquired expertise and capacity in managed care to the Medicaid population in Denver. During this year, the state implemented its 1915(b) Medicaid waiver program for enrolling Medicaid beneficiaries in managed care. With its extensive capacity for primary care delivery and its established administrative infrastructure for managed care, DHH immediately became the state's largest Medicaid managed care provider. As of 1995, DHH was one of the only Medicaid HMOs serving SSI beneficiaries as well as AFDC beneficiaries on a capitated basis. This policy was notable, given the complex needs of this population.

Currently, the Choice Care plan serves approximately 25000 Medicaid beneficiaries, all of whom are residents of Denver County. Enrollees in the Choice Care plan select physicians in one of the 10 community health centers operated by DHH as their primary care provider. These clinics are located in neighborhoods traditionally underserved by private medical care providers, and so offer easily accessible sources of care for most Medicaid-eligible Denver residents. Eight of the clinics are staffed by teams of family practice physicians and nurse practitioners, and two of the clinics are staffed by pediatricians, obstetricians, general internists, and nurse practitioners. These providers are responsible for monitoring the care received by enrollees in the plan and for making appropriate referrals to other components of the DHH system, such as the hospital, ambulatory specialty clinics, or public health clinics. Because all physicians working within the DHH system are salaried employees, the Choice Care program functions much like a staff-model HMO. In addition to their Medicaid managed care clients, the providers staffing these clinics serve uninsured and underinsured residents, and Medicare beneficiaries.

The Choice Care plan operates an extensive quality assurance program to ensure that its Medicaid enrollees receive appropriate, accessible, and timely health care. Through this system, plan administrators track indicators of preventive services utilization, prenatal care delivery, birth outcomes, service accessibility, and enrollee satisfaction (Table 12–4). DHH reports a subset of these indicators to the state Medicaid agency in response to contract requirements, and to the National Commission for Quality Assurance (NCQA) as a step toward accreditation by this body.

Table 12–4 Quality Assessment Indicators for DHH Choice Care Program

Indicator	Report Frequency
I. Primary prevention	
Pediatric immunizations	Monthly
Adult immunizations	Monthly
Family planning	
Sterilizations	Quarterly
Family planning visits	Quarterly
Teenage births	Quarterly
II. Secondary prevention	
Infant screening	Quarterly
Lead screening	Quarterly
Mammography	Quarterly
Cervical Pap smears	Quarterly
Violence intervention/prevention	Quarterly
Cholesterol screening	Quarterly
III. Tertiary prevention	
Diabetic ophthalmology	Quarterly
Asthma management/admissions	Quarterly
Care of chronic mental illness	Quarterly
Frail elderly	Annually
IV. Perinatal care	
Early prenatal care utilization	Quarterly
Teenage births	Quarterly
Vaginal births after Caesarean sections (C-section)	Quarterly
C-section rates	Quarterly
Low birth-weight infants	Quarterly
Neonatal intensive care admissions	Quarterly
V. Member satisfaction	
Member satisfaction survey results	Annually
Member grievances: quality of care	Monthly
Disenrollments	Monthly
VI. Access to health care services	
Appointment availability	Monthly
Appointment waiting time	Monthly
Utilization of emergency services	Quarterly
In network/out of network utilization	Quarterly
VII. Appropriateness of care	
Hysterectomies	Quarterly
Abortions	Quarterly
Patient transfers	Quarterly

DHH administrators report that the Choice Care plan acts as another vehicle for subsidizing nonrevenue activities within the system. Reimbursement for services to Medicaid patients totals more than $38 million annually and accounts for more than 25% of the system's annual revenue. The majority of these funds are received by DHH in the form of capitated payments for Medicaid beneficiaries enrolled in the Choice Care program. Effective management of the care received by these beneficiaries generates substantial revenues that are then used to support public health services, charity care, and other underfunded service areas. Additionally, DHH's chief executive indicates that the two managed care products together have helped the system retire a $39 million debt to the city and county of Denver, and build a $60 million revenue surplus as of 1995.

The Choice Care HMO is tightly integrated with the traditional public health services and activities provided through DHH. Medicaid enrollees may be treated in a variety of specialty public health clinics operated by DHH, including a family planning clinic; sexually transmitted disease clinics; HIV/AIDS treatment clinics; a free-standing teen health center; a tuberculosis control clinic; immunization clinics; and a network of school-based health clinics located in 11 public schools. A single medical record tracks enrollees through patient encounters in these settings as in the hospital and community health center settings. Enrollees may also move seamlessly to access other specialty services within the DHH system, such as the 90-bed alcohol treatment facility, the substance abuse outpatient treatment center, and the system's poison control and drug consultation center.

Interaction with Other Organizations

The comprehensive nature of DHH's public health and medical care system allows the organization to operate largely as a self-sufficient integrated delivery system with few dependencies on other providers. Although the system initially depended upon an alliance with an established HMO, DHH has now proven itself as an efficient and effective managed care organization on its own. As more private managed care plans begin to participate in Medicaid managed care, however, DHH has begun forging partnerships to secure its position of leadership in this market.

DHH maintains strong affiliations with the state-owned University Hospital, which serves as the state's tertiary care center and primary teaching facility for the state university's medical and allied health professions schools. Under a joint agreement for indigent care, DHH provides primary care services to all residents of Denver County, and University Hospital provides these services to metropolitan area residents who live outside the county. University Hospital provides specialty care services to all uninsured individuals in the state. Much like DHH, University operates as a state-created independent hospital authority that is independent from the direct control of the university and the state. The authority consists of a 316-bed hospital and an extensive network of specialty clinics that handled 245000 outpatient visits during 1994.

Building on the strength of their interorganizational agreement for indigent care, DHH and University Hospital joined forces in 1995 with another frequent hospital ally—the nonprofit Denver Children's Hospital—to develop a coordinated managed care network for serving Medicaid beneficiaries on a statewide basis. The three organizations have a successful history of collaboration that dates back to 1988, when they began their ongoing joint venture with the school system for operating school-based health clinics. Under the current initiative, the three hospital systems joined with a state-wide consortium of 43 federally qualified health centers in developing a coordinated managed care network that can provide coverage to Medicaid beneficiaries in all of the state's counties that participate in the 1915(b) waiver program.

Each of the four participating organizations—DHH, University Hospital, Children's Hospital, and the FQHC consortium—hold one-quarter ownership in the newly formed HMO. Under the agreement, DHH provides primary care services to enrollees residing within the city and county of Denver; Children's Hospital provides specialty pediatric services through its network of specialty clinics located throughout the Denver metropolitan area and its 209-bed inpatient facility; the consortium of health centers provides primary care services to enrollees located in areas not served by DHH and Children's Hospital clinics; and University Hospital provides adult specialty care for enrollees throughout the system. Children's Hospital undertakes much of its responsibility in the venture through the physician-hospital organization (PHO) it developed with an extensive network of private pediatric practices located in both hospital and community settings.

The joint venture HMO, called Colorado Access, allows both Children's Hospital and University Hospital to substantially increase their involvement in the Medicaid managed care market without entering into direct competition with DHH. At the same time, the collaboration offers these public and nonprofit "safety-net" providers a competitive advantage over traditional HMOs operating in the Denver market that are increasing their presence in the Medicaid managed care market. The alliance offers the partnering organizations a market share and a service-area coverage that far exceeds those of other Medicaid managed care providers.

As exemplified by the Colorado Access initiative, DHH administrators strongly support collaborative ventures among the public and nonprofit health care organizations that traditionally comprise the ranks of safety-net providers in Denver. Organizations that share a mission of public service and indigent care are identified as natural allies for the DHH system. For DHH, these organizations are limited to its familiar partners: University Hospital, Children's Hospital, and more recently the other federally qualified health centers operating in the area. Interaction with other local health care organizations is quite limited. DHH participates in a local managed care association that meets monthly to exchange information and develop consensus on policy issues, but these sessions rarely result in collaborative efforts related to service provision or program administration. Other forms of collaboration with private health care organizations appear at once infeasible and undesirable, according to DHH administrators. DHH's chief executive, Patricia Gabow, MD, reports that most of the private hospitals and managed care plans in Denver do not have the willingness or capacity to serve the vulnerable populations currently receiving care through DHH. Gabow maintains that collaboration with these organizations would be fruitless without a core commitment to community health. As an example of this conviction, Gabow points to a recent meeting with a for-profit hospital corporation, during which she turned down an invitation to "talk about our futures together" because of differences in organizational mission.

DHH's medical director for managed care also emphasizes barriers to collaboration with private health care organizations in Denver. Barbara Warren, MD, insists that DHH cannot afford to collaborate with private providers in the Medicaid managed care arena because of the competitive environment. Warren notes that DHH "faces some very significant threats to our patients being drawn off, and this undermines our ability to meet our mission to the indigent population." These threats preclude any direct efforts involving cooperation and collaboration. These administrators suggest that, despite a lack of collaboration, DHH has a strongly positive impact on the private health care market through its position as a leader and trend-setter in the marketplace. For example, the state Medicaid office now requires all Medicaid managed care plans to use a quality assessment reporting tool modeled after one developed by DHH.

Denver's formal public health system as maintained by DHH offers a compelling example of how managed care principles can be integrated with public health and medical care capacities to form an effective and efficient system of community-based care. Still, a large proportion of Denver's population receives medical care and health promotion/disease prevention services outside this formal public health system. Private health care organizations serve a majority of the area's commercially insured and Medicare beneficiaries, as well as substantial numbers of Medicaid beneficiaries and medically indigent individuals. Some of these organizations have found managed care strategies and public health practices to be compatible and even synergistic with their objectives of organizational growth and mission fulfillment. Notably, most of these organizations have developed their public health approaches independently of any formal collaboration with the public health system in Denver.

PUBLIC HEALTH IN THE PRIVATE HEALTH CARE MARKET

HealthOne Health Care System

Denver's largest private health care system, HealthOne, is a product of a series of hospital mergers taking place over the past decade. The system currently includes six acute care hospitals, four rehabilitation and psychiatric hospitals, and 60 clinics for outpatient and community-based care. The system has its origins in the merger of several nonprofit hospital systems: Presbyterian Hospital, St. Luke's Hospital, and Swedish Hospital. The resulting nonprofit system entered another merger in late 1995 with the for-profit hospital corporation Columbia/HCA, bringing three additional hospitals into the organization and establishing a unique governance structure. The new, for-profit HealthOne corporation is jointly owned—50% by the nonprofit HealthOne Foundation, and 50% by the for-profit Columbia/HCA Corporation. The system now holds approximately 33% of the total market share for inpatient care in Denver and stands as the area's second-largest employer.

Administrators of the HealthOne system report that the organization's contributions to community health issues derive from two important sources: a long-standing mission of community service and a growing recognition of the importance of health promotion and disease prevention in managed care systems. Both of these motivations remain strong even after the system's conversion to for-profit status, according to HealthOne administrators. The system's ownership structure reinforces this commitment to community health. Because of its 50% ownership of the system, the nonprofit HealthOne Foundation retains half of the seats on the system's governing board. Through this arrangement, the Foundation ensures that its mission of charity care and community service continues to be reflected in the operation of the system. Moreover, the nonprofit foundation receives a 50% share of system profits, which are then available to finance community health initiatives on an ongoing basis. This structure allows the HealthOne system to operate as a hybrid organization: a market-driven, for-profit health system governed by the community health principles of a nonprofit foundation.

HealthOne's community health initiatives include a mobile van service that provides free health screenings, physicals, and vaccinations for school-age children in Denver's public schools. The system also operates four community clinics that provide primary care services to individuals, regardless of ability to pay. Clinics are staffed by physicians participating in the system's residency programs. HealthOne also maintains an extensive community education program that offers free seminars and classes on a range of health promotion, disease prevention, and self-care topics.

With its growing involvement in managed care, HealthOne has begun to emphasize health promotion and disease prevention efforts for its commercial populations as well. These efforts stand in contrast to the hospital system's historical emphasis on inpatient care. The system now offers an extensive array of health status assessments and wellness services to employer groups and HMO enrollee populations on a contractual basis. By developing strong organizational capacities in providing wellness services such as health screening, nutrition counseling, and smoking cessation, administrators hope to improve the system's competitiveness in Denver's expanding managed care market. Administrators report that local managed care plans and employers contract with HealthOne for wellness services in order to meet their objectives of cost containment, health improvement, and patient satisfaction. HealthOne's growing expertise in wellness services also contributes to the organization's efforts to develop its own managed care products. Presently, HealthOne operates an HMO that serves employer groups as well as HealthOne employees. Plans to develop additional HMO products for serving Medicare and Medicaid beneficiaries are currently under consideration. As the dominant provider of health services to Medicare beneficiaries in Denver, HealthOne already offers several specialized health promotion and disease prevention programs for seniors, and therefore should be well positioned to develop a managed care plan for serving this population. Similarly, HealthOne's experience in serving Medicaid beneficiaries and uninsured populations through its community clinics should facilitate the system's efforts to develop an HMO for serving Medicaid beneficiaries in the state's Medicaid managed care program.

Kaiser Foundation Health Plan and St. Joseph Hospital

Kaiser Foundation's Colorado health plan exists as one of the two largest HMOs operating in the Denver metropolitan area, with more than 300000 enrollees or approximately 15% of the total metropolitan population. Like other Kaiser health plans across the country, Kaiser Colorado operates as a nonprofit, group-model HMO serving as a regional arm of the nation's largest HMO corporation. More than 400 physicians practice as part of the medical group that contracts exclusively to serve enrollees of Kaiser Colorado health plan. These physicians practice in one of 18 medical centers that Kaiser operates in the metropolitan area. Unlike some other Kaiser plans, Kaiser Colorado does not operate its own inpatient facilities; rather, it maintains a contract with the nonprofit St. Joseph Hospital for providing hospital services to members who reside in Denver. Kaiser exists as one of two private managed care organizations enrolling Medicaid beneficiaries in Denver.

As a nonprofit foundation, Kaiser Colorado operates under an organizational mission that emphasizes responsibility for community health issues. In pursuing this mission, Kaiser's involvement in public health activities is divided into community-based endeavors that reach broad segments of Denver's population, and plan-specific interventions that target only Kaiser enrollees. Given Kaiser's large market share in the Denver area, these two types of activities often overlap substantially—significant numbers of Kaiser enrollees may be served through community-based efforts, and large proportions of the community population may be served through interventions that target only Kaiser enrollees. Kaiser's community-based initiatives include an educational theater program that tours schools and community organizations year-round with information in one of four topical areas: child health and safety; adolescent health; HIV and AIDS; and issues of aging. These programs are designed in collaboration with area schools and community organizations. Second, Kaiser operates a "Tele-Health" initiative in partnership with a local telecommunications company. This program provides community members with free telephone access to a variety of prerecorded messages on issues related to health and parenting. This system of 50 prerecorded messages receives between 3000 and 4000 calls per month.

Kaiser also administers a large grant initiative that issues $270000 per year to local nonprofit and governmental organizations in support of community health initiatives. In the most recent year of this initiative, grants have been targeted specifically at projects that address issues of disease prevention and aging. The organization maintains an active program for supporting the voluntary efforts of its staff, more than half of which volunteer in the community. Through this program, Kaiser maintains a database of clinical volunteer opportunities for physicians and staff and provides matching funds of up to $100 per employee for personal donations to nonprofit or governmental organizations in the community. Finally, Kaiser serves on several community-wide task forces and planning groups that target specific health issues confronting Denver residents. These efforts include task forces on influenza and smoking cessation led by the Colorado Lung Assocation, and a childhood immunization initiative led by Denver Children's Hospital.

Kaiser supports several other community health initiatives that target specific populations of interest to the managed care community. With the support of a planning grant from the Robert Wood Johnson Foundation, Kaiser is developing a plan for serving managed care enrollees through school-based health centers in Denver. As part of this initiative, the organization is funding a three-year study of adolescents enrolled in managed care plans who have access to school health centers. Data collected will be used to examine utilization patterns among these centers. Administrators anticipate that this planning initiative may ultimately result in the development of contracts between Kaiser and existing school health centers, as well as the development of new school-based health centers with Kaiser support. These arrangements are likely to provide critical financial and operational support to the network of school-based health centers in Denver, which are currently maintained through a partnership between DHH, University Hospital, Children's Hospital, and the public school department. Consequently, this planning initiative appears likely to create new opportunities for collaboration between Kaiser and Denver's public health system. Already, Kaiser's initiative has encouraged DHH to undertake a parallel study of school health utilization among adolescents not enrolled in managed care plans.

Kaiser also maintains a wide range of health promotion and disease prevention efforts targeted specifically at its population of enrollees. These efforts include a proactive outreach program for mammography screening that is supported by direct mailings to age-appropriate enrollees and a computerized tracking system to monitor compliance. Kaiser maintains a similar outreach and tracking system for influenza immunizations among its population of seniors and enrollees with chronic diseases. Outreach programs are also targeted at members for smoking cessation and for dietary modification among enrollees identified as hypercholes-terolemic. The organization recently completed development of a health-risk appraisal protocol that will be administered to all members and used for planning health promotion and disease prevention programs and for targeting interventions to high-risk groups. Finally, Kaiser offers its members 40 different health educa-tion classes on a variety of health promotion topics. Community residents who are not Kaiser members may also attend these sessions for slightly higher fees, but participation by nonmembers traditionally is low because these sessions are not actively marketed outside the health plan membership.

Kaiser's alliance with St. Joseph Hospital is another important structure sup-porting public health activities in Denver. St. Joseph Hospital operates a 437-bed acute care facility as part of a seven-hospital system owned by the nonprofit Sisters of Charity of Leavenworth corporation. Approximately 60% of the ser-vices delivered at St. Joseph are for members of the Kaiser Colorado health plan. The hospital's chief administrator, Sister Mariana Bauder, reports that the organization's strong affiliation with the Catholic church helps to define its mission of charity care and community health improvement. The hospital's contract with Kaiser health plan plays a central role in financing many of its community health initiatives. Revenue generated through this contract, together with revenue from other payers, allows the hospital to fund programs for unin-sured individuals as well as community education campaigns. In total, the hospital reports that it spent approximately $14.6 million in community benefit activities during 1994.

St. Joseph's community health activities include a low-income health clinic operated by the hospital, which provides primary care and preventive services in a predominantly Hispanic community. Although located only blocks from a community health center operated by DHH, the St. Joseph clinic serves the unmet needs of undocumented aliens who are often afraid to seek care from public clinics. Administrators report that the demand for low-cost care in this neighbor-hood exceeds the capacity of a single clinic, so the St. Joseph clinic serves to augment the capacity of the DHH clinic. The clinic provides services using a sliding-fee scale, with individuals below poverty level receiving free care. The clinic also hosts free monthly health education classes on topics such as diabetes management, hypertension, teen pregnancy, AIDS and sexually transmitted diseases, and parenting skills. Other community health activities provided by St. Joseph include a mobile dental clinic for serving homeless individuals, and a free childhood-immunization clinic that operates every 6 weeks.

Currently, St. Joseph's administrators are in the process of establishing a joint venture with another managed care organization for operating a new HMO to serve both employer groups and Medicaid beneficiaries. This new HMO will employ private physicians that presently work in St. Joseph's Hospital but are not affiliated with the Kaiser health plan. St. Joseph's administrators hope that this new arrangement will give the hospital greater financial and clinical responsibility for the 40% of patients it serves who are not Kaiser members. This arrangement is expected to provide additional financial support for the hospital's community health initiatives, while allowing the hospital to remain competitive in Denver's rapidly consolidating health care market. The viability of this arrangement—and of the community health initiatives supported by it—seems to hinge on the ability of Kaiser and St. Joseph Hospital to coexist as both partners and competitors in the managed care market.

Other Hospital-Based Health Systems

Two other major hospital systems serve the Denver metropolitan area, both of which are nonprofit corporations with strong affiliations to religious organizations. Provenant/St. Anthony Hospital is a 364-bed acute care facility that is part of the Sisters of Charity Health Care System affiliated with the Catholic church. The hospital maintains two primary areas of involvement in community health activities: the provision of substantial amounts of charity care for individuals unable to afford needed hospital services, and cosponsorship of an annual health fair that provides disease prevention and health promotion services to individuals state-wide. The organization provides an estimated $12 to $15 million dollars annually in charity care, mainly for hospital services to patients who are seen through the emergency department. Most medically stable patients needing charity care are referred to the DHH system, where local and state provisions are in place for financing the care of Denver's medically indigent population. The organization's other major community health endeavor, the Nine Health Fair, is cosponsored by a local television station and several other organizations. The health fair travels across the state annually providing individuals with free access to health services such as breast exams, prostate exams, hemocult tests, blood pressure tests, and routine biochemical screening. Provenant/St. Anthony Hospital plays a major role in financing and performing these activities, as well as in providing individuals with physician and nurse consultations after a health assessment has been completed.

Rocky Mountain Adventist Health Care System represents the remaining hospital system serving the Denver area. The system owns one 339-bed facility in the city of Denver and two other facilities in the metropolitan area. The system operates as a nonprofit corporation affiliated with the Seventh Day Adventist church. Its mission statement reveals a substantial commitment to community health by charging the organization to "function as a catalyst in the community to enhance public health and promote individual wellness." Its relatively new administrator suggests that, traditionally, the organization has strived to accomplish this goal primarily through individual health education programming in areas such as smoking cessation and weight control. Like other organizations in the community, the system sponsors a range of health education classes, targeting health promotion and disease prevention activities. More recent efforts by the system attempt to broaden its impact on community health. The system recently implemented a health-information telephone system staffed by nurses to offer community members access to information on a wide range of health-related issues. The system also recently joined with a local health department and other community organizations in a neighboring county to conduct a community-wide health assessment and planning process.

The system's chief executive suggests that these community-based activities distinguish nonprofit health systems from the for-profit systems currently evolving in many local markets. Administrators report that a major strategic goal for the organization involves the expansion of such activities in the community in order to differentiate the system from more market-driven organizations. The planned development of an HMO product with Provenant/St. Anthony Hospital provides further motivation for expanded initiatives in community health improvement. The capitated reimbursement system entailed in this joint venture is expected to create financial incentives for the organization to enhance its capacities in disease prevention and health promotion. Once developed for the system's managed care population, administrators suggest that these capacities can then be applied to the system's community-wide initiatives in order to advance its public health mission.

Other HMO-Based Health Systems

A number of other managed care systems serving the Denver metropolitan area are actively developing and implementing public health initiatives in the form of health promotion and disease prevention programs for their enrolled populations and, to a lesser extent, for the community at large. HMO Colorado, a for-profit plan operated by the Blue Cross and Blue Shield Association of Colorado, is the state's other Medicaid managed care provider. In addition to its enrollment of over 56000 commercial enrollees, the HMO serves approximately 2500 Medicaid beneficiaries who are eligible through the state's AFDC program. For both its commercial and Medicaid populations, Colorado HMO operates an "early identification" health-screening program to identify major health risks facing enrollees at the time of enrollment in the plan. To ensure access to care for its Medicaid members, the HMO operates its Medicaid HMO product in collaboration with St. Joseph Hospital, a traditional provider of services to vulnerable populations (see section on Kaiser Foundation Health Plan and St. Joseph Hospital). Members receive care through a community-based clinic operated by the hospital and staffed by participants in the hospital's family practice residency program. This alliance allows Colorado HMO to gain experience in managing the care of Medicaid beneficiaries while also tapping St. Joseph Hospital's capacities in bilingual service provision, community outreach and education, and social and health resources for vulnerable population groups. Additionally, this alliance allows St. Joseph Hospital to further its mission of medical education by offering its residents exposure to managed care and to population-based medicine for vulnerable population groups.

Denver's largest for-profit HMO operates under the ownership of PacifiCare Health Systems, with an enrollment of approximately 200000 in the five-county metropolitan area. Formerly owned by FHP International, this HMO is the product of several HMO mergers and acquisitions during the 1980s and 1990s, culminating in the acquisition of FHP by PacifiCare in February 1997. PacifiCare's community-wide initiatives are limited to using a range of media outlets for health promotion advertising campaigns that encourage healthy lifestyles such as smoking cessation, regular exercise, and proper nutrition. The HMO's regional administrator reports that these efforts serve as both marketing tools and as avenues for improving health status in populations that PacifiCare currently serves or may serve in the future. PacifiCare also affects community health in Denver through extensive efforts to inform and educate its affiliated physicians regarding health promotion and disease prevention practices. With more than 800 affiliated primary care physicians in the Denver metropolitan area, this individual practice association HMO maintains contact and influence with a substantial proportion of the physician work force that serves this community. PacifiCare provides monthly feedback to its physicians regarding patient utilization of preventive health services and keeps physicians informed of standards of care such as optimal delivery schedules and contraindications. These efforts represent core components of the HMO's utilization review and physician profiling system, which is designed to encourage both cost containment and quality improvement among affiliated providers. Since PacifiCare-affiliated physicians also serve patients insured through other health plans as well as the Medicaid and Medicare programs, the HMO's physician outreach efforts hold the potential for influencing the care delivered to a large proportion of Denver's population.

Other for-profit HMOs serving the Denver area include MetraHealth, PruCare, CIGNA, and Qual-Med. All of these plans report growing involvement in providing health promotion and disease prevention services to their enrolled populations. MetraHealth, a managed care corporation formed by the merger of health care divisions at Metropolitan Life and Travelers insurance companies, reports that its major contributions to community health occur through efforts to encourage employers to offer wellness and worksite health benefits to employees. MetraHealth offers a range of wellness benefits that include such services as routine worksite health screenings, health education classes, and nutrition and exercise counseling. Since these benefits are optional, employers with an overriding concern for health care cost containment may choose not to finance these services for their employees. MetraHealth encourages employers to add wellness benefits to their existing plans by profiling the health and utilization experiences of employee groups and thereby offering employers evidence of outstanding health needs in their work forces. In some cases, MetraHealth agrees to underwrite part of the additional costs entailed in providing wellness benefits.

MetraHealth's administrator suggests that the company's efforts in support of wellness benefits represent both an altruistic commitment to community health as well as a strategic action to differentiate its services in a competitive marketplace. Increasingly, Denver-area employers are developing self-funded employee health plans in order to escape the need to contract with health insurers and the requirement to comply with state health insurance laws regarding mandated benefits and coverage provisions. As a provider of wellness services and third-party administrative services, MetraHealth maintains a competitive position in marketing its services to the growing number of self-funded employers. As an outgrowth of MetraHealth's strategic direction, growing numbers of Denver employees receive access to health promotion and disease prevention services at worksite and community locations.

PruCare of Colorado, the regional managed care plan of the Prudential Insurance Company, reports active involvement in outreach services encouraging the utilization of preventive services among HMO enrollees. Outreach services target three primary areas: prenatal care and infant screening; age-appropriate mammography screening; and influenza vaccination for at-risk populations. In all three areas, PruCare operates systems for tracking service utilization and for directly contacting at-risk populations by telephone or mail to encourage utilization. PruCare also maintains involvement in community health activities through its leadership role on the state association of managed care plans. PruCare's medical director has served as chair of this association, and has initiated such efforts as inviting both the state and local health departments to become members of the association and developing a collaborative, community-wide initiative for addressing the problem of teen pregnancy. Though this community-wide effort is still under development, PruCare was instrumental in enlisting the assistance of the Centers for Disease Control and Prevention and Prudential's national Center for Health Services Research.

Qual-Med, another for-profit health plan operating in Denver, initiated its emphasis on wellness services relatively recently in the Denver market. The plan began its operations in Denver in 1986, but instituted its line of wellness services beginning in January 1995. Like other organizations in this market, Qual-Med's medical director suggests that its new emphasis reflects the organization's dual objectives of improving health status in the community and cultivating a market niche as a provider of health promotion and disease prevention services. These objectives also motivate the plan's involvement in community-wide health initiatives, which include conducting health and safety fairs and giving away bicycle helmets to children. Both of these activities serve as opportunities for the health plan to market its services to non-members, as well as to promote health and safety in the community at large.

CONCLUSION

Several important trends emerge from the structures and operations of private health care organizations in Denver. First, nonprofit organizations on the whole appear extremely active in the provision of services for the medically indigent, Medicaid beneficiaries, and other populations traditionally underserved by the private health care system. These organizations uniformly point to their missions of community service as strong motivations for these activities. However, these organizations also recognize the strategic imperatives of remaining viable Medicaid providers under the state's Medicaid managed care program. These imperatives serve as the motivating factor for several of the interorganizational alliances observed in Denver's health care market. Although nonprofit organizations currently remain the dominant Medicaid providers under this system, many of the for-profit corporations are considering an entrance in this expanding market.

An emphasis on the provision of "wellness services" such as health screenings and counseling represent a second notable trend among private health care organizations. Most of these organizations report this emphasis as a relatively recent addition to their strategic orientation. Administrators at both MetraHealth and Qual-Med indicate that their organizations initially faced imperatives to emphasize the low-cost nature of their products in order to remain competitive in the managed care market. Both organizations now report success in encouraging employers to adopt wellness services as a value-added component of their employee benefits package. This trend may signal a maturation of the managed care marketplace in Denver, such that health care insurers and purchasers increasingly recognize the importance of health promotion and disease prevention activities—not only for their evaluated cost-effectiveness, but for their impact on health and well-being. These private sector efforts in health promotion and disease prevention should be recognized as important complements to the activities of Denver's formal public health system.

Given this growing emphasis on wellness services, the relatively limited interaction between private health care organizations and Denver's formal public health system (DHH) stands as a curious characteristic of this market. Although DHH administrators list competitive issues as one reason for this lack of interaction, private organizations do not perceive competition as a significant barrier to interaction. Rather, many of these organizations regard DHH as a closed system that has remained relatively insulated from the trends that are driving partnerships among private organizations. Many of Denver's private organizations indicate a willingness and a desire to work with DHH as they contemplate entering the Medicaid marketplace and acquiring the capacities to serve vulnerable population groups. Several private organizations see another possible area for interaction in the area of health data and information dissemination. Recent Colorado legislation eliminated a state health-data commission that served as a repository for a variety of health statistics produced by public and private health care organizations. Local HMOs and hospitals are currently struggling with the concept of a privately operated data repository, but several organizations suggest that this function may be an appropriate role for DHH to assume.

DISCUSSION QUESTIONS

1. In carrying out core public health functions, what potential advantages are created by the consolidated organizational structure of Denver Health and Hospitals? What potential disadvantages are implied by this structure?
2. Among the interorganizational relationships maintained by Denver Health and Hospitals, identify examples of the following forms of strategic alliances:
   - opportunistic alliances
   - shared service alliances
   - stakeholder alliances
3. Examine differences in the strength and durability of the alternative types of interorganizational arrangements identified in Question 2 above.
4. Consider the effect of marketplace competition among health care organizations in Denver in terms of its impact upon the local public health system. Are there signs that competition may affect the availability and/or quality of public health services and activities performed in the community? Why or why not?
5. Assess the nature of relationships between public and private health care organizations in Denver. What are alternative arguments that could be made regarding the optimality of these relationships from a community-wide, public health perspective?

REFERENCES

1. American Hospital Association (AHA). *AHA Guide to the Health Care Field, 1995*. Chicago: American Hospital Association; 1996:A68.

2. American Medical Association (AMA). *Physician Data by County, 1994*. Washington, DC: AMA; 1996.

3. Bureau of Primary Health Care, U.S. Health Resources and Services Administration. *Primary Care Programs Directory 1994*. McLean, Va: Health Resources and Services Administration; 1994.

4. Group Health Association of America. *1995 Directory of HMOs*. Washington, DC: GHAA; 1995.

5. U.S. Department of Commerce. *1995 Consolidated Federal Funds Report*. Washington, DC: U.S. Department of Commerce; 1997.

CHAPTER 13

Case Study: Group Health Cooperative and the Public Health System Serving Olympia, WA

Curtis P. McLaughlin, Paul K. Halverson, and Glen P. Mays

A relatively small and stable collection of health care organizations make up the local health system that serves Olympia, Washington. The most important among these providers is the Group Health Cooperative of Puget Sound (GHC), a large health maintenance organization (HMO) with a 50-year history in the Pacific Northwest region. At least five other managed care plans report operations in Thurston County; however, GHC enjoys the largest share of the roughly 25% of the population that receives care from HMOs. Two hospitals compete to serve the 180000 residents of Olympia and surrounding Thurston County, as well as the populations of surrounding counties. Providence St. Peter Hospital, part of the nonprofit Sisters of Providence system, operates a 327-bed facility in northeastern Olympia. Six miles to the west, Capital Region Medical Center operates a 110-bed facility owned by the national for-profit hospital corporation Columbia/HCA. Almost 300 nonfederal physicians practice in the county, although some rural areas of the county remain underserved because of the clustering of providers in urbanized areas. Since for many years the community was served by only one hospital (St. Peter), local health care institutions and providers maintain a long history of cooperation rather than competition. More recently, the construction of a new hospital (Capital Region) in 1985 and its conversion to for-profit status soon

The authors wish to thank individuals at the following organizations for their generous contributions of time and information: Thurston County Department of Health and Social Services; Group Health Cooperative of Puget Sound, Olympia District; St. Peter Hospital; and Capital Region Medical Center.

thereafter has introduced new competitive dynamics into the local health care market.

The Thurston County Department of Public Health and Social Services (DPHSS) serves as an important provider of personal and population-based health services in the community as well. The department provides personal health services in the areas of family planning, immunizations, sexually transmitted disease prevention and treatment, maternal and child health services, and communicable disease control. During 1996, the department served approximately 68500 active clients in its personal health care clinics, up from 18500 clients in 1989. Most of the clients served by the health department are Medicaid beneficiaries or are uninsured or underinsured. In addition, the department maintains substantial population-based health activities in areas such as health education and outreach, community health assessment, and environmental protection and monitoring. As the "umbrella" agency for county health and social services, the department also administers programs in areas such as mental health treatment, substance abuse prevention and treatment, developmental disabilities services, and child protective services.

OVERVIEW OF THE COMMUNITY

The capital of Washington state, Olympia is located on the west side of the Puget Sound, approximately 60 miles southeast of Seattle. Thurston County, which encompasses the city of Olympia, has approximately 180000 residents. Historically, the timber industry has been an important part of the local economy. Over the last decade, restrictions in access to timber in the Olympic National Forest have weakened this economy. State government is the county's largest employer. Six of the top 10 employers in the county are health care institutions. The work force is well educated, but incomes are surprisingly low on average.

HISTORY OF GROUP HEALTH COOPERATIVE

GHC opened its Olympia Medical Center in 1972 with five family practice physicians, a medical health practitioner, a physician assistant, an optometrist, a pediatrician, an internist, and a small support staff. Enrollment reached 4200 during the first year. Outpatient ancillary services included pharmacy, laboratory, and imaging.

Local providers and institutions faced pressure from some community physicians not to cooperate with GHC primary care physicians, but St. Peter Hospital welcomed them once the nuns who operated this organization were convinced that GHC would not include beds in its new facility. About four out of five patients who needed specialty services were referred the 60 miles to Seattle at GHC's Central Specialty Center, and hospitalizations were roughly evenly split between St. Peter Hospital and GHC's Central Hospital in Seattle. At that time GHC had no facilities in Tacoma, which is only about 30 miles away. Despite the distance, many patients liked the idea of being referred to the specialists in the state's largest city.

By 1980 the Olympia district of GHC had over 28000 members and had expanded to 13 physicians, 6 mental health providers, 16 other specialists, and a much larger support staff. Its facility had to be expanded twice. A small, temporary satellite facility was opened in West Olympia in 1984. A full facility, the West Olympia Medical Center, opened in 1988 as total district enrollment approached 40000.

By the end of 1994, these two medical centers served 49000 enrollees (about a 20% share of the total market, and a 25% share of the nonmilitary market) and GHC began contracting with Cascade Family Medicine in Centralia to service that small town 30 miles south of Olympia. The West Olympia site offered only pediatrics, family medicine, and optometry, but the expanded main facility now offered many specialty services, including obstetrics and gynecology, oncology, internal medicine, rheumatology, radiology, urology, and vascular surgery. The main facility also offered mental health services, urgent care, physical and occupational therapy, alcohol and drug abuse treatment, allergy treatment, audiology, contact lens services, dermatology, optical dispensing, and sports medicine. Overall, the number of medical staff (including board-certified physicians, physician assistants, nurse practitioners, midwives, optometrists, and mental health professionals) was approaching 100. Seventy percent of the inpatient days were provided at St. Peter, 19% at GHC hospitals in Tacoma and Seattle, and 11% at other hospitals. Only 24% of the specialist referrals were outside of GHC Olympia or community physicians, and most of these were to the Tacoma GHC facilities. Only 5% of referrals were to GHC Seattle.

Despite its history of being a staff-model HMO, GHC began contracting with local specialists, with agreements including capitation contracts, in the early 1980s. GHC physician contracting became substantial in 1988 with the offering of a point-of-service (POS) plan, which allowed enrollees to have a choice of GHC or community practitioners with graduated copayments. For example, in 1994 GHC began contracting with a local cardiologist and St. Peter Hospital for invasive cardiac procedures previously provided only at the University of Washington's medical center in Seattle.

UTILIZATION MANAGEMENT AND QUALITY IMPROVEMENT

By 1995, GHC Olympia was achieving an average daily census of 20 patients at St. Peter Hospital, or 100 days per thousand for non-Medicare patients. Their next target is 80 days per thousand. Part of this utilization efficiency was achieved by aggressive use of skilled nursing facility (SNF) beds, a less intensive form of inpatient care. Most admissions by the family practitioners were to the SNF rather than to the acute care hospital. Most patients who were admitted to the hospital were placed in the care of an internist who acted as the coordinator of care in the hospital, going on rounds with the specialists. The hospital did not object to this policy, since it was short of beds and also owned the SNF facility. For example, a patient with congestive heart failure would be supervised by the internist who worked directly with the cardiologist. GHC Olympia also maintained its own visiting nurse staff for cases requiring outpatient chemotherapy and other outpatient intravenous interventions. GHC's inpatient pharmacists also attended rounds with the patient care teams at St. Peter.

The decision regarding whether to continue referring patients to GHC centers in Tacoma and Seattle became one of pragmatism. Before referring cases locally, GHC administrators had to be convinced that local services were of comparable quality and cost-effectiveness. For example, cardiac surgery had been available in Olympia for five years before GHC began contracting locally. At each window of expiration for its contract with the University of Washington medical center, GHC Olympia administrators compared the university's record of quality and cost with that of the local group of providers. When these records became comparable, contracts were initiated locally.

Choices to refer locally or staff locally depended on a number of factors, including enrollee demand for services, the capacity of specialists, the capacity of the GHC Tacoma group, and the prices charged by local specialists. GHC Olympia's administrator suggested that the decision involved trade-offs among costs, clinical quality, and service quality in terms of waiting times, call schedules, and the like. Because few specialists are comfortable practicing alone, GHC recognized that it could not justify a decision to staff locally unless there existed sufficient enrollee demand for services to fill the full-time schedules of a group of specialists. This fact precluded the use of simple ratio staffing rules (e.g., 1 specialist per 10000 enrollees) in determining whether to hire new physicians for GHC clinics.

GHC Olympia has experienced marked success in its continuous quality improvement efforts. As part of these efforts, the organization has gradually moved toward the adoption of clinical pathways. For example, when GHC Olympia decided to move toward a one-day stay for normal vaginal deliveries and a three-day stay for Caesarean section patients, local physicians and nurses expressed some resistance. Rather than attempting to reach consensus on this issue prior to implementation, the organization simply began changing its standing orders and protocols to reflect the new standards. Administrators at GHC felt confident that if patients began to suffer under the new standards, then clinical staff would not follow them; however, if patients were effectively served under the standards, then staff would adopt them without resistance. The standards proved to be a success and were adopted throughout the organization. GHC Olympia's administrator suggests that most staff within the organization are less than enthusiastic about the process of continuous quality improvement. Nonetheless, most staff members appear to recognize that the results of this process have been positive in terms of reduced patient days and more efficient use of staff time. Confidence in its quality improvement successes has led the organization to seek accreditation from the National Committee for Quality Assurance (NCQA).

POPULATION-BASED HEALTH CARE

Although GHC administrators have only recently begun to emphasize population-based health care approaches in their formal strategic planning processes, the organization has used these approaches informally throughout most of its history. The structure of a staff-model HMO has long provided the organization with the ability to monitor trends in health status and service utilization across its population of enrollees. Expanding information systems are now greatly improving GHC's capabilities in this area.

An example of GHC's population-based approach to health care can be found in its strategies for diabetes management. Until recently, management of enrollees with diabetes occurred solely through medically oriented, one-on-one visits with clinicians. Over time, GHC recognized that patient learning could be enhanced by conducting group sessions with a team of clinicians that included a physician, nurse, pharmacist, and dietitian. In this setting, patients could learn from each other as well as from the clinicians, and behaviorial change could be reinforced by the perspectives of multiple people participating in the group session. Since starting the group sessions, GHC has realized greater patient compliance with clinical self-monitoring guidelines and reduced incidence of retinopathy and foot necrosis.

As another population-based strategy, GHC carefully monitors its hospital readmission rates, which tend to range between 4% and 5% of total admissions. The organization has begun targeting interventions for certain high-readmission population groups, such as enrollees with congestive heart failure and diabetes. It hopes to reduce readmissions in these groups by improving their outpatient medical management through the use of regular telephone follow-up. GHC views the improved management of high-risk population groups as a key component of its strategy to remain competitive in the growing managed care marketplace.

A third population-based strategy underway at GHC involves influenza vaccinations for senior citizens. GHC Olympia has struggled with this performance criterion, since only about 70% of its senior membership receives annual influenza vaccinations, compared with 72% for the corporation as a whole and 80% as its target. To achieve greater success, GHC Olympia recognizes the need for a larger, community-wide campaign to encourage vaccination. As part of this effort, GHC combines with the local health department in sponsoring flu shot clinics held at various community locations during influenza season. Additionally, GHC solicits the participation of other private providers by persuading them to offer reduced-cost vaccinations to community members. The organization has met with some resistance to this effort but continues to work on expanding the number of providers who participate in the program.

MEDICAID MANAGED CARE

GHC Olympia is a Medicaid managed care provider for Thurston County as well as for neighboring Lewis County. At the beginning of 1995, GHC served 1800 Medicaid beneficiaries through its capitated contract with the state Medicaid office. GHC agreed to accept up to 2500 enrollees during 1995, with the possibility of serving more beneficiaries during subsequent years as its physician capacity grows. GHC's early experience with this population suggests that expanded primary care access leads to dramatic decreases in emergency department utilization. The county-wide utilization rate prior to Medicaid managed care had been 700 emergency department visits per 1000 beneficiaries, compared with GHC's rate of 70. Within 10 months of enrolling Medicaid beneficiaries in GHC, their utilization rate dropped to 130. Clearly, some of this decrease may be attributed to differences in enrollment, since only those Medicaid beneficiaries eligible for the Aid to Families with Dependent Children program were enrolled in GHC's plan. Nonetheless, GHC's expanded primary care accessibility (clinics are open every day from at least noon to 7 PM) appears to play a major role in reducing emergency department utilization.

Another factor in GHC's success with serving the Medicaid population involves the organization's prior experience with this population through a collaboration with the local health department. Under the First Steps program, GHC provides obstetrical services for high-risk, pregnant Medicaid beneficiaries who are identified and managed by the local health department. Through this program, GHC staff gained experience in serving vulnerable population groups that face complex health, social, and economic problems. This collaborative program continues to operate successfully with the health department providing case management services to Medicaid beneficiaries who are not enrolled in managed care and GHC providing case management services to those beneficiaries enrolled in its plan.

One challenge faced by GHC in serving Medicaid beneficiaries involves the cultural diversity of this population. Prior to its Medicaid involvement, the organization had little experience with cultural diversity. Thurston County's residents are 92% Caucasian, and the largest minority population is Asian (4%–5%). GHC clinicians face a major challenge in working through the cultural differences of recent immigrants from Asia and Eastern Europe. The clinics have easy access to translators for many languages, but staff continue to experience problems in identifying the key decision makers in the extended families of these patients, and in recognizing the cultural norms and values that may affect health care delivery and utilization.

Transportation and scheduling issues present additional problems for GHC in terms of serving Medicaid beneficiaries. Because GHC emphasizes accessibility, its clinical teams are empowered to provide same-day appointments and transportation assistance for Medicaid patients who report having transportation or scheduling problems. GHC experiences a higher no-show rate in its Medicaid population compared with its other enrollees, so clinics employ a strategy to adjust their activities whenever Medicaid patients and families arrive. GHC Olympia pioneered this same-day appointment strategy as part of a continuous quality improvement approach. This strategy is now diffusing to other districts within the GHC corporation.

Medical records also prove to be problematic in the Medicaid population that GHC serves. Parents usually keep track of initial immunization records for their children, but not the records of subsequent immunizations. This problem is compounded by the high turnover rates among Medicaid beneficiaries—12% per month due to eligibility changes and patients opting in or out of managed care programs. GHC is developing an immunization tracking system to address this problem.

HEALTH SERVICES RESEARCH

GHC staff participate in research on community health problems through GHC's Center for Health Studies, which is located within the Seattle corporate headquarters. Some of these projects are funded externally, such as studies sponsored by the Centers for Disease Control and Prevention of immunization approaches or pediatric helmets for bicyclists. However, most of the research is funded internally. This work includes efforts to develop clinical guidelines, clinical pathways, and data-reporting structures for the Health Plan and Employer Data and Information Set (HEDIS) collected by NCQA. For example, the guideline clearinghouse, a part of the Division of Clinical Planning at GHC, issued clinical practice guidelines in 1995 for childhood immunizations, breast cancer screening, tobacco cessation, prostate-specific antigen screening, cervical cancer screening, and acute dysuria or urgency in women. Additional guidelines were also under development for diabetics' foot and eye care, Caesarean section (C-section), depression, and a number of other conditions. GHC develops these guidelines to be science based and consistent with the practitioners' belief in appropriate care.

The pilot site for the smoking cessation effort had been the eight-physician West Olympia clinic. A survey of patients in this clinic showed that the tobacco consumption rate was 28% rather than the expected 17% based upon state-wide rates. The research at this site showed that the most successful interventions involved conversations with providers about primary care interaction and providing a broad range of support mechanisms to everyone who expressed interest in stopping. These support mechanisms included provider encouragement; setting target quit dates; and providing self-help information, support groups, follow-up on quit dates, and nicotine replacement therapy when necessary.

The Olympia GHC also served as the pilot site for a C-section reduction effort. This study found that management of labor guidelines had been inconsistent and that rates paid to contract physicians for normal deliveries were too low. The objective for the project had been to reduce C-section rates from 18% to 13% during the first quarter of 1995; however, the actual rate achieved was an impressive 8.9%.

Clearly, the health services research efforts undertaken by GHC's Center for Health Research have motivated substantial improvements in quality and efficiency at GHC Olympia. GHC administrators express some worry that reductions in government funding for health research, combined with increases in price competition within the managed care industry, will limit the organization's ability to sustain its health services research capacity.

INTERACTION WITH THE LOCAL HEALTH DEPARTMENT

GHC and the Thurston County Department of Public Health and Social Services maintain a history of communication and cooperation that dates back to the early years of the HMO. As a nonprofit institution, GHC shares an orientation toward community health improvement and public service with the local health department. These shared objectives have led the two organizations to jointly sponsor community-wide initiatives for school immunizations and senior influenza vaccinations. The two organizations have also assisted each other periodically when medications and medical supplies have run low in one or the other organization. Administrators attribute some of this cooperation to Olympia's small-town environment, in which people's paths cross regularly. GHC's administrator suggests that the 20% to 25% local market share achieved by GHC provides additional incentives to work with the health department on community health issues. Given this large market share, any collaborative efforts that achieve improvements in community health are likely to have a substantial positive impact on GHC's membership. By the same token, quality improvement efforts undertaken by GHC hold the potential for affecting the health status of a large proportion of the total community population. For example, GHC's successful efforts to improve senior influenza vaccination rates (to 70% of the at-risk population) can be seen in the relatively high rates for the community as a whole (50%). Therefore, the local health department faces strong incentives to work collaboratively with GHC in carrying out its health promotion and disease prevention objectives.

A prime example of collaborative community health efforts in Olympia can be found in the community health clinic that is jointly operated by GHC, the local health department, and St. Peter Hospital. The three organizations formed a consortium to organize the clinic and to pool the resources necessary for operation. Staff from the three organizations, and especially from the family practice residency program at St. Peter, provide most of the clinical services that are delivered through this clinic. Services are provided free of charge or using a sliding-fee scale for individuals without health insurance coverage. As part of its long-standing mission of charity care in the community, St. Peter Hospital assumed much of the responsibility for initiating and sustaining this effort. Through its relationships with St. Peter Hospital and the local health department, GHC has expanded its involvement in community health efforts.

GHC also works with the health department on a number of community-wide planning and policy development projects. Along with the hospitals and other community organizations, GHC was a major contributor to a community-wide health needs assessment conducted in 1994 under the leadership of the local health department. The assessment included a complete inventory of health resources in the community, a profile of community health status indicators, and a consensus-building process for developing priority areas for improvement. GHC continues to be a major participant on the community committees that were formed to develop and implement actions to address the identified priority areas. GHC plays a leadership role on the committee that has targeted the problem of pediatric immunization in the community. GHC also collaborates with the health department for disaster planning, especially in the area of earthquake preparedness.

One area of conflict between GHC and the local health department involves the HMO's processes for handling laboratory work. Approximately 20% of GHC's laboratory services are conducted at a central facility in the Seattle area. Some reportable diseases for Thurston County GHC members are therefore detected in and reported to King County's health department rather than DPHSS. This system potentially inhibits the ability of DPHSS to receive prompt notification of diseases, and to begin tracking and investigational efforts in the event of potential outbreaks of communicable diseases. Although a solution to this problem has not yet been found, GHC and the health department continue to explore possible remedies.

GHC's Olympia administrator observes that most of the interactions that occur between GHC and the local health department are initiated by the latter. Given the department's primary focus on public health issues and GHC's primary focus on medical care delivery for its enrolled populations, this arrangement seems entirely appropriate. In many areas, the local health department may be at a better vantage point for identifying community health issues and strategies for addressing issues through collaboration. Nevertheless, GHC has initiated some of the collaborative efforts, such as a jointly sponsored childhood immunization effort in local schools and community centers and the jointly sponsored influenza vaccination campaign for seniors. For these issues, GHC clearly recognized the need for a community-level effort in order to improve the health of its enrolled members.

CONCLUSION

As the dominant managed care provider in Olympia, GHC impacts the local community health system on a number of different levels. GHC engages in a number of collaborative efforts with the local health department and with other community health providers, including a joint venture for operating a homeless health clinic, jointly sponsored programs and services for pediatric immunization and influenza vaccination, contractual agreements for providing obstetrical services to high-risk pregnant women served by the health department, and participation on a number of community-wide planning and policy development councils. GHC also affects the quality, accessibility, and efficiency of health care delivered in the community through internal activities such as its utilization review and quality improvement initiatives, population-based health care interventions, Medicaid managed care program, and health services research efforts. The impact that these internal activities have on community health in Olympia derives not only from the large proportion of the population that GHC has enrolled in its plans, but also from the stature and influence that GHC has achieved in the local medical community. As a recognized leader in adopting quality improvement strategies in health care delivery, GHC acts as a catalyst for improving health care practices in the larger community of public and private providers.

DISCUSSION QUESTIONS

1. Assess the strategic attributes of the interorganizational relationships maintained between GHC and the local health department. What do these relationships imply about GHC's organizational mission and culture? What do these relationships imply about the managerial orientation of the local health department?

2. What parallels may exist between GHC's involvement in community health initiatives and its endeavors in utilization management, quality improvement, and population-based health care? What are some common strategic considerations that might lie behind these alternative types of activities?

3. Identify the unique organizational and community attributes that appear to influence the interorganizational relationships forming among the health care organizations in Olympia. Consider both facilitating attributes as well as barriers.

4. Compare GHC with the managed care plans described in the Denver case study (Chapter 12) in terms of organizational contributions to community health. Speculate on the organizational, managerial, and marketplace factors that may account for notable similarities and differences.

CHAPTER 14

Case Study: A Public Sector HMO in Portland, OR

Glen P. Mays

The local public health system serving Portland, Oregon, maintains a relatively long history of involvement in managed care. During the early 1970s the county health agency developed a program for providing low-income uninsured individuals and families with prepaid managed health care, with the cooperation of several private health maintenance organizations (HMOs) and hospital systems. The state's implementation of a fully capitated Medicaid managed care program in 1994 led the local health department to join with an academic medical center and a coalition of community health centers in developing an HMO that could compete with private organizations in the Medicaid market. Despite the competitive interaction that occurs in the Medicaid marketplace, the local health department has achieved notable success in maintaining collaborative relationships with many of the private health systems operating in Portland. This chapter examines the nature of the relationships between the local public health agency and the many other public and private health care organizations serving Portland and Multnomah County.

OVERVIEW OF THE COMMUNITY

Portland and the surrounding Multnomah County are located in the northwestern corner of Oregon, just across the Columbia River from the state of Washington. More than 1.6 million people reside in the Portland metropolitan area, making

The author wishes to thank individuals at the following organizations for their generous contributions of time and information: Multnomah County Department of Health; Oregon Health Sciences University Hospital; Legacy Health Systems; Providence Health System; Portland Adventist Medical Center; and HMO Oregon.

233

the area Oregon's largest city. Approximately 625000 people reside in Multnomah County, which encompasses the urban core of the metropolitan area. An expanding and diversifying local economy has produced a steadily declining unemployment rate since the early part of the decade, with unemployment in 1995 for the metropolitan area standing at 3.8%. Multnomah County's per capita income of $23815 in 1995 is somewhat lower than in neighboring suburban counties, but is close to the national average. An estimated 13% of the county population lives below the federal poverty level. Census data from 1990 indicate that 6% of the population are African American, 4.7% are Asian, and 3.1% are of Hispanic origin. Almost 83% of county residents have attained 12 or more years of formal education.

Health statistics for the county suggest that the area confronts many of the same health problems that plague other large metropolitan areas. Approximately 6.1% of births in 1996 were low birth weight (less than 2500 grams). Births to teenage women (age 10 to 17) comprised almost 4.6% of the total births in 1996. The teenage pregnancy rate in Multnomah County has declined during the last three years but remains at 23%. More than 18% of pregnant women in Multnomah County did not receive prenatal care during their first trimester.

Three private, integrated health care systems and a public university hospital system provide the bulk of inpatient care and a substantial amount of ambulatory care for the Portland area. The Sisters of Providence Health System, a nonprofit corporation affiliated with the Catholic church, operates two medical centers in Multnomah County with a combined inpatient capacity of over 700 beds.[1] The two facilities managed over 34000 inpatient admissions and 900000 outpatient visits during 1994. Another nonprofit system, Legacy Health System, operates two hospitals in the county with a combined capacity of 739 beds and a volume of almost 25000 admissions and 354000 outpatient visits in 1994. Kaiser Permanente Northwest, a regional arm of the nation's largest HMO, has historically been a major provider of inpatient care in Portland as well. Since the 1995 closure of its 216-bed facility in central Portland, the nonprofit organization operates only one hospital in a suburban area outside Multnomah County. Increasingly, Kaiser contracts with Legacy and Providence for hospital services needed by its more than 300000 enrollees in the Portland area. The Oregon Health Sciences University operates a 350-bed hospital facility in Portland, which includes a children's hospital and a number of tertiary and quaternary care departments. This facility serves as the major teaching hospital for the university's medical and nursing schools, and had more than 17000 inpatients and 275000 outpatient visits in 1994. In addition to these facilities, Portland is served by a 270-bed hospital affiliated with the Adventist church, a Shriner's hospital for children's orthopaedics, and a Veteran's Affairs medical center.

Approximately 2754 active nonfederal physicians practice in Multnomah County, leading to a ratio of 464 physicians per 100000 people.[2] As in many urbanized areas, a maldistribution of physicians leaves some areas of the county underserved. A network of federally qualified community health centers operated by the local health department provides access to ambulatory health services in many of the county's underserved areas. In addition, a network of seven nonprofit health centers provides primary care services to low-income residents of the Portland metropolitan area. This private network had more than 25000 patient visits during 1993.[3]

Including Kaiser's group-model HMO and the managed care products operated by Legacy and Providence, more than 15 managed care plans operate in Multnomah County. In total, approximately 53% of the population in the Portland metropolitan area are enrolled in HMOs (National Research Corporation. 1994. Unpublished data). Almost 54% of Medicare beneficiaries and 90% of Medicaid beneficiaries are served by these plans.[4,5]

OVERVIEW OF THE PUBLIC HEALTH SYSTEM

The Multnomah County Health Department (MCHD) has long been a major provider of personal health services to Portland residents. The department operates seven primary care clinics; four dental clinics; a range of specialty health clinics in areas such as tuberculosis control and international health; and a network of school-based health clinics in area public schools. Community-based clinics are staffed by teams of physicians and nurse practitioners, while school-based clinics are served by teams of advanced-practice nurses. The department also operates specialized programs in areas such as human immunodeficiency virus prevention and education and substance abuse services. The majority of patients served through the health department's personal health programs are the uninsured, underinsured, and Medicaid beneficiaries. In addition to programs for personal health services, the department performs a wide range of population-based public health activities and support services, including community health education, environmental monitoring and inspection, translation services, laboratory services, vector control, vital and health statistics collection, and jail health services. In total, the department operates with a $108 million budget and 815 full-time equivalent staff.

HISTORY OF MANAGED CARE IN THE PUBLIC HEALTH SYSTEM

MCHD began its most recent involvement in managed care during the early 1990s as the state of Oregon developed its plans for reforming the Medicaid program. As the state worked during 1991 to finalize the controversial list of priority health conditions to be covered under Medicaid, the local health department began its first formal discussions with the Oregon Health Sciences University (OHSU) hospital regarding a collaborative effort in managed care. The health department already had some experience as a managed care provider under an existing state program that allowed primary care organizations (PCOs) to contract with the state on a partially capitated basis for providing a basic set of primary care services and case management to Medicaid beneficiaries. Both MCHD and OHSU recognized that the state would soon be moving to a policy of mandatory, fully capitated managed care enrollment for Medicaid beneficiaries, and that this policy could radically alter their organizations' roles and responsibilities as the dominant providers of health services to this population in Portland. In January of 1993, the neighboring Clackamas County Public Health Division joined MCHD and OHSU in their collaborative planning for Medicaid reform. Soon thereafter, the Oregon Primary Care Association, a state-wide network of community health centers, also requested to join the planning group. The group began strategizing the development of a jointly operated, fully capitated HMO that could serve Medicaid beneficiaries under Oregon's pending application with the U.S. Health Care Financing Administration for an 1115 waiver to institute state-wide Medicaid managed care. This waiver was approved in August of 1993 as a five-year demonstration program, and one month later the planning group's application as a fully capitated Medicaid health plan was approved by the state Medicaid agency.

Rapid approval of the state's managed care initiative and of the planning group's joint Medicaid health plan (CareOregon) created severe time pressures for MCHD and its partners to develop the appropriate infrastructure to operate as a capitated plan. Under the group's proposal, HMO enrollees would receive inpatient and specialized outpatient services from OHSU's medical center, and they would receive primary care and case management services from a network of providers comprised of health department clinics, affiliated community health centers, and OHSU clinics staffed by residents and faculty. The service network would consist of 17 organizations with 43 primary care clinics serving 11 Oregon counties. The partnership faced a daunting challenge in rapidly establishing an organizational structure that would support this arrangement. Three alternatives were considered by the participating organizations: (1) establishing CareOregon as an administrative unit of OHSU's hospital, (2) establishing the HMO as a unit of Multnomah County's health department, and (3) creating a separate corporate entity for the HMO that would be jointly owned and governed by the participating organizations. Participants recognized that housing the HMO within a university hospital might conflict with the HMO's emphasis on primary care. The participating organizations also recognized that sufficient time did not exist for establishing a separate corporate entity for the HMO (since start-up was planned for early 1994). Consequently, the decision was made to establish the HMO as a unit of county government under the administrative authority of the health department. This strategy would allow the HMO to take advantage of the administrative machinery already in place within the health department for managing the delivery of primary care services, such as its systems for scheduling, billing, and quality assurance. This strategy also required Multnomah County to administer a health plan that operated beyond county boundaries, since the network included community health centers located across the state. The legality of this arrangement was debated with the state attorney general's office and ultimately upheld.

The Multnomah County Board of Commissioners approved the plan to administer CareOregon through the health department in December 1993. By January 1994, mission and vision statements were adopted for the health plan, and enrollee information materials were produced in English, Spanish, Russian, and Vietnamese. The next month marked the official start-up of the state's Medicaid managed care program for beneficiaries who are eligible for the Aid to Families with Dependent Children program. This same month, the collaborative CareOregon health plan began serving its first enrollees. The plan began with 9500 enrollees who "rolled over" from their membership in PCOs that the health department and the community health centers operated under Oregon's existing managed care program. By the end of 1994, enrollment in CareOregon had doubled.

CURRENT CHALLENGES AND OPPORTUNITIES

Since its first year of operation, the CareOregon health plan has continued to expand its enrollment. In January 1995, the state extended the managed care program to include the aged, the blind, the disabled, and foster children who are eligible for Medicaid. Roughly half of the plan's enrolled population reside within Multnomah County, and a full 85% reside in the three-county Portland area.

In the Portland area, CareOregon competes with 12 other HMOs that serve Medicaid beneficiaries. HMO Oregon, a plan jointly operated by Oregon Blue Cross and Blue Shield and Legacy Health System, maintains the largest Medicaid beneficiary enrollment in the area with almost 25000 enrollees as of mid-1995. CareOregon ranks second in enrollment with approximately 20000 enrollees, with Kaiser Permanente's plan (13625) and Providence's plan (13294) also serving substantial numbers of beneficiaries (Figures 14–1 and 14–2). MCHD administrators attribute much of CareOregon's solid market position to its unique abilities to serve vulnerable populations. MCHD is known in the community for its long history of providing access to quality health services for Medicaid and medically indigent populations. Administrators suggest that MCHD's unique skills and reputation also create challenges for CareOregon to remain competitive in the Medicaid marketplace, because of the potential for adverse risk selection. As an example, MCHD's extensive capacity for providing language translation services appears to encourage larger proportions of recent immigrants and other non-English speaking beneficiaries to enroll in CareOregon. More than 35% of

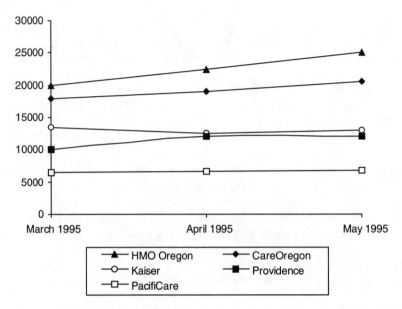

Figure 14–1 Medicaid Enrollment Trends in the Portland Area's Top Five HMOs, Spring 1995. *Source:* Reprinted from Oregon Office of Medical Assistance Programs, 1995.

CareOregon enrollees speak a language other than English at home. These enrollees may require more provider time for successful care management, and they may be at greater risk for certain health conditions than the average Medicaid beneficiary.

As a county health department, MCHD maintains contracts with several of its competing Medicaid HMOs for the provision of core public health services to their enrollees. A clause in the state Medicaid contract encourages HMOs to subcontract with health departments for these types of services, rather than to provide these services internally.[6] Some—but not all—of the Medicaid HMOs operating in Multnomah County choose to contract with MCHD for services such as tuberculosis control, sexually transmitted disease control, and maternity case management. This situation is problematic for MCHD, because enrollees of noncontracting plans must be turned away when they seek these services from health department clinics. MCHD administrators admit that this policy is very difficult to implement because of the traditional health department philosophy of open access to services.

MCHD administrators report that the health department's involvement in the Medicaid managed care market has allowed the organization to accomplish three critical public health tasks that would not have been possible if the department had simply let the private sector assume full responsibility for this market. First, by

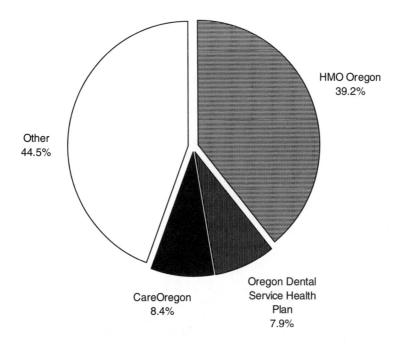

Figure 14–2 Statewide Medicaid HMO Market Share, Spring 1995. *Source:* Reprinted from Oregon Office of Medical Assistance Programs, 1995.

participating in the Medicaid market, MCHD has maintained its capacity for clinical services provision that is still needed to serve the substantial numbers of county residents who are not eligible for Medicaid or any other public or private health plan. Without revenue from the Medicaid managed care market, MCHD would have been unable to sustain its current levels of service for these uninsured and underinsured residents. Second, by competing with private plans in the Medicaid HMO market, MCHD has been able to "raise the bar" of standards regarding service quality and accessibility, since private HMOs must offer an HMO product that is competitive with the CareOregon plan in order to remain viable. In order to attract and retain Medicaid enrollees, private plans must strive to maintain comparable levels of service with MCHD in areas such as appointment availability, waiting times, and the provision of transportation and other support services. The CareOregon plan allows MCHD to ensure that a basic level of service is available from at least some plan in the community, while also encouraging other plans to offer similar levels of service.

An additional opportunity created by MCHD's involvement in Medicaid managed care relates to the health department's visibility and authority within the health care community. CareOregon's competitive market position secures MCHD a level of credibility, visibility, and authority among the major health care providers and insurers that few other local health departments are able to achieve in their communities. MCHD administrators report that they are able to use this visibility and authority to call attention to community health issues, to mobilize collaborative efforts to address issues, and to influence the strategic actions of other health care organizations. As an example, one year after the launch of CareOregon, MCHD received membership on an influential local health systems committee comprised of representatives from the major integrated delivery systems in Portland. MCHD's administrator now uses this committee to initiate community-wide planning and collaborative projects. The group has attended conferences on community health improvement efforts together, and continues to meet on a monthly basis.

CONCLUSION

MCHD plays a major role in Portland's Medicaid managed care market, largely because local administrators do not believe the private sector is ready to assume all of the health care responsibilities currently performed in the public sector. By operating a public sector HMO, the local health department maintains a direct role in ensuring access to care for vulnerable population groups within a larger, state-wide policy initiative to privatize health services and to expand health care coverage through managed care. MCHD administrators recognize that their current involvement in managed care may ultimately prove to be a temporary bridge between public sector and private sector health care provision; if a system emerges to ensure that the full community can be served through the private sector, then the need for a public sector HMO may disappear. However, MCHD administrators do not believe that this situation will emerge in the short term.

In contrast, administrators perceive that CareOregon's role in health care provision must expand rather than diminish in the foreseeable future to secure its continued viability. MCHD administrators are currently exploring the potential for CareOregon to begin participating in the commercial HMO market as a strategy for ensuring the economic viability of its Medicaid HMO and of its other public health services and activities. Currently, CareOregon stands at a disadvantage to other Medicaid HMOs that also operate commercial products, because these other plans are able to engage in marketing and advertising activities for their commercial products that also help the performance of their Medicaid products (the state forbids HMOs from marketing or advertising their Medicaid plans). These plans are also able to use their commercial products to provide financial support to their Medicaid products, which often entail greater financial risk. Expanding CareOregon's coverage to non-Medicaid eligibles might allow the public sector health plan to compete on a more equal footing with private plans, and may therefore secure the long-term financial viability of the plan.

Whether or not CareOregon expands to serve commercial enrollees, MCHD administrators recognize that the current administrative structure for the health plan may need to change in response to market imperatives. The decision to establish the CareOregon HMO as an administrative unit of the county health department was primarily one of expediency. Long-term viability for the plan may require a new administrative structure that allows greater flexibility for actions such as contracting, alliance building, financing, and personnel management.

DISCUSSION QUESTIONS

1. Assess the organizational and community considerations that might lead a local health department to adopt the strategy of operating its own managed care plan for Medicaid beneficiaries. What advantages and disadvantages might this strategy offer in terms of performing core public health functions?

2. Examine the nature of the competitive relationships between the local health department and the other Medicaid managed care plans operating in Portland. How do these relationships compare with those described in the Denver case study (Chapter 12)? Assess the opportunities as well as the challenges created within the public health system as a result of these competitive relationships.

3. Discuss the merits and the difficulties of continuing to operate the CareOregon health plan as part of the county health department, compared with alternative organizational arrangements that might be adopted for the plan. What reasons could be given for the decision to reorganize the plan within the university hospital? What reasons might support the creation of a separate organizational structure for the plan?

4. Consider the advantages and disadvantages of serving commercially insured individuals through the CareOregon health plan, from the perspective of the health department. How might this strategy affect the organization and operation of the health department? How might this strategy affect interorganizational relationships existing among the health care organizations serving Portland?

REFERENCES

1. American Hospital Association. *AHA Guide to the Health Care Field, 1995.* Chicago: American Hospital Association; 1996:A68.

2. American Medical Association (AMA). *Physician Data by County, 1994.* Washington, DC: AMA; 1996.
3. Multnomah County Health Department. *Annual Report: 1994 through 1995.* Portland, Ore: Multnomah County Health Department; 1996.
4. U.S. Health Care Financing Administration. *Medicare Managed Care Monthly Report, March 1997.* Baltimore, Md: Health Care Financing Administration; 1997.
5. U.S. Health Care Financing Administration. *1996 Medicaid Managed Care Enrollment Report.* Baltimore, Md: Health Care Financing Administration; 1996.
6. Oregon Department of Human Resources, Office of Medical Assistance Programs. *Oregon Health Plan Administrative Rules.* Salem, Ore: Oregon Department of Human Resources; 1995.

CHAPTER 15

Case Study: Reconfiguring Memphis' Public Health System for Managed Care

Glen P. Mays

Like many states and communities across the nation, Tennessee's move to managed care for Medicaid beneficiaries creates daunting challenges for the local public health system serving Memphis. A unique strategy adopted by the local health department allows the agency to maintain its substantial involvement in providing personal health services to vulnerable populations in Memphis, while largely avoiding the trappings of exclusive health maintenance organization (HMO) contracts and competitive relationships. This chapter examines the processes by which this strategy was adopted and implemented, and profiles its early experience.

OVERVIEW OF THE COMMUNITY

Memphis and Shelby County lie on Tennessee's western border along the Mississippi River. The county's population of 846584 is large and racially diverse, with African Americans comprising 44% of the population.[1] The transportation industry has traditionally driven the area's local economy, and firms such as Federal Express have a large presence in this expanding and diversifying economy. Despite steady economic improvement over the last five years, poverty is a persistent problem for this community, as more than 18% of citizens live below the federal poverty threshold. More than 75% of the population have

The author wishes to thank individuals at the following organizations for their generous contributions of time and information: Memphis-Shelby County Health Department; Regional Medical Center; LeBonheur Children's Hospital; Baptist Memorial Hospital; Methodist Hospital; St. Francis Hospital; St. Joseph Hospital; TLC Family Health Plan; Complete Health Plan; Southern Health Plan; Access MedPlus; PruCare of Memphis; and the Community Health Agency of Memphis.

completed at least 12 years of education, but less than 25% have completed four or more years of college.

Many of the most pressing health issues confronting the Memphis community have roots in poverty, according to the local health officer. Out-of-wedlock births have begun to decline in the community, but they still comprised 50% of all births and 73% of births to minority women during 1995. More than 19% of births to Memphis residents were to women between 10 to 17 years old. Approximately 10.5% of all resident births were low birth weight, and infant mortality stood at 14.4 per 1000 live births. As in many communities, heart disease, cancer, and cerebrovascular disease top the list of leading causes of death. Other leading causes of death include accidents (fifth), homicides (eighth), and human immuno-deficiency virus/acquired immune deficiency syndrome (tenth).

Health resources in Shelby County are substantial. Local hospitals include six general acute care facilities, two children's hospitals (one general acute care facility and one specialty facility), and a Veteran's Affairs medical center. The county-affiliated hospital, Regional Medical Center, assumes responsibility for the majority of indigent care in the community. The Med, as this facility is called, managed over 36000 admissions and almost 210000 outpatient visits in its medical complex during 1994.[2] Two nonprofit hospitals, Methodist Hospital and Baptist Hospital, dominate the commercial market for inpatient and specialty services. St. Francis Hospital, a facility formerly affiliated with the Catholic church and currently owned by the for-profit hospital system Tenet, stands as the area's fourth largest hospital in terms of market share. St. Joseph Hospital exists as the single remaining Catholic hospital in the area, and primarily serves the elderly population in inner-city Memphis.

The managed care market in Memphis and Shelby County continues to grow, spurred on by the 1994 launch of TennCare, the state-wide managed care program for Medicaid beneficiaries and the uninsured. The commercial managed care market is dominated by health plans that are operated by established insurance corporations such as CIGNA, Prudential, and the state's two Blue Cross and Blue Shield associations. The Medicaid market created by TennCare, however, has consisted largely of a collection of newly formed plans and small affiliates of out-of-state plans. Only lately have plans such as Prudential begun to participate in this market. Currently a total of six plans serve the almost 300000 TennCare beneficiaries in Memphis, including one sponsored jointly by the county-affili-ated hospital and a faculty practice plan of the University of Tennessee at Memphis medical school.

A total of almost 1600 nonfederal physicians practice in Shelby County.[3] A number of low-income and minority neighborhoods continue to be underserved by health care providers. Two nonprofit health centers (a federally qualified health center and a "look-alike" center) help to fill the gaps in access by providing services to uninsured and underinsured populations of Memphis.[4]

In addition, the Memphis-Shelby County Health Department serves as a major provider of personal health services to both TennCare beneficiaries and to uninsured populations. The department, which is jointly funded and administered by the City of Memphis and the County of Shelby, operates six full-time primary health care centers and seven part-time specialty clinics at various community locations. Clinics are staffed with teams of physicians, nurse practitioners, public health nurses and licensed practical nurses, and dentists. Services provided through these clinics include well-child care, sick-child care, prenatal care, acute and chronic disease care for adults, dental care for children, nutritional education and counseling, and family planning services. During calendar year 1994, the full-time clinics provided 153000 patient visits, and part-time clinics provided an additional 142000 visits. The department's part-time specialty clinics include school-based clinics, a pediatric primary care evening clinic, and targeted clinics for immunization, sexually transmitted diseases, and human immunodeficiency virus (HIV).

In addition to clinical services, the department carries out a wide range of responsibilities in providing population-based health services, assessing health problems and risks, and developing health policies and plans for the community. These responsibilities include operating programs in health promotion and disease prevention, environmental inspection and monitoring, vector control, pollution control, epidemiology, laboratory services, and vital statistics management.

MANAGED CARE AND THE PUBLIC HEALTH SYSTEM

Implementation of the state-wide TennCare program in January 1994 forced Memphis' local health department into the managed care market. With only nine months of planning, the state created a program that enrolled the entire population of Medicaid beneficiaries into health plans that contracted to serve these beneficiaries on a capitated basis (a fixed fee per enrollee regardless of services used). In addition to the state's 850000 Medicaid beneficiaries, the program also allowed individuals within 400% of the federal poverty level to enroll in TennCare plans, although some are required to pay sliding-scale premiums based upon income. As a major provider of primary care services to Medicaid beneficiaries and the uninsured, Memphis-Shelby County Health Department could not avoid the effects of such sweeping changes in state policy and programming.

Given its substantial primary care capacity and its expertise in serving vulnerable population groups, the department began to attract offers from providers and insurers seeking to form health plans that could compete in the TennCare market. One of the first organizations to approach the health department was the county-affiliated hospital. The Med had already begun planning the formation of a TennCare HMO in collaboration with a physician group from the University of

Tennessee at Memphis (UT) medical school that practiced and taught within the hospital. Administrators at the Med sought to establish an exclusive contract with the health department for providing primary care services to enrollees of the new HMO. Such a contract would require that all TennCare beneficiaries served by the health department be referred to the Med and to members of the University of Tennessee practice for inpatient and specialty services. Exclusive contracting was not an attractive prospect for the local health department director, who felt that TennCare enrollees understandably may desire to take advantage of the expanded choices created under TennCare and therefore enroll in plans that offered access to private providers and hospitals. The health director wished to preserve the department's historical role in providing primary care and public health services to the full spectrum of vulnerable populations in Memphis, and not just to the enrollees of a single HMO. The director summarized the health department's philosophy by noting, "We are a public agency that serves all the people who need our services, and if people want to use our clinics but want to use another managed care organization, we think that should be an option."

The Med proceeded with its plans to jointly own and operate an HMO with the UT group practice, and ultimately established two of its own primary care clinics in areas that largely do not compete with the health department's clinics. The health department has since been approached by other managed care plans with offers for exclusive contracts, but all have been turned down. Rather than establish exclusive arrangements, the health department began to pursue subcontracting arrangements that would allow the department to serve the TennCare enrollees of multiple managed care plans. As of 1995, the health department had successfully established nonexclusive subcontracting agreements with five of the six managed care plans that were approved to serve TennCare beneficiaries in Shelby County.

Under the nonexclusive subcontracting arrangements, the health department provides both case management and primary care services to TennCare enrollees who choose the health department as their primary care provider (PCP). The health department receives a capitated per-member-per-month payment for each enrollee who selects the health department as his or her PCP (see Appendix B for an example of a subcontracting agreement). In exchange for this fee, the health department agrees to provide all medically necessary primary care services specified in the contract. An example of these services is shown in Exhibit 15–1. Primary care services are delivered by physicians and advanced practice nurses at the department's six full-time primary care clinics. Additionally, for enrollees who are students at the two Memphis high schools where the department operates school-based clinics, services may be received at these sites.

Interestingly, once a decision is made by a health department PCP that an enrollee needs hospital services, the health department physician does not follow the patient in the hospital and manage the care in the inpatient setting. Rather, the

Exhibit 15–1 Example of Primary Care Services Provided by Memphis-Shelby County Health Department under Capitated Contract

---

1. Office visits
2. Physical exams (including Early and Periodic Screening, Diagnosis, and Treatment)
3. Injections (excluding allergy serums)
4. Immunizations
5. All outpatient laboratory work
6. Home visits
7. Hospital visits
8. Nonscheduled physician's services (24-hour on-call services)
9. Nursing home visits
10. Health education in physician's office
11. Nutrition counseling in physician's office
12. Mental health counseling in physician's office
13. Radiology performed in physician's office
14. Family planning services

---

health department establishes subcontracting arrangements with private physicians that have admitting privileges at the hospitals affiliated with the enrollee's managed care plan. These subcontracting physicians agree to follow health department clients in inpatient settings and serve as links between the health department PCPs and the hospitals. The health department PCPs hold responsibility for deciding whether or not to pursue higher levels of care outside the primary care setting; however, the subcontracting arrangements with private providers allow these PCPs to consult with outside providers for difficult and unclear cases.

The capitated reimbursement arrangements that the health department operates within create clear financial incentives for the department to manage the delivery of primary care services effectively and efficiently. Indeed, the health department assumes a measure of financial risk for health plan enrollees who choose the department as their PCP, since it must meet the costs of providing all necessary primary care services, even if these costs exceed the monthly capitation fees paid by the managed care plans. Health department administrators report that their organization is well suited to this arrangement, given its experience in working within constrained governmental budgets and its historical emphasis on preventive care. These administrators maintain that their public health clinics have long faced a need for efficiency under the often limited governmental appropriations for public health services. These clinics have also achieved substantial expertise in providing and encouraging the utilization of disease prevention and health promotion services. This expertise ranges from getting pregnant women in for timely prenatal care to providing health education to clients and community members on topics such as nutrition, family planning, and sexually transmitted disease control. The department's extensive capacity for community outreach reinforces its ability to act as an efficient and effective primary care case manager under managed care systems.

The department's role as an efficient case manager for TennCare health plans does not go unrewarded under the department's subcontracting arrangements. Several plans allocate a percentage of their premium revenue to "service pools," which are then used for capitation payments to primary care subcontractors and for fee-for-service payments for designated services such as hospital services. At the end of each quarter, funds remaining in the service pools are disbursed to subcontractors on the basis of their efficiency in managing the services required by their enrollee populations. In this way, even though the health department is not capitated or "at-risk" for hospital services, the department still receives financial incentives for serving as an effective "gatekeeper" for services in these settings. Health department administrators report receiving substantial bonus payments from TennCare HMOs because of their ability to efficiently manage services such as emergency department utilization and hospital inpatient stays.

CURRENT CHALLENGES AND OPPORTUNITIES

The health department's transition to a primary care case management role under managed care has required some organizational retooling. To effectively manage the care received by enrollees and to interface easily with managed care plans, the department has undertaken major improvements to its patient tracking and billing systems. Building the necessary information systems has proven to be a substantial effort for the health department in terms of rapidly securing funding, space, and expertise for these new systems.

The health department has also faced challenges to its relationships with other public and private providers as it has moved into managed care. The health department and county-affiliated hospital have enjoyed a long history of collaboration as the major providers of indigent care in the community. The move to managed care under TennCare has complicated some of these collaborative efforts as patients have been divided up into competing managed care plans. For example, for several years prior to TennCare, the Med and the health department operated joint case management and referral systems for adult chronic disease management. Adults admitted to the Med with acute manifestations of chronic diseases such as cardiovascular disease, cerebrovascular disease, and diabetes would be treated and then referred to the health department's chronic disease management programs operated through its community clinics. Hospital physicians would work closely with health department physicians for the long-term management of these conditions, maintaining strong communication links and arrangements for referrals and consultations. Managed care has strained these types of interorganizational links by prohibiting many of the referral arrangements that traditionally occurred between the two organizations. Many of the TennCare patients treated at the Med are members of the hospital's own HMO and must be referred to clinics operated by the University of Tennessee physician group. Likewise, many of the TennCare patients managed by the health department are members of HMOs that do not contract with the Med for hospital services. Consequently, the strong inter-organizational program for chronic disease management has largely fallen apart in the wake of TennCare.

At the same time, TennCare has created opportunities for the health department to establish new linkages with the private-provider community. As a subcontractor for managed care plans that use private hospitals such as Methodist, Baptist, and St. Joseph, the health department faces an imperative to establish and maintain solid working relationships with the medical staffs at these facilities. Through these relationships, the health department has new avenues for influencing clinical and community health practices in these organizations and for enlisting the support of these organizations in public health initiatives. In this way, TennCare has established the potential for stronger ties between public health and the private hospital and physician community in Memphis.

TennCare has also created additional incentives for collaboration between public and private sector organizations in some instances. For example, the contracts that a local children's hospital maintained with TennCare HMOs created financial incentives for efficiently managing the utilization of emergency department services and specialty physician services. These same incentives were faced by the health department in its subcontracting arrangements with TennCare HMOs. In response to these shared incentives, the two organizations (which are conveniently located adjacent to each other) established a pediatric clinic staffed by health department clinicians, which allowed patients presenting at the hospital emergency department to be conveniently triaged for nonemergent primary care services. This jointly sponsored endeavor allows both organizations to more efficiently manage the care of their TennCare enrollees and thus make use of the financial incentives established by the HMOs.

CONCLUSION

The local public health system serving Memphis and Shelby County has managed to adapt rapidly to a changing health care environment that has invested heavily in the concept of managed care. The local health department continues to respond to the short-term dynamics of this reform, but the long-term equilibrium of this system remains uncertain. Will the health department's role as primary care case manager under managed care prove to be a long-term solution or a short-term transition in the larger movement toward enhanced efficiency and expanded access in health care? Health department staff predict a continuing need for the department's direct involvement in the provision and management of personal health services for vulnerable populations in the community. The department's effectiveness and efficiency in this role lead many of the managed care plans also to see an ongoing need for health department involvement in this area. Hospitals and private providers in this community are less confident about a continuing need for this health department role, however.

It is not at all clear that the private sector is ready to assume additional direct responsibility for the care of economically disadvantaged groups currently served in the public sector, even under the realigned incentives of TennCare. Ongoing financial difficulties at the county-affiliated hospital, which have been exacerbated by TennCare reforms, make this proposition increasingly imperative but no less vexing. What does appear clear is that the current public health system and its linkages between public and private providers should provide a structure for anticipating and addressing the question of additional private sector involvement in ensuring access to health care.

DISCUSSION QUESTIONS

1. Assess the strategic attributes of the relationships maintained between the local health department and the Medicaid HMOs in Memphis. Which of the three strategic alliance models (opportunistic, shared service, and stakeholder) most adequately captures the health department's approach to these organizations? Explain.
2. Compare Memphis-Shelby County Health Department's response to Medicaid managed care with those taken by local health departments in Denver (Chapter 12) and Portland (Chapter 14). Identify the similarities in these alternative approaches, as well as the differences. What factors (organizational, political, economic, and demographic) might account for the different approaches taken in these communities?
3. What are the potential advantages that accrue to Memphis' local health department by avoiding exclusive contracting with Medicaid HMOs? Consider specifically the potential impact of exclusive contracting on the department's ability to carry out core public health functions. What are the potential benefits that are forgone by avoiding an exclusive HMO relationship?
4. Examine the sample contract between a local health department and an HMO shown in Appendix B.
   - Are there provisions of this contract that might be more easily met by local health departments than by other types of primary care providers?

- Are there provisions that might pose more difficulties for local health departments than for other types of providers?
- Identify contract provisions that could potentially support and/or interfere with the performance of core public health functions.

REFERENCES

1. Memphis and Shelby County Health Department. *1995 Vital Statistics.* Memphis, Tenn: Memphis and Shelby County Health Department; 1995.

2. American Hospital Association (AHA). *AHA Guide to the Health Care Field, 1995.* Chicago: AHA; 1996.

3. American Medical Association (AMA). *Physician Data by County, 1994.* Washington, DC: AMA; 1996.

4. Bureau of Primary Health Care, U.S. Health Resources and Services Administration. *Primary Care Programs Directory 1994.* McLean, Va: Health Resources and Services Administration; 1994.

CHAPTER 16

Case Study: The Local Health Department's Role in Milwaukee's Managed Care Market

Glen P. Mays

Milwaukee was one of the nation's first communities to implement a mandatory managed care system for serving Medicaid beneficiaries. Interestingly, early failures in this system appear to have helped motivate many of the innovative interorganizational arrangements that are now emerging between managed care plans and community health organizations. After an unsuccessful attempt at operating a health maintenance organization (HMO) in cooperation with a network of community health centers, the local health department in Milwaukee has gradually reduced its involvement in the direct provision of personal health care services. At the same time, the agency has developed innovative strategies for ensuring access to health services through partnerships with private health care providers. The relatively long history of Medicaid managed care in Milwaukee has also allowed many private HMOs to develop and improve upon targeted systems of care for vulnerable population groups. This chapter examines the evolving roles of the local health department within Milwaukee's maturing managed care market.

OVERVIEW OF THE COMMUNITY

The city of Milwaukee lies at the heart of a four-county metropolitan area located on the western shore of Lake Michigan in southeastern Wisconsin. The

The author wishes to thank individuals at the following organizations for their generous contributions of time and information: Milwaukee Health Department; Children's Hospital of Wisconsin; Froedtert Memorial Lutheran Hospital; Sinai Samaritan Hospital; St. Francis Hospital; St. Joseph Hospital; St. Michael Hospital; St. Mary Hospital; Wisconsin Independent Physicians' Group; Genesis Health Plan; Prime Care Health Plan; CompCare Health Services Insurance Corporation; Wisconsin Health Organization Insurance Corporation; and Managed Health Services Insurance Corporation.

area's 1.4 million residents make Milwaukee the nation's 32nd largest metropolitan area. Historically, the area's economy has consisted largely of heavy manufacturing industries that produce products ranging from X-ray equipment to motorcycles. As in many "rust belt" cities of the Midwest, the steady shift to a service economy has produced some unemployment and income loss for residents. The city of Milwaukee has 630000 residents, of whom approximately 83% are Caucasian, 14% are African American, and 4% are Hispanic. The area's unemployment rate stood at 4.2% in 1994 and has remained below the national average for more than a decade. Per capita income has also remained above the national average, and stood at $20325 in 1994.

Milwaukee's relatively numerous health care providers are rapidly organizing into three integrated delivery systems. This process has been aided by the closure in 1995 of the county-owned Doyne Hospital, a process that removed 350 hospital beds from the community's total supply of over 6000 beds. All of the city's 10 remaining hospitals are private, nonprofit corporations, and most of these are affiliated with one of the three emerging health care systems in the area.

Milwaukee has a long history of managed care in both the commercial and Medicaid populations. Almost half of the area's population are enrolled in HMOs. Milwaukee's experience in Medicaid managed care began in 1984 under a demonstration waiver from the U.S. Health Care Financing Administration. All of the city's women and children who received the cash assistance program Aid to Families with Dependent Children (AFDC) were enrolled in managed care plans over a six-month period. By 1993, approximately 115000 Medicaid beneficiaries received care through the six plans that participated in the program. These participating plans include several of the large, for-profit corporations that dominate the commercial managed care market, such as CompCare Health Plan, the state's oldest HMO with 160000 total enrollees and a network-model structure that includes 805 primary care physicians; Prime Care Health Plan, the largest HMO in the state with almost 200000 enrollees and 986 primary care physicians in its network; and Family Health Plan Cooperative, the area's only staff-model HMO, serving almost 110000 enrollees with its 88 staff physicians and additional 200 contract physicians.[1] The area's mature Medicaid managed care market has also allowed the emergence of several specialized managed care plans that have developed care delivery and management approaches that are tailored to the Medicaid population. For example, the Wisconsin Independent Physicians' Group (WIPG) formed as a nonprofit managed medical provider network in 1984 specifically to serve the Medicaid population. WIPG has pioneered several health education and outreach initiatives for this population, including programs in prenatal care coordination and child health screenings that have served as models for the community and state. Similarly, Genesis Health Plan began operation in 1994 as an independent practice association (IPA) HMO that was formed specifically to serve the Medicaid population. This plan has emphasized the provision of social support services such as free transportation and translation services, and has established itself as a community resource by providing reduced-fee and free care to uninsured community members who are not eligible for Medicaid.

A collection of three federally qualified community health centers and one additional health center "look-alike" provide access to personal health services for Milwaukee's uninsured and underinsured populations, and to the city's Medicaid populations who are not enrolled in HMOs.[2] Some centers also maintain contracts with HMOs for serving their Medicaid enrollees. This network of private community health centers, together with the area's collection of Medicaid HMOs and nonprofit hospitals, has allowed the city's health department to move away from the direct provision of many types of personal health services. Through its four health clinics, the Milwaukee Health Department (MHD) currently provides only specialized personal health services in areas such as sexually transmitted diseases, immunization, and tuberculosis control.

THE PUBLIC HEALTH SYSTEM'S ROLE IN MANAGED CARE

Wisconsin's experiment with Medicaid managed care in Milwaukee forced the local health department to rethink its role in the provision of personal health services. After considering possible options, such as terminating involvement in the Medicaid program or joining the provider panels of existing HMOs, health department administrators decided to establish their own managed care plan in collaboration with the three federally qualified health centers. Two years after the 1984 start-up of this jointly sponsored HMO, the endeavor failed due to financial difficulties. Despite its ultimate failure, the organizations' efforts to jointly operate a public sector HMO helped to smooth the transition to a private HMO market for Medicaid beneficiaries. The community health centers that participated in this initiative developed relationships with private providers and insurers that allowed them to continue on as Medicaid providers through agreements with private HMOs. The health department learned through this experience that it may no longer be efficient or effective to directly provide certain types of health services under the new system of managed care.

Consequently, the health department has steadily decreased its involvement in the direct provision of personal health services. Currently, the department carries out its responsibilities in providing primary care services to uninsured individuals largely through contracts with the three health centers and with the University of Wisconsin's medical center and clinic. The department now directly provides only categorical public health services that continue to be inadequately accessible from private providers in the community, such as immunizations, sexually transmitted disease services, and tuberculosis control services. Without a large responsibility in direct clinical services provision, the department relies heavily on its relationships with other providers in the community to carry out its larger mission of ensuring the availability and adequacy of health services.

Relationships between the health department and the managed care community have undergone steady improvement over the past five years. A measles epidemic in Milwaukee during 1989 and 1990 exposed substantial gaps in the local health care system, and created tension between the public health and managed care communities. During this epidemic, the vast majority of cases came from children enrolled in HMOs. The health department provided free immunizations to more than 20000 patients during the outbreak, including 11000 HMO enrollees who failed to receive immunizations from their private providers. Milwaukee HMOs experienced the severe financial consequences of this epidemic through the 232 hospital admissions and three fatalities that resulted.

The outbreak generated animosity between the managed care and public health communities, but it also created clear incentives for closer relationships. In the wake of the disaster, the health department successfully negotiated contractual arrangements with the Medicaid HMOs that allowed the department to receive reimbursement for immunizing HMO enrollees who seek care at health department clinics. This agreement on immunization soon led to a similar arrangement allowing the department to be reimbursed for conducting lead screenings among age-appropriate HMO enrollees who present at health department clinics. Negotiations are now underway for the provision of sexually transmitted disease services and tuberculosis screening and treatment. Clearly, HMOs prefer their enrollees to seek care within their networks of private providers in order to improve care coordination and management and to contain costs. The health department contracts suggest that Milwaukee HMOs are recognizing the challenges of managing care among traditionally underserved populations, and are willing to explore creative solutions in order to improve health among their enrollees.

The health department's success in establishing service contracts with Medicaid HMOs created opportunities for forming additional relationships around community health issues. Milwaukee's health director used the HMO contracts for immunization as a rationale for inviting HMO participation on a community-wide immunization planning group. Using financial support from the Centers for Disease Control and Prevention and the Robert Wood Johnson Foundation, the group—made up largely of public and private health care providers—is planning the development of a computerized immunization-tracking system for the community. HMOs have made substantial contributions to this effort given the expertise many of these organizations have in information systems, and given the potentially large role they may play in contributing and using data for the proposed system. The health department also enlists the participation of HMOs on a community environmental health task force. This effort is developing linkages between private health care providers and the health department's environmental inspection and abatement programs, so that when HMOs or other private providers detect environmental health issues such as lead poisoning, the health department can be enlisted as part of a coordinated intervention. HMOs are also serving alongside the local health department on community-wide task forces in areas such as violence prevention, teen pregnancy, infant mortality, and the federal Healthy Start initiative for early childhood development.

THE PRIVATE SECTOR'S ROLE IN PUBLIC HEALTH

Milwaukee's managed care market for Medicaid beneficiaries has achieved a level of success and stability that appears to support innovation and creativity among the organizations participating in this market. A number of managed care plans have begun to experiment with interventions that extend beyond traditional approaches to medical management, and that begin to address basic public health goals of health promotion and disease prevention at the community level. One of the most notable organizations in this regard also exists as one of the largest Medicaid managed care providers, the Wisconsin Independent Physicians' Group.

WIPG began as a nonprofit IPA formed in 1984 to operate as a provider organization under the newly established Medicaid managed care demonstration project. The IPA originally formed around physicians at the local children's hospital, but soon expanded so that the organization could serve adults as well as children enrolled in the Medicaid program. This need to expand forced the IPA to become independent from a single hospital, and therefore allowed the organization to contract with a range of different hospitals serving the community. Both physicians and specialists were included as members of the IPA. Increasingly, physicians and administrators within WIPG realized that the organizational structure of an IPA restricted the plan's ability to manage the care of its patients to the realm of physician services. To more effectively and efficiently manage the full range of care needed by patients, WIPG reorganized in 1990 as a managed medical provider network. This reorganization allowed WIPG to assume responsibility for managing all health and support services required by its enrollees, including inpatient and outpatient hospital care, alcohol and substance abuse services, mental health services, pharmacy, and transportation. WIPG established a primary care gatekeeper model to manage this care, with each enrollee assigned to a single primary care physician of the enrollee's choice who coordinates the delivery of all needed services.

Currently, WIPG serves approximately 49000 Medicaid beneficiaries in Milwaukee, or almost 50% of the total number of AFDC-eligible Medicaid beneficiaries in the county. The organization does not currently serve any commercial enrollees, although it has done so in the past and its administrator anticipates involvement in the commercial market in the future. More than 800 physicians are currently members of the WIPG network, one-quarter of which practice in primary care disciplines.

Throughout its history, WIPG has played a major role in developing community-based interventions for health promotion and disease prevention in the Medicaid and medically indigent populations of Milwaukee. One of the most notable efforts began in 1987 as the organization began to notice a rise in the number of premature and low birth-weight infants among its plan membership. In response to this trend, the plan established a prenatal support program to address the social issues believed to be at the root of these perinatal health problems. The program consists of community health nurses hired to perform health risk assessments in the homes of pregnant plan members. The assessment includes observations of the social conditions of members, such as the adequacy of housing, food, plumbing, clothing, and household and neighborhood safety. Two home visits are made to each member, during which nurses also conduct a full family and patient medical history and a health education session that includes counseling on nutrition, smoking, sexually transmitted diseases, and the use of alcohol and other drugs. Additional home visits are performed for at-risk members who miss office visits with their obstetrician. In response to the assessments, the nurses and primary care physicians can ensure that members receive access to needed social services such as housing and weatherization assistance, clothing and food assistance, drug abuse treatment, and transportation and child care assistance. Clinicians ensure access to many of these nonclinical services by making contacts with the applicable public and nonprofit social service agencies operating in the community. For example, WIPG ensures free child care to its enrollees during their health care visits through a collaborative effort with a local nonprofit day-care center.

A 1990 evaluation of WIPG's prenatal support program suggested that the program was successful and cost-effective in improving birth outcomes. This success motivated WIPG's administrator to lobby the state Medicaid office to implement the program state-wide for all Medicaid beneficiaries. In 1994, the program was added as a standard benefit to all Medicaid beneficiaries in the state. As a result, WIPG's program became the designated prenatal support program for all Medicaid beneficiaries in Milwaukee county. The program can now receive referrals from any community physician that serves Medicaid beneficiaries.

WIPG has played a leadership role in developing other types of community-based health interventions as well. In conjunction with Prime Care, another large HMO that serves both commercial and Medicaid enrollees in Milwaukee, WIPG developed an innovative system for ensuring the delivery of early childhood health screenings (known as Early and Periodic Screening, Diagnosis, and Treatment or EPSDT exams in many states). The two organizations developed a health-screening checklist that reminds physicians of the series of diagnostic and screening services that must be performed on a periodic basis under state Medicaid requirements. The checklist is placed in the medical record of each Medicaid-eligible child enrolled in either of the two HMOs, and clinicians can use the list to track the delivery of scheduled screening services. As an additional incentive, WIPG does not reimburse its physicians for well-child visits unless the child is up-to-date on the EPSDT screening schedule. WIPG administrators suggest that interventions such as this checklist are quickly diffused into the larger population of local physicians serving Medicaid beneficiaries, because many of the physician practices that are members of WIPG also maintain contracts with other Medicaid HMOs. Therefore, interventions that change physician behavior may affect not only the care received by WIPGs Medicaid enrollees, but also the care received by enrollees of other plans that contract with these same physicians. This trend is an interesting feature of a managed care market comprised largely of IPA-model HMOs with overlapping provider panels.

WIPG also plays a major role in developing community- and state-wide policies for improving access to care under the Medicaid managed care program. WIPG's administrator is currently working to secure support from local government officials and other Medicaid HMOs for the establishment of a jointly funded childhood immunization initiative. Under the proposed initiative, a case worker would use a computer-based immunization tracking system that is currently under development to check the immunization status of Medicaid-eligible children each time their parents visit the county welfare office to apply for or receive benefits. The parents of children not up-to-date on immunizations would receive counseling and assistance in setting up an appointment for immunizations. In another effort, WIPG's administrator is working to encourage state administrators and legislators to expand the state's Medicaid managed care program to cover the state's medically indigent population under an 1115(b) waiver from the U.S. Health Care Financing Administration. Through these types of policy development efforts, WIPG plays an important role in shaping the local public health system, and a role that extends far beyond the traditional responsibilities of a managed care organization.

Many of the other managed care plans in Milwaukee have begun to experiment with community-based initiatives in health promotion and disease prevention as a strategy for improving health outcomes and reducing long-term health risks among their enrolled populations. For example, Genesis Health Plan, a small for-profit plan that began operating as a hybrid IPA and staff-model HMO in 1994, has placed emphasis on establishing primary care clinics in low-income ethnic neighborhoods and in staffing clinics with members of the ethnic community that it serves. Through this strategy, the plan hopes to improve access to services for traditionally underserved populations and thereby improve health status in these populations. Genesis also places emphasis on providing easy access to support services such as transportation and language translation services. Additionally,

Genesis works to establish its clinics as health resources in the community by providing reduced-fee and free care to uninsured community members who are not eligible for Medicaid. Genesis' founder and administrator reports that these community health activities are motivated in part by belief in the cost-effectiveness of these activities, and in part by a desire to be a good corporate citizen. So far, the plan's for-profit mission has not come in conflict with its community service mission. In fact, the plan's early success in Milwaukee has encouraged the organization to consider exporting its managed care model to other states that are developing Medicaid managed care initiatives.

CONCLUSION

Milwaukee's public health and managed care systems have achieved a relatively high degree of collaboration and integration since Medicaid managed care was originally introduced in 1984. In the years since this introduction, private and public sector health care providers have tested a range of different approaches for the delivery of medical care and public health services. Some of these approaches—such as the health department–sponsored HMO and the early private sector approaches to childhood immunization—have proven to be unsuccessful. Out of these early failures emerged collaborative, interorganizational approaches to community health issues that appear to be achieving some success. A number of these efforts have occurred under the leadership of the local health department, including the contracts with HMOs for immunizations and lead screenings and the community-wide task forces. However, the initiatives launched by WIPG and Genesis exemplify the many other efforts that have been developed in the private sector.

The private sector's growing role in covering traditionally underserved population groups in Milwaukee has enabled the local health department to scale back its involvement in personal health services delivery during the last decade. The local health director reports that this trend has allowed the local health department to devote more attention to core public health functions such as health assessment and policy development, but that it has also intensified the need to perform evaluation and oversight activities regarding services provided through the private health care system. The extent to which remaining health department services can be effectively transitioned to the private sector remains an open question. Proposals such as that supported by WIPG to include the medically indigent in the Medicaid managed care system may ultimately allow such a transition to occur. What appears certain is that the level of communication and collaboration already existing between the local public health and managed care systems will ensure that future initiatives will be well reasoned and well planned.

DISCUSSION QUESTIONS

1. Identify the major types of structural alliances that exist between the Milwaukee health department and the private Medicaid HMOs serving the community. Assess the potential advantages and disadvantages of these structures in the context of the Milwaukee community. What (if any) alternative alliance structures might be feasible and desirable in this context?

2. What are the potential advantages and disadvantages of adopting the Milwaukee health department strategy of diminishing involvement in the direct provision of personal health services? Compare this strategy with that of the local health department in Portland (Chapter 14), noting similarities as well as differences. What factors might account for key differences in strategy?

3. Examine the strategies implemented by the WIPG organization for serving Medicaid beneficiaries. What factors (organizational, political, economic, demographic) might motivate a private managed care plan such as this organization to adopt these types of strategies? Might other types of managed care plans in other types of communities be expected to develop and implement these types of strategies? Why or why not?

REFERENCES

1. Metropolitan Milwaukee Association of Commerce (MMAC). *Business Resource Guide for Metropolitan Milwaukee*. Milwaukee, Wis: MMAC; 1995.
2. Bureau of Primary Health Care, U.S. Health Resources and Services Administration. *Primary Care Programs Directory 1994*. McLean, Va: Health Resources and Services Administration; 1994.

CHAPTER 17

Case Study: Privatizing a Community Hospital in Rocky Mount, NC

Curtis P. McLaughlin

Nash General Hospital was established in Rocky Mount, North Carolina in 1971. By 1995, it had grown to three separate units: 300-bed Nash General Hospital, Nash Day Hospital (which opened in 1984), and Coastal Plain psychiatric facility. Coastal Plain was acquired from a private firm in 1991 and began taking Medicare, Medicaid, and uninsured patients under its public ownership. The Nash General hospital facility is owned by Nash County, which issued the bonds for its construction and renovation and leased it in May 1978 to Nash Health Care Systems, the county's private nonprofit hospital authority under two consecutive 10-year leases. Nash Health Care Systems was virtually debt-free and made no financial demands on the county. Consolidated statements of revenue and expenses compiled by Deloitte and Touche showed an excess of revenues over expenses of $8.48 million in 1993 and $6.05 million in 1994. The hospital was considered to be modern and in good repair. The excess revenues tended to be reinvested into the facility.

In 1994, the Nash County commissioners solicited approval for a school bond issue of $35 million for school construction and renovation. That referendum was defeated at the polls. Some of the leadership against the referendum had come from a grassroots group calling itself Friends of Fiscal Responsibility. That group acknowledged that the school system needed at least $20 million, but not the whole $35 million. Following the September 1994 referendum, Friends of Fiscal Responsibility reportedly held brainstorming sessions about how to meet school needs without further funding. One of the suggestions was that the county raise the money by privatizing Nash General Hospital. After informal discussions with some hospital industry executives, the group suggested that such a sale would raise as much as $100 million and add $197000 a year to the tax revenues of the county. There were rumors that the hospital authority had as much as $40 million in reserves, but the hospital chairman countered that with a report that it had $12 million in reserves, which was "equal to one month's budget." The value of $100 million for the hospital seemed to be accepted by those for and against privatization as a conservative value for an asset in which the county had invested some $10 million dollars over 21 years.

Privately owned hospitals were not new to the area. The competing hospital in Rocky Mount, Community Hospital, has been privately owned since its founding in 1913 as Rocky Mount Sanitarium. Then, in the early 1980s, HCA purchased Edgecombe Memorial Hospital in Tarboro, the county seat of Edgecombe County, and agreed to build a new facility called Heritage Hospital, which opened in 1985. This became a Health Trust hospital in 1987, and then was merged with Columbia/ HCA in 1995. Edgecombe County borders Nash County and includes East Rocky Mount, the poorer section of the city east of the railroad tracks. In a press interview in February 1995, Edgecombe County commissioner T.C. Cherry indicated satisfaction with physician recruitment, tax revenue, and service levels, saying, "We're in better shape than before." Indigent care charges accounted for 8.5% of Heritage's gross revenues in fiscal 1994. The owners had spent $1 million on equipment and upgrades during the last six months.

Also interviewed in February 1995, Roger Hall, executive director of Community Hospital, stated that, "Most for-profits would have an interest, assuming it's for sale. . . . The community would gain equity for the school system and an influx of money while the sale wouldn't impact quality of care or access to services. . . . There is a right way and a wrong way to approach a potential sale. Before a decision is made, we need to look at the history of corporate responsibility for potential buyers." Hall also noted that there were alternative ways of handling the privatization, including outright sale and various partnership arrangements.

ROCKY MOUNT AND NASH COUNTY

Rocky Mount, North Carolina is an industrial and agricultural city with a population of 55000. It covers 35 square miles and is located in the eastern coastal plain of the state. It is the largest city in Nash County, although a substantial portion of the city east of the railroad tracks is in East Rocky Mount in Edgecombe County, for which the county seat is Tarboro, about 12 miles away. In 1990, Nash County had a population of 77000, of whom 31% were African American and 1% Hispanic. The 1993 Nash County per capita income was $18074, compared to $15432 for Edgecombe County. The 1994 Nash County unemployment rate was 5% and the Edgecombe County rate 6.8%. In 1996, Rocky Mount city government reported that it had the following facilities: 99 churches (95 Protestant), 15 shopping centers, 3 hospitals with a total of 477 beds, 3 clinics, 162 physicians, and 34 dentists. The city maintains its own electric and water distribution systems. It shares the Rocky Mount-Wilson commercial airport seven miles away, which is served by USAir commuter flights. The nearest large airport is Raleigh-Durham, 60 miles west on the northwest side of Raleigh.

THE NEW LEASE PROPOSAL

On April 3, 1995, the hospital's attorney, Thomas Young, addressed the county commissioners for 15 minutes and emphasized the hospital's provision of $50 million of charity care over the past 23 years. He then offered to revise and renew the current lease expiring in May 1998 for 20 years, offering the incentive of a $10 million advance rent payment. County commissioners seemed uncomfortable with the 20-year commitment.

This lease proposal galvanized the local press. The issues involved had strong political overtones. The editorials in the *Nashville Graphic* seemed to strongly support the issue of privatization and criticized the "Democrat" commissioners throughout. The *Rocky Mount Telegram* seemed to take a wait-and-see attitude toward the issues, and the *Spring Hope Enterprise* opposed the sale notion. Exhibit 17–1 shows the *Graphic*'s editorial of April 7, 1995, which argues that there were savings to be made from thinning the bureaucracy and through greater economies of scale and implied that the employees of the hospital might be trying to protect a "cushy" pension plan. They were not under social security, but had their own fund instead. On the same day, the *Graphic* published an article that compared charges from 1992 discharge summaries from the North Carolina Medical Database Commission for seven high-volume procedures for Nash General, Duke University Medical Center in Durham, Pitt Memorial Hospital (the teaching hospital of East Carolina University Medical School in Greenville), and Wilson Memorial Hospital, the nearest large community hospital. The headline was "NGH rates highest in area, even tops Duke Med Center." Nash General had higher charges than Duke for four of the seven procedures—hip replacement, mastectomy, Caesarean section, and cardiac catheterization—but lower charges for appendectomy, normal newborn delivery, and hysterectomy. It was higher than Pitt for all seven and higher than Wilson for five out of seven. The article quoted Nash General spokesperson Jeff Hedgepath as saying that Nash reported day surgery separately through Nash Day Hospital, so the figures were not representative and differences in reporting methods could account for some of the discrepancies. Exhibit 17–2 shows the data presented by the *Graphic*.

On April 9, the *Telegram* interviewed Bryant Aldridge, President and CEO of Nash General, who emphasized the risks to the community in terms of indigent care inherent in a sale to a private owner. (His views are summarized in an article published in 1996 in *The News and Observer* of Raleigh, North Carolina, of which Exhibit 17–3 is an excerpt.) The *Telegram* noted that North Carolina law mandates that a public hospital sold to a private organization must offer the same

Exhibit 17–1 Editorial Appearing in the *Nashville Graphic*

DESERVES A HEARING

The *Nashville Graphic* spent 45 minutes on the phone Wednesday evening with a county commissioner discussing the hospital situation.

In a nutshell, he said, "I'm reluctant to hang out a 'For sale' sign." This is a position toward privatizing the hospital noticeably less warm than it was 30 days ago when he and the newspaper had spoken.

Less warm in spite of the fact that the need for the Nash-Rocky Mount School system to build new schools is no less great.

Less warm in spite of the fact that the $100 million or more that Nash County might realize from privatizing Nash General would not only help pay for new schools, but also help pay for other much needed things too.

Less warm in spite of the fact that Nash County realizes no property taxes from Nash General Hospital-owned properties.

Less warm in spite of the fact that through privatization, a thinned bureaucracy, and greater economies of scale, the hospital might be able to offer even more services for less cost.

Less warm in spite of the fact that Hospital Attorney Tom Young's offer of an up-front cash settlement of $10 million for extending the hospital lease by 20 years will, with the declining dollar, be a joke by the year 2015.

Less warm in spite of the fact that the profit picture for the hospital in the coming years appears bleak in light of the growing AIDS epidemic.

Who got to this commissioner in the intervening 30 days? Could it be the special interest called employees of the hospital who enjoy a reportedly cushy pension plan, and for that reason, are understandably nervous about any change?

Notwithstanding their legitimate concern, the idea of privatizing the hospital deserves a hearing, after which people may decide it's a bad idea. It does not deserve to be scuttled, as it could be if commissioners accept Young's offer when they next meet on April 26.

Source: Reprinted with permission from Deserves a Hearing, April 7, 1995, © 1995, *Nashville Graphic.*

---

services to the indigent that it did before the sale. Aldridge raised the issue of resale, so the *Telegram* interviewed a law professor at University of North Carolina at Chapel Hill who said that resale was not a problem and that the only way a successor corporation could avoid the indigent care requirement was to dissolve the company without a successor corporation.

The lease proposal could have been officially considered either at the commissioners' budget meeting on April 26 to hear budget recommendations from Nash County department heads or at their regularly scheduled May 1 meeting. On April 11, an editorial in the *Telegram* urged delaying the issue at least until September for more consideration.

Exhibit 17–2 Cost Comparison of Hospital Charges (All Costs in Dollars)

Procedure	Duke	Nash	Wilson	Pitt
Hip replacement	18943	26283	17498	15513
Appendectomy	6266	4887	4986	4210
Mastectomy	6397	6953	6113	5755
Caesarean section	5375	6815	5553	5246
Normal newborn delivery	2598	2441	2531	1974
Cardiac catheterization	8079	10316	8250	5364
Hysterectomy	8848	8283	6107	5867

Source: Reprinted with permission from Hospital Costs: NGH Rates Highest in Area, Even Tops Duke Medical Center, June 30, 1996, *Nashville Graphic.*

An April 13 editorial in the *Enterprise* observed:

> To get all this money, however, the citizens of Nash County are being asked to give up one of their best success stories and most important possessions—their public hospital. Built in 1971 for only $9 million, Nash General Hospital has expanded at virtually no taxpayer cost into a thriving health care complex consisting of hospital, day hospital, mental health hospital, heart center, emergency center, doctors' offices, and other health care services available to every citizen of Nash County. The hospital has provided, by its own figures, $50 million in charity care. Financially strong, it has also given financial assistance to Nash Community College's nursing program, support for the rescue squads, and provided health education for the public. . . .
>
> In all of this, Nash General Hospital remains owned by and accountable to the public. As a nonprofit corporation, the hospital's "profits" are retained as reserves or spent in expanding the county's health care services. Members of the hospital authority are appointed by the county commissioners, their meetings are open to the public, and hospital financial records are by law open to the public. Nash General Hospital has earned its share of criticism over the years and made its share of stupid mistakes, but its role as a public hospital has given the public the right to oversee and criticize its decisions. The public has no comparable rights or stake in private, for-profit hospitals, which are answerable to their stockholders. The state law governing sale of public hospitals to private, for-profit corporations provides some safeguards for the availability of services, but the law provides no guarantee those services will be either equal in quality or lower in cost. Pressures in the health care industry nationwide, for that matter, are becoming painful to all hospitals, public and private.

It never hurts to look at any idea, including selling the hospital. But the major issue must not be how much money the hospital sale can generate but whether Nash County health care needs are best met by keeping the hospital public or private. Studies may support the value of a private, for-profit hospital. But it would be absolutely wrong to lower—or risk lowering—the quality of Nash County's health care system simply to build schools the county can finance through other means. Nash County, after all, has the lowest property tax rate in the area. *(Source:* Reprinted with permission from Viewpoints: Sale of Hospital No Easy Decision, p. 4, April 13, 1995, © 1995, *Spring Hope Enterprise.)*

Exhibit 17–3 Excerpts from Profile of Bryant Aldridge

ROCKY MOUNT—When an anti-tax group urged Nash County to sell its hospital last year to raise some money, more than buildings were at stake. A piece of Bryant Aldridge would have gone to the auction block.

You can't separate the man from the medical campus.

Twenty-eight years ago, Aldridge was hired to build a new hospital for Nash County. In three years he did, on a one-time soybean field next to a highway still on the drawing board. Since then, he's helped transform what started as a community hospital into a modern health system.

The equipment and services have changed, but the hospital's original mission survives. All county residents are welcome, whether or not they have insurance. Support groups get started there. So do programs that bring compassionate people into patients' homes, such as hospice, which helps families confront death.

Turning the hospital into a profit-making venture could threaten some of that, Aldridge feared. . . .

"A lot of people out there are trying to make money buying and selling hospitals," Aldridge said, sitting in his modest office at what began as Nash General Hospital. "But selling a hospital to a private enterprise is giving up a responsibility: looking after people who cannot look after themselves."

As Nash Health Care Systems celebrates its quarter-century anniversary, it honors its soft-spoken but competitive president and his devotion to public hospitals.

"Health care is just like education. It's part of the basic infrastructure," said Aldridge, who is 62. "It should not be dictated to by how much money you have, but by what you need."

Aldridge was drawn to this work after a family friend, a doctor in his home town of Kinston (NC), said medicine badly needed good business minds.

Aldridge (Duke, 1956) was a football fullback, student leader and business student. He liked challenges and figured he could help.

After graduate school in Chicago (MHA, Northwestern, 1960), he worked at former Watts Hospital in Durham and Greenville General Hospital in South

continues

Exhibit 17–3 continued

Carolina. Nash County hired him after a $5.5 million bond issue narrowly passed to pay for a hospital that didn't have an address, or even a name.

He came with ideas and access to $3 million in federal funds. He envisioned a four-wing hospital shaped like a cross, with nurses' stations in the center, to economize on space on each floor. He wanted only single rooms, making Nash the first in the state to have what is now an industry standard.

With help from doctors and others, he went on a buying spree for beds, desks, operating room equipment, and everything else a hospital needs. "He must know every brick in the hospital," said David Webb, president of the local N.C. Area Health Education Center, which trains health workers in Nash and four nearby counties.

Running a hospital is not the flashiest of careers. But over the years, Aldridge developed a reputation for being a steady innovator in a quick-changing business. In 1983 when Congress put limits on what hospitals could charge Medicare patients, Aldridge opened a day hospital. It was cheaper to treat some people without admitting them. That approach is standard today.

When nursing shortages hit later that decade, he opposed giving newcomers perks that longtime employees might resent. But he rewarded longevity and people willing to work unpopular shifts. And he helped start a nurse training program at the local community college for an answer over the long term. "He's not looking for a quick fix," said Connie Gorham, Nash's nursing vice president who has worked with Aldridge since 1971. "His approach is to make people look for an answer over the long term."

Nash County, with an economy powered by manufacturing and some big-time agriculture, is growing like much of North Carolina. But income and employment rates lag behind state averages. The county's health needs are as diverse as its people. Some live in battered shacks on the edge of tobacco fields, others in roomy upscale homes that stand shoulder to shoulder on former farmland.

Under Aldridge's leadership, the brick hospital complex also grew, with a total budget of $154 million last year. Nash Health Care Systems acquired a struggling 29-bed mental health hospital that now provides psychiatric care and substance abuse treatment. A new rehabilitation hospital is in the works. Mindful that the Triangle hospitals would love to lure patients from his nearby county, Aldridge is fighting for state approval to open a heart surgery center at Nash with help from Pitt County Memorial Hospital (the teaching hospital of East Carolina University). Aldridge and his staff are doing their best to adapt to the demands of managed care, which encourages hospitals to discount their fees to attract patients. Internal publications brim with graphs celebrating cost-savings from shorter hospital stays and cheaper, outpatient surgery.

At times, the people of Nash County have shown affection for the man who passed up job offers to stick with what he started. When fire destroyed his home a few years ago, local people flooded his family with canned goods, pots and pans and trading stamps.

Source: Reprinted with permission from The Silver General of Nash's Hospital, pp. B1 and B7, June 30, 1996, © 1996, *The News and Observer* of Raleigh, North Carolina.

(The hospital's contribution to Nash Community College's nursing program, mentioned in the editorial, was substantial, amounting to $85000 in 1994.)

On April 20, the *Telegram* reported on an interview with Aldridge, in which he said, "I don't feel we should get into a public debate. Our board's position is that the hospital should not be sold." The article also quoted from a memo from Tom Young to Bryant Aldridge to the effect that, while the for-profit must continue to provide indigent care, it would be at a negotiated level at which there would be "no obligation to provide more as the need might increase because of demographic change or increases in the cost of such care in the future." The hospital's chief operating officer Rick Toomey also pointed to evidence from Florida that public hospitals provide more indigent care than private ones.

The public hearing on the hospital lease took place at 10 AM on May 1, 1995. Both sides were heard at this meeting, but the issue was not discussed by the commissioners, who agreed to postpone further discussion to their May 15 meeting but indicated that they would not necessarily act at that date. At the May 1 meeting, the representative of the Friends for Fiscal Responsibility asked the commissioners to postpone acting on the new lease and to pass a resolution of intent to sell. Under North Carolina law, this would require a public hearing, a bidding process requiring no less than five bids from interested companies, another public forum, and a decision on the winner. This process was supported by Roger Hall of Community Hospital of Rocky Mount. He reported that Community Health Systems of Tennessee, the parent company of Community Hospital, had sent the commissioners a letter of interest in the purchase of Nash General. He argued that private ownership did not imply reduced indigent care, noting that while Nash General's indigent load was 5% of its total business, Community Hospital's share was 11%. Many individuals spoke against privatization. Dr. K.D. Weeks, a lifelong Nash County resident with 50 years of medical experience, concluded that "to change ownership from 'our own' to a private, for-profit would be a forfeiture of our link to the past and an injustice to future generations to come."

At their May 15 meeting, the commissioners agreed by consensus that they would end discussion of the sale of the hospital and proceed to negotiating a new lease with the hospital authority. The commissioners, however, felt that the proposed term of the lease was much too long.

THE ALTERNATIVE LEASE

On May 19, Community Health Systems (CHS) sent the commissioners an unsolicited offer to lease Nash General Hospital for five years at a prepaid rental of $6 million per year. In the letter, Robert Hardison, CHS vice-president, stated that CHS was "committed to providing personalized care and efficient service to patients, with total satisfaction as a top priority" and "to providing indigent care for all citizens of Nash County on a need basis, but not to be less than now provided by both hospitals in the community." He also argued that "external influences and constraints in this industry have made it increasingly difficult for a stand-alone hospital to enjoy long-term success. CHS does have the corporate resources and expertise to back up the local administrative team to meet the individual needs of a community hospital." The letter is shown in Exhibit 17–4. The press also reported that CHS would also be willing to pay a rental of $6 million per year over a 20-year lease.

Many letters to the editor continued to appear in the local papers about these offers. One from Bill Newkirk, president of the Nash County National Association for the Advancement of Colored People, supported the hospital. He argued that the failure to maintain the facilities in the school system had been due to the objection of some people to the merger of the city and county school systems, a problem that went back 20 years, and that there were better ways to solve those problems.

THE COUNTER-OFFER

On April 24, the Nash Hospital Authority offered a revised lease proposal. The hospital authority would make a payment of $12 million in two annual installments starting in 1995 to the county in return for extending the existing lease two more years to the year 2000. In addition, the authority would pay the county an annual $250000 fee for five years starting in 1996, which was roughly equivalent to property taxes on the hospital. Such payment in lieu of taxes was believed by the North Carolina Hospital Association to be a first in the state by a public hospital. The lease also included a clause that would automatically extend it each year for one additional year. The window for renegotiating the lease would be the six months prior to May 2, 2000, but the new terms would not go into effect until the year 2004. The county commissioners accepted that offer in principle in a six-minute meeting. No mention was made of the Community Health Systems proposal. The commissioners also seemed to lean toward investing the $12 million as it was received, using the earned interest to forestall tax increases.

The local newspapers objected to the absence of a notice of that discussion, which came as part of the continued May 22 budget meeting. The *Graphic* even reported having checked with the North Carolina Press Association about whether this was a violation of the state's open meetings law and argued that it was.

The commissioners were scheduled to give final approval at their June 5 meeting. However, two commissioners objected to the May 1, 2004, effective termination date and the others agreed to discuss the "verbiage" in question at their July 10 meeting. At that meeting the contract was approved with one

Exhibit 17–4 Text of Letter from Community Health Systems

Dear Mr. Claude Mayo and County Commission Members

This letter is to confirm our level of interest in leasing Nash General Hospital. Our offer to lease Nash General Hospital *will be structured as a five year lease*. CHS is offering to pre-pay $30 million dollars in cash to the county for the privilege of leasing Nash General for five years. The final document will be structured in a manner to indemnify the county for any Medicare recapture that might occur as a result of this transaction.

It is hard to place a value at this point in time, not having any up-to-date finances and not having inspected the hospital, but I feel we could structure a lease that would be satisfactory to the county and would preserve and protect quality health care for the citizens of Nash County and Rocky Mount, North Carolina area. The county would be relieved of all debt associated with the hospital, and Community Health Systems would commit *to providing indigent care for all citizens of Nash County "on a need basis"* but not to be less than now provided by both hospitals in the community. Community Health Systems would be a tax-paying source for the county, paying sales, property and other appropriate taxes to Rocky Mount and Nash County. I would also like the opportunity to present additional information about our company, its background, financial position, cultural beliefs and operating philosophy. A full explanation of this philosophy which includes our *coverage of services, hospital board make up*, employees, physicians, and indigent care will be explained in our final proposal, should we be asked to provide one.

Company Background. Community Health Systems, Inc., a Delaware for-profit corporation, was formed in March, 1985 by senior hospital executives with extensive experience in building and operating successful multi-unit hospital management companies who recognized the opportunity in the non-urban health care market which was neglected by the larger hospital management companies. The company's business focus is to own, lease or manage community hospitals that are the sole or dominant health care providers in non-urban, growing communities. Since inception, CHS has grown to thirty-eight (38) acute care hospitals and two (2) psychiatric hospitals. The hospitals have a total of 3,785 licensed beds located in Alabama, Arizona, Arkansas, California, Florida, Georgia, Illinois, Kentucky, Louisiana, Mississippi, Missouri, North Carolina, Oklahoma, South Carolina, Tennessee, Texas and Virginia.

The company intends to grow through the continued implementation of operating efficiencies and expansion of services provided at its existing facilities, and the selective acquisition, lease or management of additional hospitals.

CHS became a publicly traded company in March, 1991. Its stock is traded on the NYSE under the symbol CYH.

Financial Position. CHS proposes to fund its obligations under this proposal with internally generated cash, currently in excess of $32 million. In addition, CHS currently maintains a $200 million revolving line of credit provided by a group of banks led by NationsBank of Tennessee.

continues

Exhibit 17–4 continued

During the past twenty-four months, CHS has raised in excess of $300 million for hospital leases and acquisitions, early debt retirement, general corporate purposes and working capital: approximately $125 million from banks and lenders, $90 million from the equity markets, and $100 million from the bond markets. The current funding capacity is indicative of the ongoing support for CHS's strategy of continued growth through the acquisition of community hospitals.

Statement of Beliefs. CHS has adopted a Statement of Beliefs summarizing our service commitment to patients, employees and physicians—the true "customers" of the company. The CHS Statement of Beliefs is as follows:

Community Health Systems is dedicated to providing personalized, caring and efficient service to patients, with total satisfaction as a top priority.

CHS recognizes the value of employees in providing quality, personalized care and encourages involvement through open communications and recognition systems.

CHS is committed to involving local physicians in partnership, both as consumers of service and as providers who play a key role in ensuring quality care.

Through quality services and innovation, Community Health Systems maintains its leadership in health care service delivery.

Operating Philosophy. The philosophy of CHS is that each community is different and that the success of each hospital depends on our assessment and plan of action to suit the "chemistry" of the local people, employees, medical staff, board, etc. Thus, CHS does not have a "cookie cutter" approach to running a hospital.

However, CHS does have the *corporate resources* and *expertise* to back up the local administrative team to meet the individual needs of a community hospital. CHS has been successfully built on the belief that community hospitals are not only needed, they also need to be successfully managed. The CHS concept is that the hospital gets the benefit of a "community" oriented Chief Executive Officer, a team of resources and experts for back-up and other benefits of a network of community hospitals. The external influences and constraints in this industry have made it increasingly difficult for a stand-alone hospital to enjoy long-term success. Our mission at CHS is very simple: to assume through lease, acquisition or contract management, the operating responsibility of hospitals that need access to additional resources that will assist them in becoming, or maintaining, their position as the dominant health care provider in their marketplace. Since its inception, CHS has succeeded in implementing its business plan in support of this mission. As an operating company that owns, leases and manages hospitals, CHS provides the advantage and affordability of additional resources and experts that may not typically be provided through other management services.

Finally, it is significant to the Company's success that its top executives bring to the team extensive experience in operating successful hospital management companies. CHS management directs an action plan for improvement, seeking to increase services by developing a strategic plan for each of the hospitals to meet the needs of

continues

Exhibit 17–4 continued

its individual market. The depth and expertise represented by the medical staff is assessed and additional physicians may be recruited as needed. Additional or expanded medical and surgical services, or specialized services, may be added according to the needs of each community and as approved by the governing board.

CHS is intentionally designed to be a "hands-on" hospital operating company, which is decentralized and flat in organizational structure. As well as being the proper management philosophy for community hospitals, CHS also believes that other benefits include (1) being more focused and responsive; (2) making quicker decisions and actions; (3) maintaining a modest overhead; and (4) delivering more personalized services to hospital patients, governing boards, medical staff and employees.

I trust this information will be enough to warrant further discussion in the future. We appreciate your consideration.

> Robert E. Hardison, Jr. FACHE
> Vice President
> Community Health Systems, Inc.

Source: Reprinted with permission from *Nashville Graphic.*

negative vote and one abstention. The *Graphic* stated that those who supported the lease should be voted out of office. The *Telegram* explained how it had remained unbiased on the issue. The *Enterprise* commended the commissioners, saying:

> The Friends group, and Community Health Systems, deserve some credit for putting an additional $12 million into general county coffers, because the hospital authority felt pressured to match Community's annual price offer. Fortunately, Nash General was able to take the money out of $22 million in reserves, so no damage was done to the hospital's financial position. But since Nash General is a county agency, all county officials did was to use money earmarked for health care for other purposes. Future payments, if any, must always take care never to restrict or hinder the hospital's primary purpose of providing quality care to Nash County residents.

RECENT DEVELOPMENTS

The five-year rolling lease for Nash General Hospital that renewed Nash Health Care Systems' (NHCS) franchise was quickly executed in late 1995. Claude Mayo, an insurance representative who was chairman of the Nash County Commissioners, said about Bryant Aldridge, the chief executive officer of NHCS,

"People figure if you are the chief executive of a large organization that you have to be an SOB. He's not, but he knows how to manage. When you have a winning pitcher, you don't take him out of the ballgame."

On June 10, 1996, Forstmann, Little, and Co., a private investment firm, announced its offer to purchase the stock of Community Health Systems for $1.1 billion. By the July 9, 1996, expiry date of its offer of $52 per share, Forstmann, Little announced that 97.6% of the shares of Community Health Systems had been tendered. Community Health Systems was dropped from Standard & Poor's SmallCap 600 Index and replaced by KinderCare Learning Centers. Community Hospital of Rocky Mount was the only operation belonging to CHS in North Carolina.

On January 30, 1997, Nash General Hospital announced the acquisition of Community Hospital in Rocky Mount for $12.3 million, effective February 1. At that time, Community Hospital had 50 beds and 180 employees, 65 of whom were full-time. The purchase was to be financed out of Nash General's reserves. NHCS financial staff estimated that the purchase price would be recouped through operational savings in two-and-a-half to three years.

In a prepared statement, Aldridge said that the "benefits to the patients of our area will be enormous . . . it will have a broad, positive impact from patient care to economics." He stated that NHCS would continue to operate Community Hospital as an acute care facility and would offer every employee the guarantee of a job for at least 60 days. After an unspecified transition period, all patients would be routed to Nash General. Local physicians were not affected very much by this move, since virtually all of them had admitting privileges at both hospitals. Community's employees were encouraged to apply for several jobs available at Nash General. One concern was that adequate staffing be maintained at Community until its operations were transferred.

The hospital authority and the Nashville headquarters of Community Health Systems had been negotiating for several weeks. However, the negotiations were kept secret until the day of the formal announcement. At the request of Forstmann, Little, and Co., individuals on the NHCS board and staff who were privy to the pending sale had to sign a release promising to indemnify the firm $1 million if they revealed that the negotiations were taking place. Jeff Herrin, managing editor of the *Rocky Mount Telegram*, wrote in an editorial on February 16 that

> Competition keeps managers on their toes. . . . That is why I think we're going to miss something now that Community Hospital is closed. . . .
>
> We can all appreciate Nash Health Care's position. If it didn't buy Community Hospital, what was to stop another company from stepping in and buying it? The deal made good business sense.
>
> But it should have been a matter of discussion for the public that the hospitals serve. Nash County owns Nash Health Care Systems. The

money used to purchase Community might have come from patient care revenues at Nash General, but as owners, we have a stake in the future too.

Nash County commissioners are elected directly by us. They have a considerable amount of power in determining taxes, zoning issues and future growth. But on this issue, a multi-million-dollar deal that has quite an impact on our community, Nash County commissioners had no say-so. They read about the purchase in the paper, along with the rest of us.

That needs to change. Nash County commissioners should relate to Nash Health Care Systems board members as they would any other advisory group. A decision as major as the expenditure of millions of dollars should be discussed in full by the county.

Buying Community Hospital might have seemed like a great idea to every resident in Nash County, despite the resulting loss of competition. But we should have had a chance to find that out for ourselves—before Nash Health Care Systems made the decisions for us. *(Source:* Reprinted with permission from Editorial, February 16, 1996, © 1996, *Rocky Mount Telegram.)*

On February 6, Aldridge announced that Community Hospital would be closed effective February 12. Its operating rooms would close at 7 AM on February 10 and the emergency department would close at midnight. All other Community patients would be transferred to Nash General by February 12. Nash General staff expected a 20%–25% increase in emergency department traffic after the merger. The 16-year-old Community Hospital facility and its 10-acre site was to be evaluated for other health-related uses.

On February 27, the engineer retained to evaluate the Community Hospital physical plant reported that the building would require $2.3 million in repairs to eliminate existing major safety hazards. "If state inspectors had found the code violations, they probably would have shut it down. It was a shocker." He observed that these violations came about because of "shortcuts" in the construction process. It would require replacement of room and floor supports with new steel ones and rewiring of bathrooms. In addition, the engineer recommended spending another $800000 to modernize the heating and air conditioning systems.

The possible uses of the acquired facility were presented to the NHCS board of directors at its February 27 meeting:

- Conversion to a long-term acute care facility for individuals on ventilators or with serious brain injuries would cost $3.4 million and could be done under existing NHCS licenses.
- Relocation of Coastal Plain psychiatric and counseling hospital after major renovations would cost $7.8 million.

- Conversion to a skilled nursing home or rest home facility would cost $4.46 million.
- Conversion to a rehabilitation hospital would cost about $6.07 million.
- Conversion to a wellness and fitness center, considered the least practical alternative, was estimated to cost $8.86 million.

CONCLUSION

This case study displays the contrasting points of view in the community. The three papers in the county seem to mirror positions on the right, center, and left of the political spectrum. The hospital authority form of organization removes the hospital from some of the complexities of local politics but also screens it from public view when the public's interests are at stake.

At no time did anyone outside the authority and the county commissions seem to know what the true financial position of the authority was, yet many were willing to attribute various values to it. Very large sums of money were involved compared to the operations of local government but with seemingly limited public oversight.

The decision of the county commissioners not to sell the hospital was an unusual one, seemingly related to local trust of the institution and its management. The decision of the local hospital authority to then buy the local for-profit hospital is even more unusual. The trends in the United States are in the opposite direction, and the saga of Nash General Hospital is—as always—unfinished. Many issues besides health status affect the provision of health care at the local level—taxation, race relations, political ideology, and political infighting are just a few. We should not forget that fact when looking at individual community-based public health decisions.

DISCUSSION QUESTIONS

1. Identify the major arguments for and against privatization of Nash General Hospital (through either sale or lease). Are there alternative interorganizational arrangements (see the structural models discussed in Chapter 11) that would potentially address the "for" arguments in this debate? Are there alternative arrangements that would potentially address the "against" arguments? Compare and contrast alternative interorganizational arrangements that might be considered as feasible alternatives to the privatization strategies under consideration in this case.
2. Identify and compare the predominant public health issues that are raised by the following:

- the consideration to sell Nash General Hospital
- the consideration to lease Nash General to a for-profit corporation
- the consideration to consolidate Community Hospital and Nash General

3. Compare the public health issues identified in Question 2 with those that emerge from the Medicaid managed care initiatives underway in Denver (Chapter 12), Portland (Chapter 14), Memphis (Chapter 15), and Milwaukee (Chapter 16). What similarities and differences can be identified among these issues?

4. Assess the role of the local media in defining the community health issues surrounding the hospital privatization debate in Nash County. From a public health perspective, what advantages and disadvantages emerge from the roles assumed by local media organizations in this debate?

CHAPTER 18

Case Study: Providing Public Health Services through an Integrated Delivery System in Mecklenburg County, NC

Stephen R. Keener, John W. Baker, and Glen P. Mays

Local government officials are experimenting with a variety of organizational and management strategies to address the growing demand for public services with static and even shrinking public resources. By the 1980s, most city and county governments had used some form of privatization strategy to deliver services or develop infrastructure in a manner characterized by improved efficiency and sustained quality.[1] When the services under consideration move from leaf collection or public transportation to the provision of public health services, the stakes are raised, because potential benefits and costs may be realized not only in the local treasury but also in the community's health status.

On October 1, 1995, the local public health officials of Mecklenburg County, North Carolina initiated a five-year agreement with Carolinas HealthCare System that endeavored both to sustain and improve the quality of public health services provided to county residents and to contain the costs of delivering these services. This newly formed alliance transferred the responsibility for providing a wide range of public health services from the county health department to a hospital-

Source: Adapted from S.R. Keener, J.W. Baker, and G.P. Mays, Providing Public Health Services through an Integrated Delivery System, *Quality Management in Health Care,* Vol. 5, No. 2, pp. 27–34, © 1997, Aspen Publishers, Inc.

The authors wish to thank individuals at the following organizations for their generous contributions of time and information: Carolinas HealthCare System; North Carolina Department of Environment, Health, and Natural Resources; and the Cecil G. Sheps Center for Health Services Research at the University of North Carolina at Chapel Hill.

based integrated delivery system. This chapter examines the quality management implications that emerged from this unique and innovative public health privatization initiative. First, the rationale and history of this initiative is presented, followed by an overview of the alliance's structure and operation. The remainder of this chapter offers an analysis of the existing approaches to quality management within the alliance and of the remaining and emerging challenges to quality management that have yet to be resolved.

RATIONALE AND HISTORY

Mecklenburg County is a metropolitan jurisdiction in the southern Piedmont region of North Carolina with approximately 580000 residents. A council-manager form of government oversees an annual budget of $940 million and 4700 employees. Growing public service needs and a comparatively static tax base led the Board of County Commissioners in 1993 to authorize the county manager to investigate privatization of a number of county services, including the health department. During this time, the Mecklenburg County health department employed 475 professionals and provided clinical preventive health services primarily to women and children in nine community locations, in addition to a full range of traditional, population-based public health services. Through privatization, the county hoped to curb the annual growth in health department expenditures while maintaining the provision of high-quality public health services in the community.

The Carolinas HealthCare System (CHS) is a quasi-governmental integrated regional health care system serving 12 counties in two states. Established in 1949 under the North Carolina Hospital Authority Act, it is technically a unit of state government but operates as a not-for-profit corporation. With an annual budget of $1.5 billion and 15000 employees, CHS consists of a tertiary care hospital, regional hospitals, long-term care facilities, a home health agency, and a network of physician practices. CHS was a natural choice for a public-private partnership because it shares a long history of collaboration with the county government. The county had privatized a number of health services to CHS over the previous 15 years, including a rest home formerly subsidized by the county, the state's largest nursing home, and the county's mental health center. Additionally, CHS's flag-ship hospital serves as the medical control for the area's emergency medical system and as a station for county social workers to enroll eligible hospital patients in Medicaid.

Both CHS and the county hoped to realize cost containment and quality improvement in the local public health system through an innovative strategy that transferred responsibility for performing most public health functions from the health department to the CHS system. The organizations hoped to achieve these objectives through four critical actions that would be taken through their alliance: eliminating duplication of services; creating economies of scale; realizing efficiencies through cost shifting; and exercising organizational agility. The alliance hoped to achieve this first action by consolidating and coordinating services that were provided independently by both CHS and the health department, such as the provision of preventive and primary care services to indigent patients. Similarly, the alliance hoped to realize economies of scale by merging operations and taking advantage of such benefits as volume discounts in purchasing supplies, shared use of equipment and clinical staff, and increased leverage in contracting.

The third action to be achieved by the alliance, cost shifting, involved the well-understood concept of spreading costs through an institution. A vertically integrated system appeared to offer unparalleled opportunities for using the cost-shifting strategy to achieve overall cost savings and quality improvement. In these systems, less profitable functions could be subsidized by other parts of the system that may benefit from these functions. In a system responsible for both public health services and hospital services, hospital services could subsidize unprofitable preventive health services, which could, in turn, improve overall hospital operation by reducing the number of non-emergent cases seen in the emergency department. The potential cost-shifting benefits of public health services could be realized to an even greater extent under managed care and capitated reimbursement arrangements, in which public health services could be used to increase system revenues by reducing the utilization of costly acute care services.

The fourth and final objective of the alliance, achieving organizational agility, would allow the public health system to remain optimally responsive to changes in the external environment. Compared to stand-alone public health agencies, a vertically integrated system could respond more effectively and efficiently to sudden changes in the health care needs of a community, due to the diversity of health resources and manpower contained within a single organizational structure. In this way, vertically integrated systems could mediate the financial and health status impacts of sudden environmental changes such as the resurgence of a communicable disease or the closure of a significant community health provider.

STRUCTURE AND OPERATION

The privatization initiative adopted by Mecklenburg County and CHS is structured around a contractual agreement under which the county pays CHS a fixed fee for providing a specified range of public health services traditionally offered by the county health department. Under the North Carolina state law, counties have broad powers to contract for a variety of services, though there are some regulatory constraints on the contracting of certain public health functions.[2,3] The agreement adopted by Mecklenburg County and CHS transfers the responsibility for providing all public health services that can legally be contracted to CHS. These services, which comprised approximately 80% of the health department's staff and resources, include:

- all direct clinical services, including maternity care; child health; family planning; dental services for children; the Special Supplemental Food Program for Women, Infants, and Children (WIC); services for special-needs children; childhood immunizations; sexually transmitted disease clinics; and tuberculosis clinics
- community services, including school health services; nursing visits to mothers and newborn; case management services for at-risk children, human immunodeficiency virus patients, and the elderly; respite care; and health education and outreach services for vulnerable and underserved populations
- support services, including administration, laboratory services, medical records, data and information processing, budgeting and purchasing, appointment scheduling and registration, and billing
- public health assessment and policy development activities, such as community diagnosis and needs assessment, epidemiologic surveillance, community-wide planning and agenda-setting, public and media relations, coalition-building, and community advocacy

A department of public health was established within CHS's Division of Education and Research to house the group of contracted services. All health department staff associated with these contracted services were offered employment with CHS at comparable salary and benefit levels. Moreover, contracted services continued to be provided in the original health department facilities, which were leased to CHS as part of the privatization agreement.

Under the agreement, the county health department maintains primary responsibility for managing and overseeing the contract with CHS, and for directly providing public health services that legally cannot be contracted out to another agency. These services, which accounted for approximately 20% of the health department's original budget, include:

- registration of births and deaths occurring in the county, and maintenance of these records
- communicable disease control services, including the identification and follow-up of people with communicable diseases, identification of contacts, and notification of those with tuberculosis and sexually transmitted diseases
- environmental health services, including inspection of food, lodging, and institutional establishments; individual on-site water supply and waste disposal systems; and lead-hazard abatement programs

The organizational location of the health department within the county government remains unchanged. The Mecklenburg Board of County Commissioners continues to be accountable for the health of the public by serving as the local board of health. The board oversees the actions of the local health director, who supervises the public health activities that remain the responsibility of the health department and monitors the contractual obligations of CHS in performing the contracted services.

The contract between Mecklenburg County and CHS takes the form of an interlocal agreement between the two governmental entities, which runs from October 1, 1995, to June 30, 2001. During the five-year term of this contract, county funding for all contracted services remains fixed at the fiscal year 1995–1996 level. This feature allows the interlocal agreement to function similarly to the capitated reimbursement contracts used by many managed care organizations. These arrangements provide a fixed fee to the contractor regardless of the level of services that is provided. Under these arrangements, contractors face strong financial incentives to improve the efficiency with which they deliver services, and to reduce the volume and intensity of services that are utilized by their clients.[4,5]

Improvements in service delivery efficiency lie at the heart of the privatization initiative's goals. The initiative is grounded on the premise that efficiencies may be gained through the four general strategies of duplication avoidance, economies of scale, cost shifting, and organizational agility. In contrast, reductions in service utilization have a more tenuous relationship with the initiative's goals. On one hand, this outcome may support the initiative's goals of improved efficiency and effectiveness in the public health system if it is achieved through strategies that improve community health, such as enhanced service coordination and improved access to preventive services and health education. On the other hand, reduced utilization may confound the initiative's goals if it is achieved through reductions in the availability and quality of public health services. These two competing incentives under capitated reimbursement arrangements give rise to the need for innovative and effective approaches to quality management within the CHS-Mecklenburg initiative.[6,7]

EXISTING APPROACHES TO QUALITY MANAGEMENT

The quality management strategies operational within the Mecklenburg initiative flow from three distinct sources. The local governance and advisory structure exists as the first and most basic system for quality management. Behind this structure, an extensive internal evaluation and monitoring system is in place, maintained jointly by a major, university-based health services research center and CHS's own research unit. A third quality management structure is administered by the state health agency, through a statewide local public health account-ability system. Together, these three structures form the mechanisms for ensuring that public health services remain available, accessible, and adequate for meeting the health needs of county residents under the CHS-Mecklenburg initiative.

Local Governance and Advisory Structures

Under the privatization agreement, the local health director retains direct responsibility for managing all aspects of the service contract with CHS, and for ensuring that all contract conditions are adequately performed. A major compo-nent of the director's performance review process, therefore, is based upon demonstrated success in contract enforcement. The health director reports di-rectly to the Board of County Commissioners, in its role as the local board of health. As elected officials, members of the board remain accountable to county residents for the health of the community under the privatization initiative.

A human services council composed of government officials, community leaders, and private citizens advises the board on issues related to health and human services within the county. Under the privatization initiative, this council acts as a vehicle for injecting informed public participation into the monitoring and evaluation efforts of the new public health system. The combined effects of these local structures enable the Mecklenburg County initiative to transfer service delivery responsibilities to an outside organization while retaining public ac-countability and local governance.

Local Evaluation and Monitoring System

Both county officials and CHS administrators are informed and supported in their quality management responsibilities by an extensive evaluation and moni-toring system maintained jointly by a university-based health services research center and CHS's own research entity. The monitoring system administered through this consortium is designed to evaluate the new public health delivery system along three dimensions: organizational structure, service processes, and community health outcomes. First, organizational structure will be monitored through an analysis of changes in the organization, location, and administration of public health services delivered in the county. For every program offered within the public health system, this analysis will include an evaluation of the scope of services, access to services, personnel responsible for providing services, staffing patterns, program funding, and program management. In addition to this descrip-tive evaluation, an analysis of productivity of labor will be conducted to examine issues of efficiency in the delivery of clinical services. The relationship between output and changes in the quality of labor will be examined according to total product, average product, and marginal product. Maintenance of discrete financial performance centers will allow accurate tracking of resource input for the contracted services.

Service process measures, a second group of measures used in the evaluation system, detect changes in service quality, utilization of services, appropriateness of care, and continuity of care. These measures may change as delivery processes change over time. Data collection will encompass those elements routinely collected by the county health department, elements routinely collected within the hospital setting, and elements collected specifically for evaluation purposes. Critical markers normally reported to the state health agency will be tracked on a regular basis to document changes in public health services delivered and clients served. This group of measures will be used to address questions such as how immunization services, prenatal care follow-up visits, and breast and cervical cancer screening services change once they are provided under the CHS system. Issues related to changes in demographics and client needs will also be examined. Changes in utilization patterns will be assessed by monitoring trends in the hospital and emergency department services rendered at CHS, such as changes in the demographics of patients served, volume and intensity of services rendered, patient case mix, and payment of bills.

The final set of evaluation measures, community health outcomes, includes indicators that must be monitored in the larger population of all county residents and over longer periods of time (one to three years) in order to assess system performance. Outcome evaluation will be specifically focused on the following indicators: immunization rates for two-year-olds; adequacy of prenatal care; low birth-weight rates; adolescent repeat pregnancy rates; interpregnancy intervals; cancer screening rates; and incidence of tuberculosis and sexually transmitted diseases. Additional outcome measures will be added to respond to changes in demographics and health threats, with priority given to areas of public concern, such as violence, substance abuse, and heart disease. Many of these outcomes are relatively resistant to short-term interventions, and therefore may require follow-up periods of 2 to 10 years to detect meaningful changes in system performance.

The evaluation and monitoring system established as part of the CHS-Mecklenburg initiative promises to provide both CHS administrators and county officials with valuable information about the performance of the initiative and its impact upon community health. Some of the indicators included in this system will offer relatively rapid feedback on the management and operation of this initiative, but others will require time lags of several years to produce valid estimates of impact, which clearly limits their value as quality management tools. Another limitation of this monitoring system is its exclusive reliance on single-institution comparisons over time. The use of cross-community and cross-institutional comparisons of quality and performance is imperative in the current environment of rapid change in health policies, resources, and practices. An evaluation effort underway at the state level promises to build upon the initiative's internal quality management efforts by offering a cross-community approach to quality assessment.

State Evaluation and Monitoring Structures

North Carolina's state health agency is currently finalizing an accountability system for evaluating the performance of local health departments in addressing the health needs of their jurisdictions. Although this system was developed independently of the privatization initiative in Mecklenburg County, it promises to offer valuable insight into the effects of the initiative on public health performance in the county, relative to the other local public health jurisdictions in the state. The evaluation tool is based on two sets of performance measures, each containing more than 30 indicators. One set of measures reflects the adequacy of local health department practices and services, such as the percentage of children eligible for Medicaid who are screened for lead. The second set of measures reflects health outcomes and risks in the community, such as the age-adjusted rates of heart disease mortality and childhood injury. These indicators are used to compute a composite score for each health department in each of the two dimensions, and then to rank-order each department on the basis of its performance scores.

The state accountability system may be used to track the performance of the newly privatized public health system in Mecklenburg County over time, relative to other systems in the state that remain county operated. This benchmarking approach may be refined to allow comparisons among only those public health systems with similar demographic and health-resource characteristics. The flexibility and multidimensionality of the state system promises to make it a valuable quality management tool not only for state policy makers and regulators, but also for those responsible for management of the CHS-Mecklenburg initiative.

REMAINING CHALLENGES FOR QUALITY MANAGEMENT

Collectively, the quality management approaches underway at local and state levels offer a promising system for ensuring the adequacy of public health services provided through the CHS-Mecklenburg initiative. Several important challenges in quality management remain to be addressed by the existing system, however. These challenges include implementing quality management for the full spectrum of essential public health practices, and integrating public health quality management approaches with other operational areas of CHS.

Quality Management for the Full Spectrum of Public Health Practices

The existing approaches to quality management within the initiative focus exclusively on the performance of personal and population-based health services, not addressing the critical public health roles in health assessment and policy development. These roles include activities in community needs assessment, epidemiologic surveillance, coalition-building, community advocacy, and community-wide planning. Responsibility for these vital functions is transferred to CHS under the interlocal agreement, but there are few existing mechanisms in place for ensuring that they are adequately performed by the contracting organization. The need for such mechanisms appears especially compelling, given the conclusion by the Institute of Medicine and other groups that these two public health functions are among the least adequately performed by public health agencies.[8-10]

The need for quality management strategies in the areas of public health assessment and policy development is also underscored by the inherent difficulties likely to be faced by an integrated health care system in performing these functions within a competitive health care market. Because of proprietary concerns, competing health systems and providers may be reluctant to share data and information that are needed by CHS to conduct community assessment activities. For similar reasons, some systems and providers may express an unwillingness to participate in community-wide initiatives and planning sessions led by CHS. These competitive pressures are likely to continue building with CHS's plans to participate in the newly forming capitated Medicaid market in Mecklenburg County.

These opportunities appear to merit targeted quality management approaches. Several validated approaches now exist for assessing organizational performance in the full spectrum of public health practices, including the areas of assessment and policy development.[9,11-13] Although difficulties in performance measurement remain,[14] the CHS-Mecklenburg initiative may benefit greatly by developing and testing new quality management approaches in these areas.

Integrating Public Health with Other Quality Management Approaches

An extensive quality management infrastructure exists for ensuring the availability, accessibility, and quality of public health services delivered through the CHS-Mecklenburg initiative, but little work has been done to date in integrating this infrastructure with existing quality management efforts in other operational areas of the system. A major objective of the initiative is to realize improvements in system efficiency and effectiveness through the integration of public health with other health care services and settings offered within the CHS system. This objective should be supported by quality management efforts that link public health practice with other functional areas within the system. These efforts might include activities such as tracking hospital admissions that are avoidable with proper utilization of public health services; comparing patient satisfaction rates among public health clients with those of other patients within the system; evaluating the proportion of all CHS patients who have some form of contact with the public health system and its community initiatives; or assessing the knowledge and attitudes of CHS physicians and staff regarding public health services and practices performed by the system.

These types of efforts may provide indications of the degree to which public health functions are integrated within the CHS system, and the extent to which improvements in system efficiency and effectiveness are realized through this integration. As the CHS system continues to expand, these integrated quality management approaches may offer strategies for assessing the public health impact of new system components, such as the new community-based primary care centers currently underway at CHS. Clearly, targeted quality management approaches, such as those currently in place, are essential for ensuring system accountability for public health performance under the CHS-Mecklenburg initiative. Nonetheless, integrated approaches to quality management may also prove valuable in realizing system-wide improvements in efficiency and effectiveness through the integration of public health with other health care services.

CONCLUSION

The CHS-Mecklenburg initiative represents a bold and innovative approach to ensuring an effective local public health system in the context of health care cost containment. The initiative is still too young to offer any definitive demonstrations of impact, but it does offer valuable insight into the quality management issues that emerge from privatization initiatives and the approaches that may be taken to address these issues. The existing quality management structures operating at both local and state levels promise to provide an effective framework for ensuring the availability and adequacy of public health services provided through the initiative. These quality management structures, like the CHS health care system itself, must continue to evolve and respond to emerging service and management needs.

DISCUSSION QUESTIONS

1. From a public health perspective, identify the major advantages and disadvantages of integrating public health within a larger hospital-based health system.

2. What alternative structural arrangements might have been employed to integrate the public health and hospital systems in Mecklenburg County? Discuss the strengths and weaknesses of these alternative arrangements.

3. Compare CHS with the public sector integrated delivery system serving Denver (Chapter 12). Note similarities and differences in the two systems' structures, operations, and political and economic environments.

4. What opportunities and challenges might the CHS system face in carrying out core public health functions once it enters the Medicaid managed care market in Mecklenburg County? How do these issues compare with those faced by the local public health agency serving Portland (Chapter 14)?

REFERENCES

1. White W. Competition: a privatization strategy. *Am City and County.* 1994;109:16.

2. North Carolina General Statutes, Chapter 153A-259.

3. North Carolina Administrative Code, Title 15A, Subchapter 25, Section 0200.

4. Rodwin MA. Conflicts in managed care. *N Engl J Med.* 1995;332:604–607.

5. Hillman AL. Financial incentives for physicians in HMOs—is there a conflict of interest? *N Engl J Med.* 1987;317:1743–1748.

6. Kassirer JP. Managed care and the morality of the marketplace. *N Engl J Med.* 1995;333:50–52.

7. Vladeck BC. Managed care and quality. *JAMA.* 1995;273:1483.

8. Institute of Medicine. *The Future of Public Health.* Washington, DC: American Public Health Association; 1988.

9. Miller CA, Moore KS, Richards TB, McKaig CA. A proposed method for assessing the performance of local public health functions and practices. *Am J Public Health.* 1994;84:1743–1749.

10. Richards TB, Rogers JJ, Christenson GM, Miller CA, et al. Evaluating local public health performance at a community level on a statewide basis. *J Public Health Manage Practice.* 1995; 1:70–83.

11. Miller CA, Moore KS, Richards TB, McKaig CA. A screening survey to assess local public health performance. *Public Health Rep.* 1994;109:659–664.

12. Studnicki J, Steverson B, Blais HN, Goley E, et al. Analyzing organizational practices in local health departments. *Public Health Rep.* 1994;109:485–490.

13. Turnock BJ, Handler A, Dyal WW, Christenson G, et al. Implementing and assessing organizational practices in local health departments. *Public Health Rep.* 1994;109:478–484.

14. Miller CA, Richards TB, Christenson GM, Koch GC. Creating and validating practical measures for assessing public health practice in local communities. *Am J Prev Med.* 1995;11:24–28.

CHAPTER 19

Case Study: Hospital Privatization as a Quality Improvement Strategy in Jersey City, NJ

Jonathan M. Metsch, Donald R. Haley, and Donald Malafronte

The health care industry is a hostile environment, and hospitals are struggling to survive. Faced with shrinking profits and financial insolvency, health care institutions are developing strategies of survival to adapt to an environment of reformation. Public hospitals are in a period of rapid change; these changes are driven by the underlying problems of the American health care system.[1] In an industry of decreasing reimbursement, capitation, and the acceptance of greater financial risk on the part of the health care provider, public hospitals are strategically positioning themselves to survive as an organization while reconstructing the ideology of their mission.

As managed care organizations increase their share of covered lives in a community, hospitals are faced with either insolvency or re-engineering in an effort to compete in a new environment characterized by capitated reimbursement and reduced utilization of health services. Los Angeles County-USC Medical Center, a public hospital system, for example, was confronted with closure under budget pressure unless the county could find $200 million to salvage the medical center.[2] Similarly, one analyst predicts that "New York City's public hospital corporation, which began in 1969, won't live to see its 30th birthday."[3] A hand-picked mayoral advisory panel recommended that New York City should abolish its municipal hospital system. The panel accused the city's Health and Hospitals Corporation of delivering inefficient, low-quality health services and asserted that

Source: Adapted from J.M. Metsch, D.R. Haley, and D. Malafronte, Privatization of a Public Hospital: A Quality Improvement Strategy, *Quality Management in Health Care*, Vol. 5, No. 2, pp. 19–26, © 1997, Aspen Publishers, Inc.

its 11 hospitals, clinics, nursing homes, and home health agencies could not compete in a marketplace dominated by managed care.[4]

These and other examples suggest that governments are looking for ways to save money. Public hospitals are being forced to drastically cut budgets, they are receiving fewer local tax dollars, and they are losing their patient base to the more efficient private hospitals. These forces are pushing the public health care system toward financial ruin.

In the changing world of health care, hospitals are adapting by developing strategies to gain market share and decrease costs and improve quality. As a result, health care providers are investing capital to form vertically integrated systems, join multihospital systems, and develop their own insurance products. However, in a culture where the theme is less government and lower taxes, the need for capital is forcing these institutions out of the public sector through privatization.

Privatization in the health care industry is on the rise because of "mounting fiscal pressures and popular concern about growth in government."[5] County governments often face the criticism of being too cumbersome to adapt to the rapidly evolving health care system.[6] The belief is that the consumer's freedom of choice and the greater autonomy of the provider will foster competition, thus maximizing quality while minimizing cost.[7] The cumbersome bureaucracies that are inherent to public institutions, however, may hinder government-owned health care organizations in their efforts to quickly adapt to competitive environments.

The objective of this chapter is to describe the privatization goals and process of one such governmental institution: the Jersey City Medical Center (JCMC). We will discuss the strategies that JCMC used to transform its organization and culture from a public institution to a privatization model and discuss lessons learned from the privatization process, its impact on quality, and the development of future strategies. As growing numbers of public institutions confront the realities of a changing health care system, it is critical that they benefit from those who have confronted similar challenges. This imperative exists not because the choices become easier, but because insight may be gained from the past which offers guidelines for the future.

PRIVATIZATION: PURPOSE AND PROCESS

The primary goal of privatization is to improve the efficiency of the institution and to increase the organization's productivity. Privatization shifts the authority and financial responsibility from the public governmental sector to the private sector by relieving the financial and administrative burden from government. This shift reportedly offers advantages in the marketplace by fostering competition and supporting the expectation that "markets work best when entrepreneurs and investors earn a profit."[8]

Over the past 15 years, JCMC has confronted many of the external and internal challenges posed by an increasingly competitive environment and a rigid governmental structure (Table 19–1). JCMC has long maintained a large inpatient-care capacity, which becomes increasingly difficult to support in an environment of growing managed care market share and reduced inpatient utilization. As is typical of public hospitals, the vast majority of JCMC admissions have been Medicaid beneficiaries and charity care patients. Most of these admissions have come from the emergency department.

The hospital filed for bankruptcy as a public hospital in 1983 and was in bankruptcy protection from 1983 to 1985. New Jersey's health care industry was rapidly changing as the state implemented controls on health care spending. For example, NJ became the first state to adopt diagnosis-related groups in 1980. At the same time that this cost-cutting strategy was started, hospitals were also ordered to impose a surcharge on insured patients to subsidize charity care. "Forced to impose exorbitant surcharges—some as high as 40%—to make up for their heavy burden of charity care, urban hospitals could no longer compete against suburban ones, whose well-insured, less acute clientele incurred fewer uncompensated costs."[9]

As a strategy to compete in a heavily regulated environment in which reimbursement will continue to decrease in response to the advancing presence of managed care, and to ease the escalating financial risk that was being imposed on the community, JCMC was privatized in 1988. Below, we highlight the three phases resulting from the privatization of Jersey City Medical Center: recovery, planning, and development.

Recovery Phase (1984–1989)

As a community institution, JCMC was established to guarantee health care to everyone who needed it. During this period of uncertain financial stability, the organization maintained its commitment to the core principles of this mission: providing appropriate, effective, and compassionate care; ensuring safe, well-equipped, and efficient facilities; supporting capable, qualified, and well-managed staff; providing sound medical education; and offering informed leadership that is responsive to changing community needs. The political environment necessitated

---

Table 19–1 Operational Characteristics of Jersey City Medical Center, 1995

Number of hospital beds	388
Number of admissions	19000
Percent of admissions from Medicaid and charity care patients	70%
Percent of admissions originating in emergency department	70%
Number of full-time equivalent staff	1850
1995 budget	$130000000

that JCMC incorporate an additional caveat. Under bankruptcy protection, it became the further purpose of JCMC to develop its self-sufficiency and fiscal integrity and to protect the locality against unwarranted financial burden.

Privatization offered one option for JCMC to maintain its commitment to mission while meeting its financial obligations. Economic theory suggests that the type of ownership may have a substantial impact on the quality, fiscal integrity, and performance of an organization. As Paul Starr suggests, "The overwhelming consensus is that private ownership is more efficient in providing private goods in competitive markets."[10] This rationale was adopted by JCMC as a primary strategic goal for the organization. During the recovery phase of JCMC, the organization prepared for privatization by stabilizing its structure and operation.

Under privatization, a host of strategies were implemented as part of a catch-up plan to get the hospital out of bankruptcy and back into business. These strategies focused on rebuilding the institution physically and culturally, and included:

- refocusing and strengthening services
- rebuilding human resources
- rebuilding and equipping the physical structure
- strengthening teaching programs
- stabilizing finances
- improving management systems
- resolving creditor claims
- terminating bankruptcy protection
- revising governance structures and processes
- redeveloping community support

In the recovery stage, primary emphasis was placed on refocusing, rebuilding, and strengthening JCMC under the imperative of financial stability. By the end of this stage, the organization was becoming financially stable, although it remained programmatically fragile. The organization then turned to the task of disenfranchising itself from the strict bureaucratic environment of a government entity. Privatization was viewed as an option that would allow the institution to rapidly adapt to a turbulent, competitive environment. As a result, JCMC was privatized, and the organization quickly moved into a planning phase for determining how best to compete in the marketplace.

Planning Phase (1989–1991)

During this stage, JCMC developed a plan for establishing a broad health care corporation, with JCMC as its centerpiece, that would extend beyond the confines of a traditional community hospital. Following privatization, affiliations with various health service providers offered opportunities for expansion and re-growth. Under the plan, JCMC continued to redevelop and support its hospital component, while also forging a network of integrated health care institutions and services. This network grew with the purpose of repositioning JCMC as a leader in the industry and a preeminent health care resource. As a result, the organization developed two missions: a network mission and an institutional mission. The network mission focused on developing and supporting JCMC as an institution through the network of integrated health services that would remain responsive to the health care needs of all community members. The institutional mission remained one of caregiving, teaching, and financial responsibility. Both of these missions continued to target all those who required health care, regardless of class, creed, race, type of illness, or ability to pay.

The goal of the institution became more precise as the plan for the strategic direction began to evolve. Recognizing its need to compete for increased market share and to positively improve its position within the community, the privatized entity invested capital in its programs and corporate culture.

During the planning process, JCMC leadership recognized that the organization's services must be easily accessible within the community in order to compete in the growing managed care environment. JCMC confronted the additional imperative that it must develop care plans and services that are reimbursable by the protocol imposed by third-party providers, and must develop a corporate culture that can adapt quickly to the unpredictability of the marketplace. As a result, the following strategies were planned to provide a foundation that will lead to the development of a fully integrated delivery system:

- implementing a system to recruit highly qualified medical staff
- developing a network of community-based services supported by a core of specialty and selected tertiary-care services
- recruiting qualified, capable, and well-managed nursing and support staff
- implementing a system to provide opportunity for personal growth and fair reward
- instituting postgraduate and continuing medical education programs that meet all the standards of respective specialty review boards
- investing in equipment that meets the advanced technical standards appropriate for a tertiary-care teaching center
- investing in continuing education for staff at all levels
- developing an improved system for community outreach
- ensuring the financial stability of the organization
- providing an environment of involved and informed leadership

JCMC began to reposition itself by strategically creating an environment to improve quality through its investment in staff, services, and alliances. This allowed a shift in corporate culture to develop. Managers were challenged and held accountable for salvaging existing programs. They recruited board-certified clinical staff and implemented a program that provided a systematic review of quality.

Administration also implemented a system that provided incentives that challenged managers to take risks. This new culture challenged managers to strive to be welcoming and responsive to the community and to identify community health care needs, to develop a motivated and appreciated work force, to be physician-friendly, and to develop benchmarking methods as a means to provide the best, most accessible care in their medical service area. As a result, this commitment to a privatization model shifting the corporate culture to one of competition in the marketplace promoted empowerment, horizontal relations, team building, and willingness to take risks.[11]

Development Phase (1991 to the Present)

The goal of the development phase, which is still in progress, is to construct an integrated delivery system as a means to gain market share and provide structure for global contracting. JCMC is "reinventing" itself and developing networks as an adaptation strategy to compete in an environment increasingly characterized by capitated reimbursement. Under managed care and capitation, health care organizations require the ability to provide a full range of health services in exchange for a fixed per-member fee.[12] As a result, the hospital becomes less of a focal point as a continuum of care begins to take form. In 1991, JCMC established Liberty Healthcare System (LHS) to provide structure and organization for the integrated delivery system. Through LHS, strategies are implemented to continue the development of networks and alliances that will move the organization toward a full vertically integrated delivery system. These strategies include:

- continuing to invest in programmatic development and expanding services
- developing transitional facilities
- creating consortia with other hospitals to maintain and develop residency programs
- forming a foundation for fundraising, board recruitment, community involvement, and corporate promotion
- developing health maintenance organization (HMO) products
- forming physician partnerships
- joining local alliances

These changes have transformed the culture of the hospital by fostering an environment of partnership with physicians through the development of primary care networks, instituting a system that provides an infrastructure to assume risk, and developing a health care delivery system that will assess the health care needs of the community (Exhibit 19–1).

These changes in organizational culture and philosophy provide a foundation for future strategies, such as further affiliations with additional residency programs, active negotiations to bring additional hospitals into the system, further physician partnerships, consolidation of services, and the creation of additional alliances for services. The goal of these future strategies is to provide a structure to develop further partnerships that link physicians, hospitals, and insurance products with capitated reimbursement so that the integrated delivery system becomes fully responsible—both financially and clinically—for the cost and quality of care it provides.[13]

LESSONS LEARNED FROM PRIVATIZATION OF HEALTH CARE DELIVERY SYSTEMS

The privatization of JCMC continues to support the development of an integrated delivery system. Although the emergence of LHS is an ongoing, dynamic activity, it is possible to suggest several lessons that may be useful to others involved in the privatization of a health care facility. Through the privatization process and the formation of an integrated delivery system, JCMC created a strategy to gain a competitive advantage in its medical service area. This competitive advantage is gained through power, pace, and position.[14,15]

Power

One of the most important sources of acquiring power as a competitive advantage is gained through the accumulation and effective combination of mass. A health care organization can acquire mass through the formation of strategic alliances and hospital consortia, through the acquisition of organizational units, and by participation in multihospital organizations. Through privatization, JCMC gained the capital to acquire several satellite hospitals, join a large regional multihospital network, and create community and auxiliary services, such as JCMC's HMO.

For example, JCMC's procurement of two tertiary-care facilities and its plans to build a new 300-bed replacement hospital promise to strengthen the system's power in the marketplace. Thus, as JCMC becomes an integrated delivery system, the organization becomes more attractive to third-party payers who have a desire

Exhibit 19–1 Components of Liberty Healthcare System

Jersey City Medical Center

- General acute care hospital
- Life safety/facilities program
- Regional perinatal center
- Level II trauma center
- Family health center
- Five-year emergency medical system (EMS) contract
- EMS communication center
- Surgical residency training center

Greenville Hospital (1989)

- General acute care hospital
- 86 beds
- 2701 admissions/year
- 241 full-time equivalent staff
- $19500000 annual budget

Meadowlands Hospital (1994)

- General acute care hospital
- 200 beds
- 11000 admissions/year
- 283 full-time equivalent staff
- $49000000 annual budget

Liberty Homecare (1994)

- Provides skilled home health care services as well as unskilled (homemaker) services

Hudson Cradle, Inc.

- Home for abandoned infants

Liberty Health Plan (1994)

- Independent practice association model HMO

Liberty Healthcare System Foundation (1991)

- Governs the development of the integrated delivery system

LHS Receivable Corporation (1993)

- For-profit corporation

continues

Exhibit 19–1 continued

- Bundles the receivables of system entities to enhance cash flow and fund balances
- Generates income stream to system by selling receivables of outside entities

Jersey Integrated Healthcare Practice (1995)

- Medical services organization
- Acquires and manages practice sites, medical equipment, nonclinical staff

Hudson Rehabilitation Institute (In Progress)

- A 30-bed, freestanding entity to be housed at Meadowlands Hospital
- Managed jointly with Mount Sinai Health System

Strategic Alliances

- Mount Sinai Health System (1995)
- St. George's University Medical School (1996)

Seton Hall University School of Graduate Medical Education (1990)

- Internal Medicine
- Pediatrics
- Obstetrics and gynecology
- Oral maxillofacial surgery
- General dentistry
- Orthopaedic surgery
- Ophthalmology

University of Medicine and Dentistry of New Jersey (1990)

- Orthopaedic surgery
- Ophthalmology

Jersey City Medical Center Faculty Practice Plans (1994)

- Liberty Medical Associates
- New Margaret Women's Health Institute
- Liberty Surgical Associates
- Liberty Anesthesia and Pain Management Services
- Liberty Child Health Services
- Hudson Laboratories P.A.

Horizon Health Center (1995)

- Federally qualified health center offering primary care services to women and children to contract with institutions that provide the comprehensive services that are geographically convenient for their covered lives. This power and presence becomes even greater with LHS's alliances and partnerships with other health care systems throughout the region.

Pace

One of the primary goals of privatization is to create an organizational culture that allows for the improved efficiency of the health care system. Thus, this shift of authority improves efficiency by eliminating the bureaucratic process imposed by governmental ownership. This improved efficiency is vital in our current health care environment, which is characterized by sudden change and unpredictability.

Through privatization, LHS created a structure that streamlines the decision-making process. The decision to join consortia and networks, acquire organizations to further the vertical and horizontal integration process, and the ability to form physician partnerships may be transacted quickly through the governing board or through the designated authority of administration. This streamlining of the decision-making process is not usually part of the structure or corporate culture of public institutions. In a competitive environment, it is imperative that health care institutions quickly establish and implement services that are attractive to their consumers and to contracting managed care institutions.

Position

"Strategies that derive their competitive advantage from the achievement of distinctive value in the marketplace"[14(p367)] can be achieved by pursuing low cost and a distinctive niche. Any health care organization offering a low-cost, quality product relative to its competition is in a strategic position to gain market share and deter potential entrants into the market.[16]

For example, direct contracting is provided through Liberty Healthcare System's HMO. This structure allows LHS to decrease its reliance on third-party payers and improve its profit margin relative to its competition. This decreased reliance on third-party payers eliminates or decreases LHS's fees paid to these payers. Consequently, the organization achieves flexibility in offering lower costs and lower charges and in improving its profit margin relative to its competition. Through the system's lower costs, network affiliations, and comprehensive services, the LHS is in a position to acquire a distinctive niche and further its goal to become "unavoidable" within its medical service area.

CONCLUSION

To compete in a capitated environment, hospitals in general and public hospitals in particular must form an integrated delivery system and join strategic alliances as a means to gain market share and ensure quality. The hospital, whether public or private, must transform its culture to strategically refocus itself from hospital to integrated delivery system and to pursue actions that will allow the system to "own" the patient, either directly through an HMO or other related insurance products.

The emphasis in health and hospital care has shifted from ownership of beds to ownership of patients. This ownership occurs directly through insurance products such as the HMO, as well as indirectly through the development of integrated groups of physicians, hospitals, and services that meet the needs of patients and insurers.

Public institutions must continue to build a commanding block of institutions, physician partnerships, and programs that are attractive to patients and important to payers. They must also maintain financial stability in order to achieve success in developing an integrated delivery system that will contend in a competitive marketplace. The organization's leadership must work toward the goal of becoming a preeminent and predominant health care provider in its service area. Preeminence entails the system's determination to enhance the scope, quality, and reputation of its services. Predominance refers to increased market share and improved financial strength through volume.

There is no longer a status quo to protect, and resources must not be wasted in the hope that things will settle back to the way they were. The only constant now is change, and only those organizations that can quickly and creatively adapt to a tumultuous environment and that are unencumbered by the past will succeed. The aim of a successful health care provider is to produce an efficient, dominant, integrated system, anchored by a more compact hospital and invigorated by other health delivery affiliates.

The ultimate goal of an integrated delivery system is to create a comprehensive health system composed of physicians, inpatient and outpatient care, home care, and preventive and wellness services that are geographically dispersed, yet efficient and fully coordinated. These partnerships may hold more potential for creating positive change in the way health care is delivered and the way costs are contained than any national mandate could.[12] This delivery system will assume and effectively manage the full risk for delivering services for a fixed payment, with one level of quality throughout the system. A fully integrated system will provide a comprehensive service continuum that is geographically dispersed, yet coordinated. It will align incentives between the physician, hospital, and insurance product.

Organizationally, the integrated delivery system will have one management and administrative support structure and a medical information system connecting all parts of the system, and costs and value will be continuously measured. Consumers will benefit from the availability of a product that is highly competitive in cost and quality, and that is more accessible within the community. To compete in a capitated environment, the goal of a hospital is to become part of a delivery system designed to improve the health of the population.[12] Due to their inherent bureaucracy and difficulty in adapting to changing environments, public hospitals are losing the battle in their attempt to compete in a competitive environment. With capitation on the horizon, privatization offers potential strategies for their survival.

Postscript

There are only two choices in the hostile environment of health services—anticipate or panic. JCMC has achieved success because it has anticipated. Anticipation must lead directly to strategy so that survival and success may continue. Events within health services today occur in milliseconds rather than days, and those involving JCMC have been no exception. The success JCMC now enjoys derives from its past efforts in rapidly transforming itself from a public hospital into a fully integrated delivery system known as Liberty Healthcare System. Currently, Liberty is engaged in negotiations to link with an emerging state-wide megasystem. These megasystems are among the newest and fastest growing organizational innovations to surface in New Jersey, and JCMC is poised to respond. Yet for JCMC/Liberty and any new partner, the priorities are clear: to secure, maintain, and enhance its mission.

DISCUSSION QUESTIONS

1. Identify the major factors that motivated officials in Jersey City to pursue a privatization strategy. How do these factors compare with the issues under consideration in the hospital privatization debate in Nash County, North Carolina (Chapter 17)?
2. What role did managed care play in the decision to privatize Jersey City Medical Center? To what extent were public health considerations (broadly defined) influential in the decision to privatize the hospital?
3. In what ways does the privatization strategy used for Jersey City Medical Center enhance the organization's ability to undertake community health activities? In what ways may this strategy limit the organization's abilities in this area?

4. As an alternative to privatization, what interorganizational arrangements (see Chapter 11) might have been employed to address the motivating factors identified in Question 1? Compare the strengths and weaknesses of these alternative strategies.

REFERENCES

1. Griffith JR. *The Well-Managed Community Hospital.* Ann Arbor, Mich: AUPHA Press; 1992.
2. Ross J. A dangerous domino. *Hosp and Health Networks.* 1995;69:34–37.
3. Hudson T. Sick & tired; reinventing the public health care system may be its only hope for survival. *Hosp and Health Networks.* 1995;69:28–32.
4. Rosenthal E. Mayor's advisors seek to dismantle hospital system. *NY Times.* August 16, 1995:A1.
5. Barry J. Privatization and environmental health service delivery. *J Environ Health.* 1994;56:33.
6. Gray BB. Shrinking county health systems change the face of public health. *Nurseweek.* 1995:13.
7. Banoob SN. Private and public financing—health care reform in Eastern and Central Europe. *World Health Forum.* 1994;15:329–334.
8. Leone R. Foreword. In: *Privatization and Public Hospitals: Choosing Wisely for New York City.* New York: Twentieth Century Fund Press; 1995.
9. Frankel D. USA: health-care reform in New Jersey. *Lancet.* 1993;341:41.
10. Starr P. The meaning of privatization. *Yale Law and Policy Rev.* 1988;6:6–41.
11. Shortell SM, Gillies RR, Devers KJ. Reinventing the American hospital. *Milbank Q.* 1995;73:131–160.
12. Davidson R. The community: where reform rolls on. *JAMA.* 1995;273:255.
13. Enthoven A. On the ideal market structure for third-party purchasing of health care. *JAMA.* 1995; 273:1474.
14. Luke RD, Begun JW. Strategy making in health care organizations. In: Shortell SM, Kaluzny AD, eds. *Health Care Management: Organizational Design and Behavior.* Chicago: Delmar Publishers; 1994:355–391.
15. Quinn JB. *Strategies for Change: Logical Incrementalism.* Homewood, Ill: Richard D Irwin, Inc; 1980.
16. Porter ME. *Competitive Strategy: Techniques for Analyzing Industries and Competitors.* New York: Free Press; 1980.

CHAPTER 20

Case Study: Privatizing the Mental Health System in King County, WA

Anne Y. Ilinitch and Curtis P. McLaughlin

In 1989 the Washington state legislature passed legislation that established a new framework for the management and delivery of public mental health care. Each county or group of counties with a combined population of at least 40000 was permitted to form a regional support network (RSN) responsible for local resource management, including planning, coordination, and authorization of residential and community services. The King County Regional Support Network (KCRSN) was established in 1990. KCRSN was charged with planning, administering, and ensuring the availability of mental health services in King County, which includes the city of Seattle. It is the largest RSN in the state in terms of population (almost half of the state), with a budget of over $80 million. It receives funds administered by the Mental Health Division (MHD) of the state Department of Social and Health Services (DSHS) and contracts with private mental health centers to provide services. MHD is responsible for certifying RSNs and licensing mental health agencies as providers. Providers worked for DSHS on a fee-for-service basis until the establishment of KCRSN, which then assumed that role. Quality assurance responsibilities are shared among DSHS, the RSN, and the providers. MHD assists with contractual noncompliance issues and provides problem-specific interventions.

The authors wish to thank individuals from the following organizations who contributed useful information to the development of this case study: Peregrine Associates; Washington State Department of Social and Health Services; King County Department of Human Services, Mental Health Division; Washington Advocates for the Mentally Ill; Deloitte & Touche; North Sound Regional Support Network; Pierce County Regional Support Network; Thurston-Mason County Regional Support Network; Mental Health North; and High Line Mental Health Services. This case study was originally developed as an integrative experience for first year MBA students at the University of Washington School of Business.

THE TITLE XIX WAIVER

The Mental Health Division of DSHS submitted a waiver request to the federal Health Care Financing Administration (HCFA) for a change in the structure of the Medicaid (Title XIX of the Social Security Act) program as it pertains to mental health services. This waiver was approved. It allowed the RSNs to add management of federal Medicaid funds to their current responsibilities for state funds. Medicaid costs were then split between 55% federal and 45% state and local funding; however, they were expected to be at 52% federal and 48% state and local by fiscal year (FY) 1995. This waiver also gave RSNs the option of shifting from traditional fee-for-service reimbursement to a capitated prepaid health plan (PHP). To contain the cost of Medicaid billings and the drain on the state budget, the level of funding for RSNs still providing fee-for-service reimbursement also would be capitated for the federally entitled population.

AUTHORIZATION TO PURSUE BECOMING A PREPAID HEALTH PLAN

In June 1993, the King County Council approved a resource management plan directing KCRSN to pursue the option of becoming a PHP. KCRSN argued to the council that becoming a PHP would allow it to consolidate management, to control expenses, and to achieve the appropriate balance between access to services, quality of care, and costs of care.

Under the fee-for-service method of reimbursement, health care providers have an economic incentive to overserve individuals, since the more times they see a person, the more revenue they generate. There may be a bias toward treating symptoms rather than the cause of the illness, and there is no economic incentive to provide preventive care. There is certainly no incentive for the provider to check whether or not the client is being served by someone else, a situation that encourages the duplication of services. Under a capitated managed care program, such as a PHP, the provider agency receives a flat rate per covered individual per day that varies with the severity of mental illness. There is no increase in funding for additional or repeated treatments. This payment system is intended to promote preventive care rather than acute care. Providers under a prepaid system would have no incentive to provide duplicate services to clients who are assigned to another provider, except in an emergency situation. Under a PHP, however, a watchdog agency is expected to monitor the quality of the prescribed treatments to ensure that the providers are not underserving their clients.

The initial oversight of mental health services in King County had been delegated by the King County Council to its appointed, voluntary citizen arm, the King County Mental Health Board. Administrative functions were performed by the County Mental Health Division, which then became KCRSN. The PHP method of contracting for services could essentially bypass the County Mental Health Board and the Mental Health Division and possibly KCRSN. Exhibits 20–1 and 20–2 indicate the criteria that an organization would have to meet to become a bidder for the PHP role.

MENTAL HEALTH ACTIVITIES IN KING COUNTY

In October 1993, the King County Mental Health Division reported that there were 157106 Medicaid enrollees in King County, 52% of whom were children, and that KCRSN had provided outpatient medical services to 8178 individuals eligible for Medicaid, consisting of 9.2% of the eligible adults and 1.57% of the children. The population of King County in 1993 was estimated to be 1590000 people. It was clear that the major risk under capitation was the latent demand for services among children. Up to this point, the constraint on services to children had been the number of providers available to treat them. There were estimates that 15000 children in King County suffered from some type of severe mental disturbance (defined as chronic mental disability, psychosis, or other behavioral disorders that require sustained treatment interventions for a year or more) and early diagnosis might lead to an escalation in long-term treatment costs. At least 60% of the severely disturbed children came from low-income families. However, low income did not necessarily equate with Medicaid eligibility, since the Washington cutoff was 61% of the federal poverty level of about $15000 per year for a family of four. The number of eligible children was expected to double as the new Medicaid requirements for screening of children, the Early and Periodic Screening, Diagnosis, and Treatment program, went into effect in Washington.

There was also an ill-defined responsibility to serve a non-Medicaid population of low-income individuals, including those drawing unemployment insurance, the working poor, and those with health insurance whose coverage had run out. There was also a high level of uncertainty about the size of the gap between those potentially eligible for Medicaid and those actually enrolled. The county estimated the total non-Medicaid group at 12% of the population, whereas the state DSHS estimated it at about 20%. There would be no additional funding from Medicaid to cover this population.

MENTAL HEALTH CATEGORIZATION

The categorization of mentally ill patients is relatively crude compared to the models used in other health care sectors. At the time of this case, four categories were in use in King County:

- Tier II long-term patients
- Tier III long-term patients

Exhibit 20–1 Sample PHP Solicitation Form Letter

Dear _____

The Medicaid payment and contracting system for community mental health services in the _____-county area of the _____ Regional Support Network (RSN) will change as of _____.

As an organization holding a full license as a mental health agency or certification as a regional support network, you are one of the potentially qualified entities that could become a Medicaid prepaid health plan (PHP) and manage mental health services to people covered by Medicaid throughout the catchment area of _____ Regional Support Network. The Coordinated Community Mental Health Plan permitted under an approved waiver from the federal Health Care Financing Administration is described in the enclosed waiver request and clarifications.

The qualifications of a PHP were outlined in the request to the federal government for approval of this program. Those qualifications are also outlined in the letter of interest. If your organization is interested and qualified to become the Medicaid mental health PHP for the _____-county service area, please complete the requested information and return no later than _____.

If only one letter of interest is received, the Mental Health Division will begin contract development with that organization. If more than one letter of interest is received from qualified organizations, a further selection process will be initiated. It is possible that the extended selection process will delay implementation in the _____ RSN service area past _____.

If you have any questions, please feel free to call me at _____.

Sincerely,

_____, Chief
Community Services
Mental Health Division

Source: Reprinted from Division of Mental Health, Department of Social and Health Services, Seattle, Washington.

- acute episodes/emergency cases
- Tier I patients with short-term treatment needs

The penetration rate (proportion of potential cases receiving care) for Tier II and Tier III cases was quite high due to the needs of these classes of patients; however, the penetration for the other two categories was unknown. By law, patients could not be prioritized by age, race, gender, or other categories—only by

Exhibit 20–2 Sample Letter of Interest

My organization is interested in becoming and qualified to become the prepaid health plan for Medicaid Community Mental Health Services for the _____-county services area of _____ RSN.

ORGANIZATION: _____

ADDRESS: _____
_____
_____

PHONE: _____

ADMINISTRATOR: _____

My organization meets the qualifications of RCW 71.24 by (indicate one):

_____ Being certified as a Regional Support Network
(Date of most recent certification: _____)

_____ Being fully licensed as a Mental Health Agency
(Date of most recent licensure: _____)

My organization meets the qualifications of RCW 48.44 as required by (indicate one):

_____ Being licensed as a Health Insuring Organization
(Date of most recent license: _____)

_____ Being certified as a Regional Support Network.

Please indicate whether your organization meets the following requirements.

___ Yes ___ No   1. A 24-hour crisis response system to resolve crises in the least restrictive manner possible, including emergency services, crisis intervention, crisis respite, investigation and detention services, and evaluation and treatment services.

___ Yes ___ No   2. Resource management services to plan, coordinate, and authorize outpatient residential and community support services administered under an Individual Service Plan (ISP) for priority populations including seven days a week, twenty-four hours a day availability of information regarding mentally ill adults' and children's enrollment in services; and access to ISP by county-designated mental health professionals, evaluation and treatment facilities, and others.

                                3. Demonstrated ability to:

___ Yes ___ No   a. Cover a full range of mental health services for children, elderly, minorities, disabled, and low-income priority popu-

continues

Exhibit 20–2 continued

	lations. In areas where a significant ethnic minority exists, as defined by department guidelines, the plan shall ensure that culturally relevant services are available and accessible to this population
___ Yes ___ No	b. Cover the full scope of waivered services
___ Yes ___ No	c. Meet the needs of the most serious and persistently mentally ill recipients, high utilizers of state and community inpatient care
___ Yes ___ No	d. Develop individualized tailored services packages for high need individuals
___ Yes ___ No	e. Design an array of services which meets the needs of specified geographic areas
___ Yes ___ No	f. Utilize existing community resources to the greatest extent possible
___ Yes ___ No	4. Collaborative agreements with the covered counties' Alcohol and Substance Abuse program, the DSHS regional office of the Division of Developmental Disabilities; the DSHS regional office of the Division of Aging and Adult Field Services; and the local AIDS Network to improve mental health services to mutual services populations, in accordance with state statute.
___ Yes ___ No	5. Admission and discharge planning agreements with state hospitals.
___ Yes ___ No	6. Linkage to a full range of residential options with the means to assess and place recipients.
___ Yes ___ No	7. Agreements with local evaluation and treatment facilities for inpatient care of covered recipients.
___ Yes ___ No	8. Submission of a comprehensive plan for children's mental health services in the covered area. This plan must incorporate the services available to children through Medicaid and non-Medicaid resources in accordance with state statute.

Signed:_____   _____
                                                          Name and Title/Date

(This form must be returned to _____, Mental Health Division, by close of business on _____.)

Source: Reprinted from Division of Mental Health, Department of Social and Health Services, Seattle, Washington.

"medical necessity," itself an imprecise term. Consequently, every patient must have access to basic levels of treatment. Exhibit 20–3 shows the standardized annual hourly limits and treatment time frames for each tier and subtier under the existing level of federal service guidelines. Subsequent allocation decisions then pertained to what other support services, such as vocational training, should be offered to the patient.

THE CURRENT KCRSN FEE-FOR-SERVICE PROCESS

Under the existing process, consumers entered the KCRSN system as Medicaid enrollees, as referrals from other social agencies, or as walk-ins. The consumer would visit a clinic and be evaluated by an attending psychiatrist, who decided whether treatment was appropriate and necessary and, if so, developed a treatment plan that also categorized the consumer into a tier and subtier. Once treatment was begun, billing occurred after each office visit. Under KCRSN, patient visits and outcomes would be stored in one or more of four separate databases:

1. the KCRSN database, which attempts to include information on patient demographics, diagnosis, treatments, and outcomes
2. the Community Hospital Admission and Registration System, a statewide hospital discharge database
3. the Medicaid management information system database maintained by the state DSHS office, consisting of Medicaid accounting data
4. HIIS, a state hospital information system

Exhibit 20–3 Washington Level of Service Guidelines: Standardized Treatment Time Frames and Annual Hourly Limits

Subtier	Description	Standardized Annual Hourly Limits	Treatment Time Frame
Ia	Brief treatment	<15	Up to 6 months
Ib	Aftercare	<15	Annual
IIa	Maintenance	>15–50	Annual
IIb	Brief intensive	>15–50*	Up to 3 months
IIc	Short-term rehabilitation	>50–80*	Up to 6 months
IIIa	Intensive/long-term treatment	>80–200*	Up to 9 months
IIIb	Exceptional care	>200	Up to 12 months

*Individuals authorized for these levels of care will be eligible for Ib authorization for aftercare. (Ib may also be the only level of care required for other individuals.)

No single common identifier was used in these four record systems, so the data could not be crossmatched for case management purposes.

DECISION TO HAVE A PREPAID HEALTH PLAN IN KING COUNTY

In 1993, King County decided to investigate the possibility of becoming a PHP. In a PHP system, subscribers pay a fixed fee to enroll in a plan. If they receive treatment, they may have to pay additional payments at the time of an office visit. Since the state was quite likely to cap payments to RSNs and PHPs at a fixed maximum and might reward those who developed PHPs, KCRSN had relatively little choice other than moving toward a PHP format. KCRSN presented two FY 1995 pro forma budgets to the county. The first showed significant losses under the existing payment system from the state and federal governments, which consisted of prospective payments per episode of illness, and fee-for-service at $70 per hour for children. An alternative budget showed a smaller loss, due to savings from the proposed PHP initiative. As the pro forma budget in Exhibit 20–4 shows, losses were expected even with the PHP process in place, because the upper payment limits set by the state and federal payers would fail to meet the allowable Medicaid reimbursements. This was despite the very low levels of aftercare being provided to the more severely ill patients. The PHP effort was to pay off in the long run through case management efforts that would reduce the case mix for adults in Tiers IIc, IIIa, and IIIb and increase the number in Tier IIa, and reduce the number of children in Tiers II and III and increase the number in Tier I. These changes could be accomplished through reductions in long-term outpatient treatment and inpatient hospitalizations through an early intervention and stabilization approach. For example, the monthly premium rates per enrollee in the North Sound RSN contract for the period July 1994 to June 1995 were:

Tier	Adult	Child
Tier I		
Categorically needy	$ 2.34	$ 1.73
Medically needy	2.36	2.16
Disabled	4.52	3.59
Tier II	456.00	491.00
Tier III	1598.00	1486.00

The HCFA waiver and the contract both addressed the issue of case mix by establishing a maximum consideration rate that the compensation per enrollee could not exceed, regardless of how skewed to the high side the case mix became. This was intended to control the tendency of the PHP to classify cases into the higher categories, similar to the concern about "DRG (diagnosis-related group) creep" in hospital services. For North Sound RSN's contract, the first one developed, this average monthly rate had been set at:

Type of Tier I Patient	Adult	Child
Categorically needy	$ 13.73	$ 15.69
Medically needy	10.05	8.71
Disabled	118.90	53.56

The categorically needy population included those eligible for Medicaid due to their participation in other programs such as Aid to Families with Dependent Children, whereas the medically needy were those who qualified for Medicaid only, and the disabled included those who had qualified under Social Security for Supplemental Security Income (SSI) based on their disabled status and, therefore, also qualified for Medicaid. Many chronically mentally ill patients had qualified as disabled for SSI and were at the same time in the Tier II and Tier III categories, which is why the maximum monthly payment for the disabled was so much higher than for the other two populations.

Exhibit 20–4 1995 Fiscal Year Pro Forma Budget of KCRSN, Assuming PHP in Effect

Revenue		
Medicaid PHP-related		
Federal Medicaid adult	$21945782	
Federal Medicaid children	12758295	
State Medicaid adult	20282008	
State Medicaid children	11791051	
Medicaid administrative (5%)	3338857	
Other RSN activities	5591479	
Subtotal		$75707472
Other RSN programs		
Block grants and other support	$5033761	
Reserve funds	2200000	
Total revenue		$82941233
Expenses		
Adult care Medicaid and crossovers	$21147406	
Adult care non-Medicaid	7240637	
Child care Medicaid	24548346	
Child care non-Medicaid	4091682	
Board and domiciliary services	3750463	
Evaluation and treatment centers	6691389	
RSN crisis and commitment services	3923311	
Other RSN services	4840861	
County administrative costs	4147062	
Reserves	8044324	
Total expenses		$88425481
Budgeted loss		$5484248

When Washington state submitted its waiver request to HCFA in 1993, its actuarial consultants, Milliman and Robertson, Inc., had estimated the statewide FY1994 payment rates at:

	Adult	Child
Tier I		
Categorically needy	$1.60	$1.15
Medically needy	1.35	1.81
Disabled	3.92	2.56
Tier II	357.00	457.00
Tier III	1193.00	1445.00

and the maximum Tier I monthly payment rates for the same period at:

	Adult	Child
Categorically needy	$7.86	$10.28
Medically needy	7.68	9.45
Disabled	75.42	38.69

That same report estimated the same data by RSN. For King County and North Sound RSNs these estimates were:

	Adult	Child
Tier I		
Categorically needy		
North Sound	$2.31	$1.47
King County	1.22	0.66
Medically needy		
North Sound	2.16	1.81
King County	1.22	0.97
Disabled		
North Sound	3.84	2.91
King County	3.63	1.51
Tier II		
North Sound	411.00	470.00
King County	352.00	569.00
Tier III		
North Sound	1230.00	1446.00
King County	1164.00	1723.00

The comparable maximum allowable Tier I rates for the two counties were calculated to have been:

	Adult	Child
Categorically needy		
North Sound	$13.41	$14.99
King County	7.97	8.24

Medically needy		
North Sound	11.09	12.43
King County	12.80	6.96
Disabled		
North Sound	93.03	50.26
King County	94.67	39.30

All enrollees were considered to be in Tier I unless specifically diagnosed and given a treatment plan that would warrant a Tier II or Tier III classification.

IMPLEMENTATION PROBLEMS

The tier definition tended to differ from analysis to analysis depending on whether the analysis was ex-post or ex-ante. The actuaries who prepared the waiver estimates used 1992 data and classified as Tier I recipients those who received 15 or fewer standardized hours of rehabilitative mental health services in 1992, those receiving 15–80 hours as Tier II, and those receiving more than 80 standardized hours per year as Tier III. The North Sound RSN capitated care contract defined Tier I as all Medicaid recipients who resided within the RSN's service area. Tier II patients were defined as the chronically mentally ill, severely emotionally disturbed children, and those who were "seriously disturbed" and at risk of becoming chronically mentally ill. Tier III patients would have to meet the Tier II requirements and were also expected to be high utilizers of services, including inpatient psychiatric care, to have experienced more than one jail or detention episode in the past year, to be homeless, to have experienced two or more out-of-home placements in the past year if under 21, to require interpreters (including the deaf), or to be involved with multiple counseling agencies, including those for alcohol/substance abuse, school problems, acquired immune deficiency syndrome case management, child protective services, and so on.

One can see how these ex-ante and ex-post conflicts could continue if a mental health center made a diagnostic classification and treated a patient and then a behavioral health care management company challenged that classification and authorized payment only at a lower level. Such a difference of opinion with the auditors could bankrupt a PHP or health center very quickly.

Given this information, the Metropolitan King County Council authorized KCRSN to proceed with seeking PHP status, and the procedure was for the state DSHS to go out for bids to existing agencies in the area. Exhibits 20–1 and 20–2 show the bidding procedure. So far, the only bidders for PHP status had been RSNs, and until Peregrine–Northwest, a for-profit provider of both outpatient and inpatient services to the state and county, began indicating that they were thinking of bidding, the county had not even considered competitive bidding. When they heard that Peregrine–Northwest might team up with a behavioral health care management company, KCRSN also sought an alliance with a behavioral health management company.

PRIVATIZATION OPTIONS

The state could encourage both for-profits and nonprofits to bid; however, the ground rules allowed only existing mental health agencies to bid, and Peregrine–Northwest was the only for-profit in this category in King County. Senior staff at the county level were open in their distrust of having for-profit firms as the lead contractor. The distrust of for-profit agencies was couched in terms of concern about whether or not they would use other allocation criteria that would lead to the curtailing of basic services to certain segments of the population in order to maintain their desired profit margins. This concern was certainly heightened by reports that for-profit health maintenance organizations and managed care organizations were setting arbitrary limits on treatments and discriminating against those enrollees who incurred higher mental health care costs.

This issue of discrimination has been heightened by the fact that there are relatively little cost data on specific treatments. Unlike the DRG system used to classify and cost medical hospitalizations, the *Diagnostic and Statistical Manual of Mental Disorders*[1] has not been associated with cost-collection or rate-setting scales. This is primarily due to the variability of outcomes experienced in the delivery of mental health services and the lack of record systems that link treatment data to outcome data.

PROVIDER AGENCIES

Mental health care in King County was provided by a network of autonomous health care service centers that operated as critical care outpatient clinics or short-term intervention inpatient clinics. The 1989 state law delineated the role of this network of providers as a more economical care system to meet the short-term needs of people with mental illness who had previously been treated in state hospitals. Providers contracting with the state under the initial fee-for-service reimbursement model submitted bills to the Medicaid program for both federal and state funds. Providers excluded by an RSN could appeal to the state. All of the accepted providers were nonprofits except for Peregrine–Northwest.

Exhibit 20–5 shows audit information on 16 of the 20 or so providers to KCRSN during FY 1992. It is clear that there was a great deal of variability in costs per patient within the three tiers.

Exhibit 20–5 Audited Cost per Patient for Selected King County RSN Providers

Agency	Number of Tier I cases	Average cost per Tier I case	Number of Tier II cases	Average cost per Tier II case	Number of Tier III cases	Average cost per Tier III case
A	396	$428	468	$3001	227	$16846
B	158	467	317	5422	152	13195
Peregrine–Northwest	270	410	317	4406	189	14703
D	271	397	260	3153	143	11248
E	221	318	413	2628	132	3025
F	908	260	373	1676	80	2950
G	256	379	307	2417	34	4995
H	29	596	126	4583	9	3852
I	93	696	95	3094	8	12006
J	177	590	136	2056	4	5112
K	174	358	125	1174	31	2207
L	39	665	74	3044	3	3402
M	19	575	30	3297	12	9547
N	55	428	38	2154	3	18613
O	82	240	22	1622	3	5667
P	90	43	143	170	28	547
Total cases	3238		3244		1058	
Average cost		$369		$3025		$10827

PEREGRINE–NORTHWEST

Peregrine Associates, established in 1991, is a small subchapter-S corporation (that is, profits flow to the shareholders and are taxed as ordinary income). It is affiliated with Northwest Mental Health Services, Inc., and the Northwest Evaluation and Treatment Center, two providers that served King County's mental health patients. Peregrine executives sit on the boards of directors of these companies and provide management direction for both of them. Peregrine was established by the founders of these two organizations as a way to provide them with executive management services, while the employees assumed actual ownership through an employee stock ownership plan (ESOP). Peregrine has a demonstrated ability to get Medicaid-eligible people onto the Medicaid rolls and has shown good cost-control skills. Peregrine was seriously considering bidding for the PHP administration contract because its leaders felt that they could offer higher-quality mental health services at a significantly lower cost, maximizing the return to the owners of the company. Exhibit 20–6 compares Peregrine–Northwest's cost structure with that of the 15 nonprofit organizations shown in Exhibit 20–5. Peregrine–Northwest had a somewhat higher pretax profit ratio, but approximately the same after-tax profit ratio.

Northwest Mental Health Services and Northwest Evaluation and Treatment Center are wholly owned subsidiaries of United Northwest Securities, Inc., the holding company through which the ESOP is offered (see Figure 20–1). Northwest Mental Health Services was established in 1987 and employs 150 persons. It was currently under a fee-for-service contract to King County to serve more than 850 people with severe mental illness, primarily in the south King County area. The company provides patients with inpatient services through a contractual arrangement with the Department of Psychiatry at Valley Medical Center in Renton.

Northwest Evaluation and Treatment Center, established in 1984, is a residential facility providing acute psychiatric services to involuntarily detained and committed mentally ill adults who reside in King County. The Center employs 50 full-time staff and is currently under contract to the county to provide services for

Exhibit 20–6 Cost Ratios for Selected King County Providers in Exhibit 20–5

	Total of 15 nonprofits		Peregrine– Northwest	
Net revenues and support	$77079000	100%	$9597000	100%
Excess of revenue over expenses before tax	1955000	2.54%	361000	3.9%
Income tax	0	—	123000	1.3%
Revenues				
Donations and grants	11624000	15.0%	0	—
KCRSN contract	50380000	65.4%	8155000	85.0%
Private patients	9515000	12.3%	1442000	15.0%
Other sources	5550000	7.2%	0	—
Expenses				
Salaries	53841000	69.9%	5326000	55.5%
Facilities	4327000	5.6%	656000	6.8%
Professional contract services	5872000	7.6%	1694000	17.7%
Inpatient program expenses	686000	0.9%	0	—
Interest expense	573000	0.7%	0	—
Depreciation	1269000	1.6%	100000	1.0%
Other expenses	8558000	11.1%	1468000	15.3%

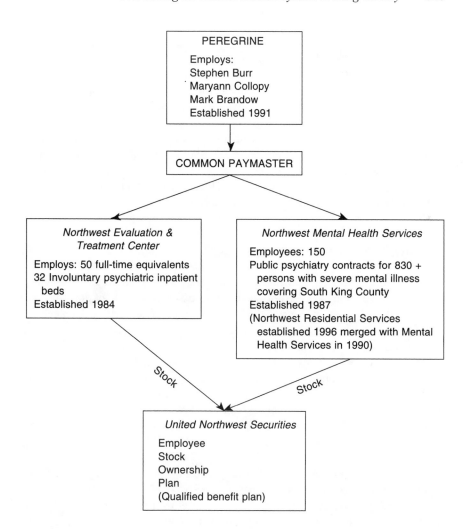

Figure 20–1 Organizational Structure of Peregrine–Northwest Corporate Network. Courtesy of Peregrine, Seattle, Washington.

up to 32 involuntarily committed inpatients on an ongoing basis. Northwest Evaluation and Treatment Center provided inpatient hospitalization services under a capitated payment state contract calling for payment of about $250 per patient per day, whereas state hospital costs were averaging about $600.

Peregrine's three founders believed that their collective, hands-on experience, both as providers and as administrators in the present system, would enable them to add value to King County's mental health program in the role of executive administrator of a PHP. Peregrine had acquired a reputation with the county for providing quality care through its clinics. The company had also gained additional respect from its record of running its clinics profitably and for its careful management practices. The only portion of the PHP skills requirement the company lacked was the risk management part, since the Northwest Evaluation and Treatment Center contract, while at a fixed rate, called for a fixed number of beds to be filled.

Peregrine's management recognized that enrollment in traditional, fee-for-service indemnity mental health plans was declining, and that independent health providers who relied on this type of business would be at an increasing disadvantage. Managers and their associates believed that they would have to redefine their role and methods of operation if they were to continue to be players in the mental health care system.

THE ROLE OF THE STATE DSHS

In addition to the requirements listed in the letter, DSHS would consider a number of other factors, namely efficiency, the cost-effectiveness of the proposed PHP, and the relationship between the RSN and the proposed PHP with respect to allocation of funds. Finally, DSHS would consider the proposed PHP's relationships and links to other mental health service systems.

DSHS had not yet faced a competitive bidding situation. In all instances so far, the RSNs and the counties had not faced competitive bids, and no selection procedure was utilized. If DSHS were to receive a bid to become a PHP from a qualified mental health agency other than an RSN, it would have to establish a structure within state guidelines for competitive bidding. According to the director of MHD, any competitive bidding process would take 90–120 days to complete.

Heretofore, the only designated PHP administrators in the state had been RSNs: Pierce County (Tacoma) RSN, North Sound RSN, and Thurston-Mason (Olympia) RSN. Pierce County RSN started functioning as the PHP in October 1993. No other bidders had been considered in awarding the contract. It was receiving $450 per month per enrolled patient under 21 and $520 per month for adults. These figures were derived from a utilization review, provider surveys, and state actuarial data. The number of enrolled patients was estimated prospectively monthly from the data on the number of people eligible for Medicaid in the catchment area. Pierce County RSN contracted in turn with six mental health care providers: three mental health centers with major hospitals and three other specialty agencies, one concerned with Hispanic patients and two concerned with children.

The chief of the Washington state MHD outlined her concerns and the issues to be addressed if a non-RSN were to bid to become the PHP for a given area. She questioned whether a non-RSN would have the necessary system linkages that a functioning RSN would have. For example, a non-RSN as PHP would have to initiate and establish the relationships and working agreements necessary to fulfill contract terms such as 24-hour crisis response. Another concern of hers was the climate after a competitive bidding situation: could the RSN that had lost the bid be an unbiased supervisor for the new PHP in the area of quality assurance? Secondly, there could be problems in getting the other providers to cooperate with the new PHP who was a former competitor of theirs. This conflict of interest could also be exacerbated by the passage of Initiative 601, which limited all state spending to population growth and inflationary increases. The governor had already requested all state agencies to prepare a 2% budget cut scenario.

PEREGRINE'S DILEMMA

Peregrine management felt that it could both cut costs and increase capitated enrollment under a PHP system. They believed that many patients were currently receiving unnecessary, duplicate treatments from more than one provider under the fee-for-service system. It was difficult to track down this duplicated service, with the visit data in many separate databases. However, if Peregrine won the bid, it could check all the databases and build a common patient record file.

Peregrine could save money by assigning cases to the more effective and efficient providers and dropping those who were not performing well. Additionally, if the patients stayed within the Medicaid mental health system for at least two years, Peregrine could benefit from investments in prevention, thus reducing the number of episodes of severe mental illness.

With revenue based on Medicaid enrollment under the capitation alternative, Peregrine felt that it could do a superior job of finding and placing on the Medicaid rolls patients who were not currently enrolled nor receiving treatment. It felt that there were many patients eligible for Medicaid who had not been enrolled yet. However, it was probable that total payments would be capped eventually, even under the capitation system, that enrollment would not be a completely open-ended source of revenue, and that the state would put a budgetary limit on its liability somehow.

There was also the issue that KCRSN might choose to bid for the business to preserve its franchise, to maintain control of the system, and to provide employment security for its current employees, although it was estimated that its employment level might drop by as much as 50% anyway if it became the PHP but did not have to process individual payment claims. Therefore, it would be likely that KCRSN would be in the position of being a competitor in the bidding process, as well as being in part judge and jury for the process. Any potential PHP contractor could also form alliances with other potential bidders to fulfill all the functions expected of the PHP contract, including ones with KCRSN.

When asked what new challenges Peregrine might face if it became the PHP, the Pierce County RSN director quickly cited the political factors affecting resource allocation in a region. There were pressures from advocacy groups such as the Washington Alliance for the Mentally Ill and from the King County Council, whose members might favor certain mental health centers or patient subgroups. The biggest challenge, however, would be the threat of miscalculating the costs involved and having to incur losses for the life of the contract. Some of that risk could be passed on to subcontractors and some of it could be covered by a reinsurance policy, but the risks would remain high.

KCRSN felt that it could safely assume the risk associated with being a PHP and still provide the quality of service demanded by the patients and their advocates. Utilization review was the key to achieving this. There was, however, one loophole to capitation that concerned most policy analysts: the capitation did not include or cover inpatient services, which were funded separately through direct contracts between the state of Washington and the institutions. Therefore, observers were concerned that the PHPs might tend to meet their resource utilization targets by transferring the most resource-intensive cases to the state institutions.

PEREGRINE'S CHOICES

It was clear that the mental health bureaucracy, particularly at the county level, was hoping that Peregrine would not bid and that it could continue all the functions that it had carried out before. Yet Peregrine's managers were concerned that if they did not bid and KCRSN became the PHP, it might reduce the number of providers, and Peregrine–Northwest had no guarantee of a seat at the table— especially since some county staff had already expressed irritation with Peregrine for threatening to force competitive bidding. Peregrine's managers not only felt that they could do the PHP job and do it properly at a profit, they also believed that winning the PHP contract might be the only way to ensure the firm's survival.

CONCLUSION

This case study illustrates a number of issues discussed earlier in this book. The mental health programs in the state of Washington were already moving from being government agencies to quasi-governmental status. The change undertaken at the time of the case moved the programs even further toward privatization through a contracting mechanism. However, there are still major issues of accountability to be addressed, as well as whether the private for-profit sector should have a role in the mental health managed care arena. There is also the issue of whether access can be significantly improved when the budget is cut.

Peregrine–Northwest's dilemma is whether a for-profit provider of services to KCRSN should bid against that agency. In fact, that agency appears to be both judge and jury in the bidding process, leaving Peregrine–Northwest in a very uncomfortable position. It is clear that the agency realizes the threat to its jobs and its budgets and is opposed to bid from a for-profit, although it may be willing to partner with one. There is no apparent recourse to a higher accountable authority in this situation, and the conflicts of interest are clear and not uncommon.

Another question is whether the definitions of illness and the categories of coverage in mental health are sufficiently clear to make contracting an effective method of control. This is especially true in this case, where there is great uncertainty about the number of patients eligible and their ultimate cost. Capitation may or may not make sense in such a fluid situation.

Neither the payer nor the providers know what the effects of changed access for children will mean. EPSDT screening may produce so many cases that it will swamp the capacity and the budgets of the existing system. Access and cost are on a collision course, and the agencies involved are urged, and sometimes mandated, to act rapidly on managed care and privatization with very incomplete information and underdeveloped public health policy guidance.

DISCUSSION QUESTIONS

1. Compare the public health issues raised by managed care initiatives in the mental health arena to those raised by initiatives in the medical care arena, such as the initiatives underway in Denver, Olympia, Portland, Memphis, and Milwaukee (see Chapters 12–16). To what extent are the issues similar or different?

2. Describe the potential advantages and disadvantages for the local mental health system that might result if Peregrine were to win the PHP contract for King County. Describe the advantages and disadvantages that might result from KCRSN winning the contract. Structurally, how might the local mental health system differ under the two alternative scenarios? Make sure to comment on possible differences in interorganizational relationships under the two scenarios.

3. As an alternative to a competitive bidding process, what types of interorganizational arrangements might be developed to meet the objectives of both Peregrine and KCRSN in securing their roles in a PHP initiative? Compare and contrast these alternative arrangements in terms of their feasibility and desirability from the perspectives of each organization.

REFERENCE

1. American Psychiatric Association. *Diagnostic and Statistical Manual of Mental Disorders*. 4th ed. Washington, DC: American Psychiatric Association; 1996.

PART IV

Managing the Public's Health: Policy Implications and Conclusions

The chapters in Part IV examine public health policy and management implications created by the trends in managed care and privatization discussed in this book. Chapter 21 focuses on the managed care market and assesses the adequacy of policies for ensuring access and quality within managed care plans. Chapter 22, a more personal view, expands the discussion by reflecting upon market-based health care delivery in general, and speculating about the limits of this approach. The final chapter identifies some potential strategies that both public and private organizations may use in managing the public's health amidst the turbulence created by managed care and privatization.

CHAPTER 21

Ensuring Quality and Access under Managed Care

Pam Silberman

Ever since the demise of the Clinton administration's universal health care plan in 1994, the private market has attempted to restrain decades of upwardly spiraling health care costs. Rather than rely on regulation to control rising health care costs, businesses have turned to various forms of managed care. Health care providers, in their efforts to become more efficient, have merged, consolidated, downsized, and changed the locus of services from institutional settings to the community. Further, formerly not-for-profit institutions, seeking capital to compete in the new health care market, have converted to for-profit status. These changes raise the question of what will happen to quality and access to care when billion-dollar proprietary corporations control the health care system. The purpose of this chapter is to consider some of the challenges to ensuring quality and access within the world of managed care, describe the mechanisms available to meet this challenge, and suggest ways to improve these mechanisms given the reality of a market-driven health care system.

THE CHALLENGES OF MANAGED CARE

In the last three years, there has been an unprecedented growth in the enrollment in managed care plans. Managed care, with its emphasis on reducing hospitalizations, eliminating unnecessary utilization, and controlling costs, has been seen as the solution to escalating health care costs. Health maintenance organizations (HMOs) in particular have been shown to be successful in reducing

Source: Adapted from P. Silberman, Ensuring Quality and Access in Managed Care: How Well Are We Doing? *Quality Management in Health Care*, Vol. 5, No. 2, pp. 44–54, © 1997, Aspen Publishers, Inc.

health care costs. A Towers-Perrin study[1] of the nation's biggest companies showed that these companies experienced no increase in their HMO costs in 1996, compared to a 4% increase, on average, for employees covered by traditional indemnity insurance or other forms of managed care. A study by Foster Higgins showed similar results. While it is still open to debate as to whether these savings represent one-time savings due to the shift from indemnity plans to other forms of managed care,[2,3] businesses have nonetheless jumped onto the HMO/managed care bandwagon. By the end of 1995, approximately 28% of U.S. workers were enrolled in HMOs, 25% in preferred provider organizations (PPOs), and 20% in point-of-service plans.[4] The total number of Americans enrolled in HMOs, for example, has increased from 36.5 million in 1990 (according to Erin Carlson, American Association of Health Plans [AAHP], in a conversation in May 1996) to approximately 58 million in 1996.[5] Enrollment in PPOs and other less tightly controlled forms of managed care has grown to approximately 81 million.

Enrollment in Medicare risk contracts is also growing. Managed care plans have been an option in the Medicare program since 1972, with the current risk-contract payment mechanism in place since 1982. Until recently, few enrollees have chosen to enroll in traditional managed care plans. In the last year, however, enrollment in HMOs grew by 25%, now 10% of all Medicare beneficiaries.[6] Traditionally, those who chose to enroll tended to be healthier and use fewer services than those who remained in the traditional Medicare system. As a result, the Medicare system actually lost money on its managed care enrollees.[7,8] A number of recommendations have been made to address these issues, including, but not limited to, restricting disenrollment to once a year (to prevent individuals from opting back into the traditional Medicare fee-for-service plan once they become ill); revising the adjusted average per capita cost (AAPCC) payment system to capture more of the savings; or developing a competitive bidding system.[9] Despite the Medicare system's rather dubious financial experience in Medicare managed care, Congress and the Health Care Financing Administration (HCFA) still view managed care as a viable way to reduce Medicare expenditures. With approximately 21% of the federal budget being spent on health services in 1994,[10,11] and data showing that the Medicare Hospital Insurance Trust was likely to run out of funds earlier than expected,[12,13] there was increased interest in expanding enrollment in managed care by both the White House and Congress. In December 1996, for example, HCFA announced the Medicare Choices demonstration project, intended to give Medicare beneficiaries additional managed care options.

Similarly, states have also turned to HMOs and other forms of managed care in their efforts to control rising health care costs. Health and hospital spending accounted for 9% of state budget expenditures in 1991, and welfare spending, which included Medicaid, accounted for another 14%.[14] Medicaid spending has been one of the fastest growing state expenditures, increasing by 28% between

1990 and 1992. The numbers of enrollees in Medicaid managed care grew from 750000 beneficiaries in 1983 (3% of the Medicaid population) to 7.8 million people in June 1994 (23% of the Medicaid population).[15] By June 30, 1996, 13.3 million Medicaid beneficiaries were enrolled in managed care plans in 48 states (35% of the Medicaid population). Of the 13.3 million, more than half were in fully capitated HMOs, 18% in prepaid health plans (generally partially capitated plans that cover a less comprehensive range of services, such as mental health coverage), and 31% in primary care case management systems that provide a monthly management fee to the primary care provider to manage the patient's care but pay providers on a fee-for-service basis for the services rendered.

In addition to the recent expansion in managed care, there are several other trends toward privatization that merit discussion. First, there has been an increased number of consolidations and mergers in the health care industry. Columbia/HCA has purchased all or part of 342 hospitals over the last eight years;[16] Healthsource bought the health care indemnity business of Provident Life and Accident Insurance Company; United Healthcare bought MetraHealth (the merger between Metropolitan Life Insurance Company and Travelers); and U.S. Healthcare bought Aetna Life and Casualty, to name just a few of the recent mergers and acquisitions.[17] Second, formerly not-for-profit health care organizations are being purchased, have converted, or are entering into joint ventures with for-profit corporations. In 1982, for example, 18% of managed care providers were proprietary. This grew to 67% by 1988.[18] By May 1996, 398 of 574 HMOs were for-profit organizations, according to AAHP's Erin Carlson. Dan Fox, from the Milbank Memorial Fund in New York, reported that "easier access to capital for expansion was a major reason for these activities; selling stock yielded more money with fewer constraints than issuing tax-exempt bonds. The financial incentives for top managers was another reason."[19,20]

MECHANISMS TO ENSURE ACCESS AND QUALITY

There are at least three formal systems to oversee quality and access to care and otherwise ensure that enrollee needs are being met within managed care plans: state HMO and insurance laws; federal HMO laws (governing federally qualified HMOs or managed care plans that serve Medicaid or Medicare enrollees); and voluntary accreditation processes.

State Oversight Mechanisms

Most states regulate HMOs and other forms of managed care through their Department of Insurance, although some of the states shift some or all of this responsibility to the Department of Health. State regulatory oversight generally falls into eight areas: marketing and enrollment, access to care, quality, utilization review, complaint or grievance mechanisms, data-collection requirements, insolvency protections, and enforcement mechanisms. A majority of states, for example, have statutory or regulatory requirements that:

- prohibit HMOs from issuing any materials that are false, misleading, or deceptive
- require "adequate" access to personnel and health care facilities
- require plans to have specific quality assurance plans and to take corrective action when problems are found
- mandate that HMOs have specific grievance procedures
- require plans to collect, analyze, and report to the state certain utilization, enrollment, and grievance data
- mandate that certain information be provided to enrollees and the public at large, including covered and excluded services, how to obtain services, how to file a complaint, and the enrollees' financial obligations
- have mechanisms to solicit enrollee participation in HMO policy decisions
- have a system to ensure the HMO's financial solvency and to hold the enrollee harmless for a carrier's failure to pay the provider
- have a variety of enforcement mechanisms to ensure that HMOs comply with their statutory and regulatory requirements (see Note 1)[21]

While all states have some level of oversight, the array of protections in any given state is not always comprehensive. Thus, the National Association of Insurance Commissioners (NAIC) decided to develop model statutes governing managed care organizations and other networks. NAIC has finalized five model statutes to be used by the states to ensure access and quality of care. The model acts have been developed with the input of state agency personnel, managed care organizations, insurers, and consumer groups. The proposed model acts cover quality assessment and improvement,[22] provider credentialing,[23] utilization review,[24] provider network adequacy and contracting,[25] and grievance procedures.[26] (See Note 2.) In addition, NAIC is also developing model standards governing data collection and reporting and confidentiality, but these standards are less fully developed.

Federal Oversight Protections

The U.S. Department of Health and Human Services also has responsibility for overseeing certain managed care organizations, including federally qualified

HMOs and those plans enrolling Medicaid or Medicare enrollees. There were 294 federally qualified HMOs in this country in 1996, according to AAHP's Erin Carlson. In addition to the typical requirements found in state statutes or regulations, federally qualified HMOs must provide a comprehensive set of benefits (described in the federal statute); enroll persons broadly representative of age, social, and income groups within the service area; base the premiums on a modified community rating system; and report specific information on utilization patterns, availability, and accessibility to the secretary.[27]

Plans that participate in Medicaid managed care arrangements must meet additional requirements. For example, services should be made available for Medicaid enrollees to the same extent as for non-Medicaid enrollees, and at least 25% of the enrollees must be commercially insured (that is, not be Medicaid or Medicare enrollees).[28] In addition, the HCFA requires additional quality assurance mechanisms. States that enroll recipients in managed care plans should have a formal written quality assurance program for managed care organizations, and must make compliance with this program part of the contract with any managed care organization. States must annually assess quality of care, including an independent external quality review. Managed care organizations need to conduct focused care studies on clinical care or delivery systems, and utilization review systems must examine both under- and overutilization.[29]

HCFA imposes similar requirements on Medicare risk-bearing plans to ensure financial solvency, quality, and access.[30] For example, plans may not enroll more than 50% Medicare and Medicaid recipients. Additionally, the plans must enroll at least 75 Medicare recipients, and must have at least 5000 total enrollees (or 1500 in rural areas). Medicare risk contracting plans must enroll individuals on a first-come, first-serve basis designed to prevent plans from "cherry-picking" healthy enrollees; submit marketing materials to HCFA to ensure that materials are not deceptive or misleading; provide the full array of Medicare services (although plans can provide additional services or reduce the level of copayments or deductibles); and participate in quality assurance programs.

Voluntary Accreditation Organizations

In addition to the oversight provided by state and federal agencies, many HMOs and managed care organizations seek accreditation by nongovernmental organizations. For example, the National Committee on Quality Assurance (NCQA) has reviewed almost 50% of all HMOs in the country. NCQA's accreditation process examines 50 different areas of plan operation, including quality improvement mechanisms, credentialing, members' rights and responsibilities, preventive health services, utilization management, and medical records.[31] The Joint Commission on Accreditation of Healthcare Organizations (Joint Commission) also reviews health care networks,[32] and the Utilization Review Accreditation Commission has moved to begin accrediting PPOs, noted Lisa Sprague, legislative affairs director of the Association of Managed Health Care Organizations in a phone conversation in May 1996. Managed care organizations are not required in most states to obtain this accreditation, but the competition from other accredited HMOs has compelled many of these organizations to do so.

HOW WELL DO OVERSIGHT MECHANISMS PROTECT CONSUMER INTERESTS IN QUALITY, ACCESS, AND HEALTH STATUS IMPROVEMENT?

. With this broad array of formal oversight structures and the stated focus on keeping people healthy, why should we be concerned about the quality of care within managed care organizations? Does managed care pose more of a threat to consumers than under the more traditional fee-for-service indemnity system? Studies that have compared the HMOs with fee-for-service indemnity plans have generally found that consumers were more satisfied with access to, and quality of, care in fee-for-service plans, while HMO enrollees were more satisfied with the plan's cost, paperwork, and coverage of preventive care.[33] Other studies that have focused on access or health outcomes have found mixed results in the Medicaid population,[15] although comparable or more positive results for the general commercial and Medicare populations.[34-37]

Despite the initial positive quality-of-care findings and the vast system created to monitor managed care arrangements, there are at least three reasons why continued vigilance is needed. First, the payment methodology employed by many managed care companies, which shifts the risk of caring for patients onto the provider, gives providers a financial incentive to withhold necessary care. The increased emphasis on cost containment, coupled with the transformation of the managed care industry from a largely nonprofit industry into one controlled by billion-dollar corporate giants, has the potential to change the focus of the health care industry from managing care to managing costs. Second, the formal oversight mechanisms are not always adequate to ensure quality, access to care, and other consumer protections. Some states are missing key consumer protections, and others have passed laws that are too vague to be enforceable. Even when the necessary laws are enacted, federal and state agencies often lack the resources to properly monitor and ensure compliance. Third, our current data systems are largely inadequate to ensure quality of, and access to, care. Data that are collected generally measure the process and structure used to provide care, but not the health outcomes of the care provided. Even the limited outcome data that are collected are not always comparable across plans. Further, information that is collected is not routinely made available to consumers.

Financial Pressures To Withhold Care

Managed care organizations that shift the risk to providers through capitation or other systems that reward providers for "efficiency" also place financial incentives on providers to withhold necessary care. As Jerome Kassirer wrote in an editorial in the *New England Journal of Medicine*, "The incentive to remain employed is so strong that many physicians in a capitated system may not provide all the services they should, may not always be the patient's advocate, and may be reluctant to challenge the rules governing which services are appropriate."[38] This is particularly troublesome when the financial system is set up to discourage overutilization, but not to discourage or monitor underutilization of services.

The benefits of managed care systems—including the focus on prevention and keeping a person healthy—are also likely to be eroded because of the need for publicly traded companies to yield high returns to the investors. Most health promotion and disease prevention efforts take years, or even decades, before seeing positive health impacts,[39] but enrollment in most managed care companies is not that stable. A study of managed care enrollees in Miami, Los Angeles, and Boston in 1994 showed that the average length of time that most members were enrolled in managed care plans was less than three years.[18] For Medicaid recipients, the average length of time is less than one year.[40] Further, with few exceptions, preventive care usually increases medical expenditures rather than reduce net health care costs.[39,41] Thus, managed care companies are likely to lose money by investing in prevention. How willing will companies be to make that investment in prevention if their primary driving force is the bottom line?

Small subpopulations with special health care needs are the most likely to suffer in this transition to a profit-driven managed care system. Presumably, competition in the marketplace will force managed care companies to correct access or quality problems that affect large numbers of enrollees. However, problems that affect a smaller subpopulation, especially those with large medical needs, can more easily be ignored. The results of a study of children with special needs enrolled in Medicaid managed care plans bears out this point.[42] The study showed that access to primary and preventive services appeared to be as good or better than for similar children under fee-for-service plans, but that the managed care organizations made few efforts at early identification or treatment of developmental, behavioral, or emotional problems unless they could specifically offset future hospital costs. Thus, individuals with special needs may have less access to special therapies or other treatments that are likely to improve functioning or quality of life, but which do not lead to direct cost savings through reduced use of other services. In fact, a health plan would benefit financially by discouraging enrollment by individuals with large medical needs.

Formal Oversight Mechanisms Not Always Adequate

Although states have an array of laws designed to protect enrollees in managed care plans, they are not always sufficient to ensure access, quality, or improved health status. For example, only four states require HMOs to maintain minimum ratios of physicians to patients, while 11 states set maximum travel times or distances.[21] Unlike the Medicaid managed care requirements, only eight states require external reviews of the quality of care provided under the plan, nor do they have systems to regulate physician-hospital organizations that assume full or partial risk from employers.[43]

Sometimes, the laws are on the books but are so vague as to be unenforceable. The NAIC Provider Network Adequacy and Contracting Model Act, for example, requires plans to develop their own methodology and "target standards" to ensure adequacy and accessibility of provider networks. The model act does not include specific provider-patient ratios, minimum driving distance, or waiting time to obtain an appointment. Even though the model act theoretically gives the commissioner the authority to require corrective action if he or she determines that a carrier's access plan does not ensure reasonable access, given the vague nature of the access standards, a court may not uphold a commissioner's decision to require corrective action. Other laws are drawn so narrowly as to be almost useless. Barbara Morales-Burke, the Deputy Insurance Commissioner for Managed Care in North Carolina, testified to a legislative study commission that "current HMO statutes allow the Commissioner to suspend or revoke an HMO license only for very specific and very serious violations of the law. Our ability to issue cease and desist notices to HMOs and to fine them in lieu of suspension of revocation is tied to these same specific, very serious violations. In other cases, we have no option but to try to reason with companies over an issue in an attempt to win their cooperation. In essence, our choices are between a club and a fly swatter."[44]

Even when the laws exist, questions arise as to whether states or the federal government have the resources to monitor and properly enforce the laws. A General Accounting Office (GAO) study of state oversight of Medicaid managed care plans found in the early 1990s, for example, that states were doing an inadequate job monitoring quality, access to care, and oversight of provider financial reporting, disclosure, and solvency. GAO concluded that states needed to institute a set of safeguards to protect consumers, including better quality assurance mechanisms, outside review of medical records, monitoring subcontracts and utilization data, and better state and federal oversight.[45,46] Given the recent expansion in the commercial HMO enrollment and number of licensed managed care organizations, a similar question arises about the ability of state regulatory agencies to adequately monitor managed care activities.

Inadequate Data Collection and Reporting

Both consumers and employers have reported that they are interested in information to measure health care outcomes, especially standardized health care information that would allow them to compare the performance of health plans or health providers.[47] The leading national effort to collect this type of standardized information is NCQA's Health Plan Employer Data and Information Set (HEDIS). It was created primarily to meet employer demands for information to compare competing health plans. HEDIS 3.0, which went into effect in 1997, collects information about quality of care, member access and satisfaction, membership and utilization, finance, and health plan management and activities. The quality measurements include information on childhood immunization rates, well-child visits, initiation of prenatal care, check-ups after delivery, breast and cervical cancer screenings, flu shots for older adults, beta blocker treatment after heart attacks, treatment of children's ear infections, ambulatory follow-up after major affective disorder, diabetic retinal exams, and changes in self-reported health status for senior Medicare risk plan members.

Although HEDIS is an important first step to measure health plan performance, there are several problems with the HEDIS measures. First, most of the performance measurements are largely structural or process measures. Few of the measurements actually address health outcomes. Sometimes, process measures may be appropriate substitutes for more sophisticated outcome measures (such as using immunizations as a proxy for preventing certain communicable diseases). However, relying on process measures is not always a good indicator of outcomes. (The percentage of women receiving mammograms, for example, may not be a good proxy for the five-year survival rate after the breast cancer has been discovered.) Further work is needed to develop appropriate measures of chronic care and of mental health and substance abuse treatment, as well as to develop appropriate risk adjustment methodology.[48]

Second, data are not collected in a uniform manner across plans. Plans are given the choice of collecting the required data through claims data or a combination of claims data and chart review. Depending on how data are collected, they can yield vastly different results. HEDIS data need not be audited by an independent third party; thus there is no system to correct mistakes in data collection.

Third, and perhaps most important, plans are not required to collect this information, nor are they required to distribute the information to the public. Although some managed care organizations collect and disseminate this information, this is not routine for all plans. This is a problem that is not unique to managed care organizations. Employers who are able to obtain information comparing health care plans do not routinely share the information with their employees, nor does HCFA routinely provide beneficiaries with performance-related information collected for participating Medicare risk plans.[47]

WHERE DO WE GO FROM HERE?

Although this chapter highlights the concerns that are raised with a market-driven health care system, some opportunities to improve health status have been created as a result of recent changes. One of the major advantages of a competitive health system over a more regulatory approach is that a market-driven system can more easily adapt to changing needs. In addition, the move to managed care has helped to reduce escalating health care costs, has provided greater coverage of preventive services, offers opportunities for greater coordination of care, and has helped to reduce unnecessary services.[49] Thus, the question is not necessarily how to turn back the clock and undo recent market changes, but how to improve the current system to maximize patient outcomes.

We often assume that state or federal regulators can provide all the protections necessary to ensure the adequacy of our health care systems. Although they play a critical role in protecting the public's interest in high-quality, accessible health care services, regulatory oversight by itself is not sufficient. State and federal regulators may lack necessary resources and are often subject to political pressure, which minimizes their effectiveness. Some of the most exciting developments in measuring quality, access, and utilization have come not from regulatory bodies, but from demands from the business community. However, a system that relies solely on the market is also insufficient. As noted earlier, large purchasers of care may have the clout necessary to force managed care companies to correct access or quality problems that affect large numbers of enrollees. However, these purchasers, or the market as a whole, do a much poorer job addressing problems that affect a smaller subset of the population. The Joint Commission, NCQA, and other nonprofit accreditation bodies also play an important oversight role. Once again, however, these systems are inadequate to provide all the protections needed. The accrediting bodies lack the enforcement mechanisms needed to ensure that the plans provide the required quality of, and access to, care. At best, they can deny accreditation to plans that fail to meet the accreditation standards. In most states, however, there is no requirement that health plans have NCQA or Joint Commission accreditation. And few businesses consider NCQA accreditation to be very important in choosing health care plans.[50] The lack of accreditation therefore will not prevent the carriers from continuing to offer or provide services.

Thus, there is no singular system that can provide all the oversight necessary to ensure quality, access, and efficiency.

While no one system can provide all the necessary safeguards, a combination of systems can. There are four major changes needed to ensure that the current, profit-driven health care system meets the health care needs of the individuals it serves. First, states should enact a comprehensive array of laws to oversee managed care organizations. Both the NAIC Model Acts and the federal Medicaid managed care requirements are good starting points, but states may need to go beyond these recommendations to include data and enforcement mechanisms specific to meet individual state's needs. To make these standards meaningful, regulatory agencies should be equipped with the staff and financial resources to properly monitor the performance of managed care organizations. An alternative to enhanced state or federal oversight would be to require NCQA or Joint Commission accreditation (which is now only voluntary), although this would not remove all oversight responsibility from state or federal agencies.

Second, health plans should be required to submit certain information to a third-party data repository. This could be the state regulatory agency, NCQA, or another body set up to collect state health data. Information should be comparable across plans, publicly available, and should include:

- enrollment and disenrollment numbers (disenrollment figures may be especially useful to alert regulatory agencies of potential access or quality concerns)
- data on utilization of key services (including primary care visits per 1000 enrollees, specialist visits per 1000 enrollees, percent of enrollees seeing a primary care provider in the last year, hospital admissions and days per 1000 enrollees, mental health and substance abuse outpatient visits per 1000 enrollees, and any other services that the state has reason to believe may be underutilized by enrollees)
- consumer satisfaction information, including information on provider communications skills, access to care, and continuity
- access information, including the average waiting time to get an appointment, and travel time to primary care providers
- the reasons for and number of grievances filed, and how they were resolved
- process and outcome information, which should reflect some of the state's major health care problems (such as infant mortality, heart disease, or diabetes), as well as measurements to gauge the quality of, and access to, care

To the greatest extent possible, states should rely on the existing HEDIS quality measures, so as to minimize a plan's data-collection requirements. However, the state should not be limited to HEDIS measures if there are particular health problems in the state that need to be more closely monitored.

Third, information should be made more available to consumers. Employers have some opportunity, albeit limited, to obtain information comparing coverage, quality, access, utilization of services, and costs among plans—but the information is almost non-existent for consumers. The systems that have been established to date, particularly NCQA accreditation and the HEDIS 3.0 system, were created largely to address the needs of the purchasers of care. While consumers have similar interests to those of the purchasers, different data may be needed to properly address their needs. For example, consumers are particularly interested in hearing the experiences of other people who are "like them."[51] Moreover, consumers are interested in information about costs of care, choice of providers, coverage, provider communication skills, access to various types of care, continuity of care with their chosen provider, and quality. In addition, consumers are interested in information about individual providers and treatment options. For a market-based system to work, individual consumers (as well as large purchasers of care) need information to compare competing health plans. In August 1996, NCQA began publishing *Quality Compass*, a report containing comparative information on HEDIS 2.5 performance measures and accreditation status for 226 health plans. The data are available for purchase from NCQA, but the costs make the data unaffordable to most individual consumers.

Finally, alternative systems of accountability should be established. Large purchasers of care (including state health plans, large businesses, and the Medicaid agency) already have the ability to negotiate needed changes in a plan's operation when problems arise. Small employers, through purchasing cooperatives, have a system to band together to obtain this same control over costs, quality, access, and coverage that large purchasers already enjoy. Only consumers lack a system to be able to demand needed changes in a health plan. Thus, systems should be created to involve the consumers more directly in the operation of the plans. One system already in place in eight states is to mandate enrollee representation on all HMO governing boards.[21] Minnesota, for example, requires that HMOs in operation for at least a year should have at least 40% of the board made up of enrollees elected by other enrollees.

In addition, other models have been developed within the Medicaid managed care context to involve consumers in the oversight of managed care arrangements.[52] Several states have developed "ombudsprograms" with the authority to resolve complaints and to report systemic problems to the attention of plan personnel, the state regulatory agencies, or the legislature. Other states have employed consumers directly in gathering consumer satisfaction information, and still others have involved consumers in plan-level grievance systems. Without these systems to ensure quality and accessibility, the current emphasis on cost containment and the need to generate profits will inevitably lead to poorer health outcomes.

NOTES

1. The Center for Health Care Rights analyzed all of the states' HMO statutes and regulations in place prior to March 1994 and published an overview of state laws with recommendations of how to improve consumer protections in state laws, together with a detailed description of the HMO statutes and regulations in all 50 states.

2. The Quality Assessment and Improvement Model Act requires carriers to have quality assurance systems that measure, assess, and improve processes and outcomes of health care. The quality management tools must include procedures to identify and take corrective action on quality problems. The program must focus on practices and diagnoses that affect a large number of the plan's covered persons or that could place covered persons at serious risk and use a range of methods to analyze quality, including but not limited to information on over- and underutilization of services, health status measures, outcomes evaluations, enrollee satisfaction, and grievances. The carrier must have mechanisms to compare findings with past performance, measure the performance of participating providers, and utilize treatment protocols and practice parameters with appropriate clinical input. The carrier's quality assurance system must also report any persistent pattern of problematic care provided by a provider to the appropriate licensing authorities; should have a system to allow members to comment on the quality assurance process; and should integrate public health goals with the health services being offered under the plan.

   The Health Professional Credentialing Model Act requires carriers to obtain information on the providers' practice histories, education and training, license/certificate/registration to practice, current level of professional liability coverage, status of hospital privileges, drug enforcement agency registration certificate and any prescribing restrictions, and specialty board certification (if any). Providers must be recredentialed no less than once every three years.

   The Utilization Review Model Act includes provisions intended to ensure that decisions about clinical necessity are based on objective, clinically appropriate standards, ensure that decisions are reviewed by clinical peers, and protect member confidentiality. The Act also requires plans to measure under- and overutilization, and sets specific requirements for notices of adverse determinations. In addition, the NAIC Model Utilization Review Act contains protections to ensure that carriers do not retroactively deny payment for emergency department care rendered, if a prudent person would have considered it an emergency at the time.

   The Provider Network Adequacy and Contracting Model Act requires plans to develop methodology and targets standards to ensure adequacy and accessibility of provider networks, including provider-patient ratios (for primary care and specialists), driving distance or time, average/expected waiting times, and the ability of the plan to cover emergency services on a 24-hour, 7 day/week basis. The Act does not include specific standards that plans must meet, but does give the Commissioner of Insurance (or appropriate state official) the authority to require corrective action if he/she determines that a carrier has not contracted with enough participating providers to ensure that covered persons have accessible health care services in a geographic area. In addition, a carrier's access plan must include the carrier's network and referral procedures; the process to monitor sufficiency of the provider network; a description of carrier's efforts to address the needs of special populations; how the health carrier assesses covered person's health care needs and satisfaction; and provisions to ensure coordination and continuity of care. Further, the plan must be made available to the public.

The provider contracting provisions require plans to include information on credentialing, confidentiality, grievance procedures, utilization review procedures, maintenance of records, quality assurance, and payment methodologies. Provider contracts must also include provisions prohibiting them from discriminating against members on the basis of race, color, national origin, gender, age, religion, marital status, health status, or health insurance coverage. Carriers retain the right to approve or disapprove participation of individual providers contracting with the intermediary for inclusion in or removal from the carrier's own network plan but may not discriminate against providers because they treat high-risk populations or are located in areas that include populations or providers serving higher-risk populations. Provider contracts may not include gag clauses, or any provisions that prohibit or discourage a health provider from protesting or expressing disagreement with a medical decision of the health carrier.

Grievances can be filed by a member, representative, or a provider about complaints over availability, delivery, and quality of health services; adverse utilization review decisions; or any other matter between an enrollee and the health carrier. NAIC requires carriers to establish utilization review committees or panels, and that adverse decisions be reviewed by a health professional who is a clinical peer to the provider who recommended the course of treatment under consideration. The NAIC model act mandates a first-level review by the carrier (which includes the right to submit additional information), a second-level de novo review (with a right to be present before the carrier), and a right to contact the commissioner for assistance. The act also includes specific time limits to hold the review and render the decision, including provisions for expedited reviews in certain situations. NAIC also requires carriers to keep a record (registry) of all grievances, including the date of review, and resolution at each level. The report must also include the number of covered lives, total number of grievances, number referred to the second level of review, and number appealed to the commissioner.

REFERENCES

1. Freudenheim M. Survey finds health costs rose in '95: up 2.1% for workers, reversing '94 decline. *NY Times*. January 30, 1996:D1.

2. Levit KR, Lazenby HC, Sivarajan L. Health care spending in 1994: slowest in decades. *Health Affairs*. 1996;15:130–144.

3. U.S. General Accounting Office (GAO). *Managed Health Care: Effects on Employers' Costs Difficult To Measure*. Report to the Chairman, Subcommittee on Health, Committee on Ways and Means, U.S. House of Representatives (GAO/HRD-94-3). Washington, DC: GAO; 1993.

4. Winslow R. Employee health care costs were steady last year: but big rise for retirees may prompt companies to cut back coverage. *Wall Street J*. January 30, 1996:A2.

5. Freudenheim M. Health care in the era of capitalism. *NY Times* April 7, 1996:E6.

6. Jeffrey NA. Sign of the times: Medicare users turn to HMOs. *Wall Street J*. October 20, 1995:A1.

7. U.S. General Accounting Office. *Medicare: Increase in HMO Reimbursement Would Eliminate Potential Savings* (GAO/HRD-909-38). Washington, DC: GAO; 1989.

8. Brown R, Bergeron JW, Clement DG, Hill GW, et al. *The Medicare Risk Program for HMOs—Final Summary Report on Findings from the Evaluation*. Princeton, NJ: Mathematica Policy Research; 1993.

9. Prospective Payment Review Commission. *Joint Report to the Congress on Medicare Managed Care*. Washington, DC: Government Printing Office; 1995.

10. Burner ST, Waldo DR. National health expenditure projections, 1994–2005. *Health Care Financing Rev.* 1995;16:234.

11. Congressional Budget Office. *The Economic and Budget Outlook: An Update.* Washington, DC: Congressional Budget Office; 1995.

12. Pear R. Shortfall posted by Medicare fund two years early: a surplus was expected. Deficits to continue growing unless system to care for the elderly is changed. *NY Times.* February 5, 1995:A1.

13. Rich S. Medicare nearer to red, report says: CBO projects hospital trust fund will be insolvent by 2001. *Washington Post.* April 29, 1996:A4.

14. Winterbottom C, Liska DW, Obermaier KM. *State Level Databook on Health Care Access and Financing.* 2nd ed. Washington, DC: The Urban Institute; 1995.

15. The Kaiser Commission on the Future of Medicaid. *Medicaid and Managed Care: Lessons from the Literature.* Washington, DC: Henry J. Kaiser Family Foundation; 1995.

16. Segal D. Health care giant towers over region: Columbia/HCA adds to chain of hospitals. *Washington Post.* March 11, 1996:A1.

17. Freudenheim M. Managed care empires in the making: companies build networks to stay a step ahead of a hard-charging field. *NY Times.* April 2, 1996:D1.

18. Davis K, Collins KS, Schoen C, Morris C. Choice matters: enrollees' views of their health plans. *Health Affairs.* 1995;14:99–112.

19. Fox D, Isenberg P. Anticipating the magic moment: the public interest in health plan conversions in California. *Health Affairs.* 1996;15:202–209.

20. Hamburger E, Finberg J, Alcantar L. The pot of gold: monitoring health care conversions can yield billions of dollars for health care. *Clearinghouse Rev.* August-September 1995:473–504.

21. Dallek G, Jimenez C, Schwartz M. *Consumer Protections in State HMO Laws. Volume 1: Analysis and Recommendations.* Washington, DC: Center for Health Care Rights; 1995.

22. National Association of Insurance Commissioners (NAIC). *Quality Assessment and Improvement Model Act.* Washington, DC: NAIC; 1996.

23. National Association of Insurance Commissioners. *Health Professional Credentialing Model Regulations.* Washington, DC: NAIC; 1995.

24. National Association of Insurance Commissioners. *Utilization Review Model Act.* Washington, DC: NAIC; 1996.

25. National Association of Insurance Commissioners. *The Provider Network Adequacy and Contracting Model Act.* Washington, DC: NAIC; 1996.

26. National Association of Insurance Commissioners. *Grievance Procedures Model Act.* Washington, DC: NAIC; 1996.

27. 42 USC §§ 300e-1 et seq.

28. 42 CFR §§ 434.20 et seq.

29. U.S. Department of Health and Human Services (HHS), Health Care Financing Administration. *A Health Care Quality Improvement System for Medicaid Managed Care: A Guide for the States.* Washington, DC: HHS; 1993.

30. 42 CFR §§ 417.400 et seq.

31. National Commission for Quality Assurance (NCQA). *1996 Standards for Accreditation of Managed Care Organizations.* Washington, DC: NCQA; 1996.

32. O'Leary D. Evaluating quality in managed care networks. *Health Care Manage: State of the Art Rev.* 1995;2:71–77.

33. Davis K, Collins KS, Schoen C, Morris C. Choice matters: enrollees' views of their health plans. *Health Affairs.* 1995;14:99–112.

34. Miller RH, Luft HS. Managed care plan performance since 1980. A literature analysis. *JAMA.* 1994;271:1512–1519.

35. Retchin SM, Clement DG, Brown B, Brown R, et al. How the elderly fare in HMOs: outcomes from the Medicare competition demonstration. *Health Serv Res.* 1992;27:651–669.

36. Greenfield S, Rogers W, Mangotich M, Carney MF, et al. Outcomes of patients with hypertension and non–insulin-dependent diabetes mellitus treated by different systems and specialties: results from the medical outcomes study. *JAMA.* 1995;274:1436–1444.

37. Oberlander JB. Managed care and Medicare reform. *J Health Politics, Policy, and Law.* 1997;22: 595–631.

38. Kassirer JP. Managed care and the morality of the marketplace. *N Engl J Med.* 1995;333:50–52.

39. Sisk JE. The cost of prevention: don't expect a free lunch. *JAMA.* 1993;269:1710–1715.

40. National Commission for Quality Assurance. *Medicaid HEDIS: An Adaptation of NCQA's Health Plan Employer Data and Information Set 2.0/2.5.* Washington, DC: NCQA; 1995.

41. Russell LB. The role of prevention in health reform. *N Engl J Med.* 1993;329:321–325.

42. Fox HB, McManus P. Preliminary analysis of issues and options in serving children with chronic conditions through Medicaid managed care plans. Presented at the annual meeting of the National Academy for State Health Policy; August 1994. Portland, Me.

43. Group Health Association of America (GHAA). *PHOs and the Assumption of Insurance Risk: A 50 State Survey of Regulators' Attitudes toward PHO Licensure.* Washington DC: GHAA; 1995.

44. Morales-Burke, B. Testimony to the North Carolina State Health Care Reform Commission. March 27, 1996.

45. U.S. General Accounting Office. *Testimony to the Subcommittee on Health and Families and the Uninsured Committee on Finance, U.S. Senate.* Washington, DC: Government Printing Office; 1992.

46. Inglehart JK. Medicaid and managed care. *N Eng J Med.* 1995;332:1727.

47. U.S. General Accounting Office. *Health Care: Employers and Individual Consumers Want Additional Information on Quality.* Report to the Ranking Minority Member, Committee on Labor and Human Resources, U.S. Senate (GAO/HEHS-95-201). Washington, DC: GAO; 1995.

48. Prospective Payment Review Commission. *1995 Annual Report to Congress.* Washington, DC: Government Printing Office; 1995.

49. Brown RS, Clement DG, Hill JW, Retchin SM, et al. Do health maintenance organizations work for Medicare? *Health Care Financing Rev.* 1993;15:7–23.

50. Segal D. HMOs: how much, not how well. *Washington Post.* Jan. 19, 1996:F1.

51. Lubalin J, Schnaier J, Forsyth B, Gibbs D, et al. *Design of a Survey To Monitor Consumers' Access to Care, Use of Health Services, Health Outcomes, and Patient Satisfaction. Final Report.* Submitted to Office of Program Development, Agency for Health Care Policy and Research, Dept. of Health and Human Services. Contract No. 282-92-0045. Research Triangle Park, NC: Research Triangle Institute; 1995.

52. Perkins J, Skatrud J. *Making the Consumers' Voice Heard in Medicaid Managed Care: Increasing Participation, Protection and Satisfaction.* Report to the Center for Health Care Strategies for Robert Wood Johnson and Pew Charitable Trust; 1996.

CHAPTER 22

Public Health, Privatization, and Market Populism: A Cautionary Note

Dan Beauchamp

Despite the progress in promoting the public's health and ensuring the quality of care provided within communities over the past 30 years in the United States, public health has always been a precarious value within the United States. Ensuring quality and promoting the public's health involves saving tens of thousands of statistical lives through burdening many powerful corporate interests, limiting or regulating markets, and even regulating the behavior of millions of private individuals. Public health has always been something of an alien ethic in a capitalist land.[1] In recent years, these tensions and conflicts have become all the greater, leading to a strong move toward privatization, including the following:

- A sustained attack on programs in health care and other forms of spending for the medical assistance for the poor and disabled, due to the need to reduce the federal budget deficit and to make the nation more competitive.

- A drive to actually roll back regulations for the health care and public health sector. The 1995–1996 Republican "Contract with America" was largely an argument against many public health measures as primary obstacles to the challenge of making America more competitive in world markets and as an appropriate democratic ideal. Thus, it would submit public health regulations to cost-benefit standards and lengthy budgetary reviews, to interminable legal challenges, to the requirement that significant losses to private property through public health legislation be compensated, and to fully funding all federal initiatives that require state action or compliance, from seat belt legislation to improvements in epidemiological surveillance.

Source: Adapted from D. Beauchamp, Public Health, Privatization, and Market Populism: A Time for Reflection, *Quality Management in Health Care*, Vol. 5, No. 2, pp. 73–79, ©1997, Aspen Publishers, Inc.

- A drive to make the public sector more market-like in its incentives. A leading example is the long struggle to link Medicaid spending and managed care or preferred providers. A more recent example is the use of managed care for Medicare. This drive is actually quite old and can be traced back to the 1970s and to leading Democrat theorist Charles Schultze and his Godkins Lectures at Harvard.
- A nationwide move to privatize the public sector in order to increase efficiency and to reduce public expenditure, the most famous examples being the conversion of Blue Cross plans in many states to for-profit entities, and the conversion of the Health and Hospitals Corporation, a collection of 11 public hospitals in New York City serving the poor, to a private organization.
- The move to incorporate aspects of what has been public health responsibilities into newly formed and spreading health care networks and community corporations, managed care delivery systems, and so forth, including data collection, preventive services such as immunization and prenatal care, and even school health, changing the very nature of the local health department.
- The drive to place the health care sector under market-like standards for compensation and rewards, or vastly higher salaries for executives, and much lower or no benefits for those at entry-level positions.
- The spreading use of the market and market forces to accomplish what politics cannot accomplish: lowering health care spending through competition, breaking up the professional and political power of specialists and hospitals, and even providing a new path toward universal health.

These separate processes need to be seen as part of a larger pattern of politics, which I call "market populism." It is market populism that is the most serious threat to public health in many decades, and the rest of this chapter will explore the meaning of this new era in American politics and its implications for public health.

THE MARKET AND DEMOCRACY

To understand market populism, we first need to understand the relationship between the market and democracy. In 1984, the distinguished political scientist Charles Lindblom, then president of the American Political Science Association, delivered a series of informal talks before the regional political science associations. These talks later became a famous article, "The Market as Prison."[2] In the article, Lindblom argues that with markets, democracies face a deep paradox. Markets, among the many institutions in a democratic society, are uniquely difficult, even intransigent, to change. This is because attempts to regulate them, even in the name of the public welfare and health, trigger an economic backlash, including unemployment, higher costs, and public complaint. Lindblom readily agrees that business leaders too often overstate the economic pain of safety rules, a higher minimum wage, or stronger pollution controls. Nevertheless, the grip of the market's welfare on the mind of the political class is so strong and pervasive as to imprison democratic leadership and their policies. The people's welfare is predicated on, and subordinate to, the market's welfare.

Lindblom locates the triggering mechanism for the market backlash or "punishments" in hidden and decentralized incentives or inducements. As he argues, the huge private sector in democracies is led by unseen market incentives that operate more or less inexorably to force managers and entrepreneurs to seek to reduce all costs and to treat regulation as just another cost. It is this automatic side of the way markets work—invisibly, as Adam Smith would have it—that makes it difficult for democratic leaders to anticipate and counter business objections to government regulation. What is hidden has become the mysterious and powerful "market forces"—forces that amplify business disaffection into national, politically seismic events. Market leaders are powerless to do anything but fight back.

This is not to say that privatization and other market-led initiatives never present powerful advantages to the public or to political leaders. Public budgets can be reduced. Efficiency can be encouraged. Innovations in the delivery of services can result. Powerful professional interests can be effectively countered. Yet these advantages are nearly always purchased at great price. Extensive regulation is required to unleash market forces. The cost of a unit of service may decline, but the whole market for health care (for example) can expand under market pressures, which increases public obligations. The health and safety of the whole community can gradually disappear. And most of all, there is a steady and inexorable loss of democratic responsibility and control over the conditions that protect whole communities, and not just those who are traditionally pushed out of markets.

MARKET POPULISM

To understand these forces, we need to go further than Lindblom; what we are seeing is a new form of populism that has turned the market prison into a positive virtue.[3] Instead of simply making the market's welfare the top priority of our politics, today increasing numbers of people are directly attacking the public sector and government and advocating the market as a replacement institution. And this new populism is being launched to defend the general population from a new enemy: big government. What we have here is not a movement that just places the public sector under the shadow of the market's welfare; we have a public sector that is being transformed and made an adjunct to the market sector to better advance the interests of the general population. Ours is the age of market populism.

Populism as a political movement has been on the American scene since the end of the 19th century.[4] Originally it meant the revolt of agrarian and small-town interests fearful of big corporate monopolies like the railroads, the big land interests, and the utilities. It has occasionally included labor, although the alliance of labor and the farmer has always been fragile and suspicious. Generally, populism has come to mean mobilizing power on the part of the "ordinary people,"[5] those who see themselves as having a limited voice in Washington and other corridors of power. While populism was originally an angry voice raised against the economic power of corporations, it has increasingly become the angry voice raised against the federal government. Populists on the left and right argue that effective change must be accompanied by a massive and organized redistribution of power away from Washington and the federal government and to the people. There are a variety of outbreaks of populism in contemporary American politics. One is economic populism, represented most clearly by Jesse Jackson. The second is cultural populism, represented by such leaders as Reverend Pat Roberts. The recent rise of Pat Buchanan represents something of an amalgam of economic or old-time populism and cultural populism. But Newt Gingrich and the House Republican majority represent something very different, a peculiar form of economic populism that I have called "market populism." The market populists ride the wave of public confusion and mistrust of government and the public blame heaped on Congress and the president for gridlock. Market populists not only trust the market, they embrace it. The market does it better than government. The market is the plain people's friend. Market populists have a tactical alliance with cultural populists; both are linked together in a joint strategy that is benefiting from the fear and unhappiness with the stalemate in American politics.

Market populism is the effort, primarily on the part of conservatives (and many Democrats), to offer the market as the primary alternative institution to government, and to use the market to return power to the people. In their campaign, these advocates are aided considerably by the perception that markets are a force for change and are difficult to resist by those opposed to change. Also, markets deliver the goods in the form of an ever-increasing array of choice and variety in life.

Ironically, the major force driving these changes was the Clinton health care reform plan. The decision by the Clinton administration to put managed care at the center of its health reform debate was likely the single most important event triggering the shift. The Clinton plan's biggest impact was to send the signal that the market, not government, was to be in charge of the health care system of the future. To be sure, before the arrival of the Clinton plan, business coalitions across the nation were trying to move aggressively to embrace managed care as a solution to their health care cost woes. But the truly big push came from Clinton's plan.

A second and equally important factor was the resentment against government fanned by Republicans and many Democrats. I see the new age as less an incursion by a powerful market into the realm of health and the community than a raid on the community and the health sector by politicians advocating market populism, seeking gains for their corporate sponsors, and money for their own campaign coffers. Thus, the Cooper Plan—a plan by Congressman Jim Cooper (D-Tenn), a member of the House of Representatives who ran for the Senate in 1994 and was defeated—was less an alternative to the Clinton plan than a staking out of a position on the Democratic right that would guarantee huge contributions from the newly forming managed care industry. A third factor in the rise of market forces as solutions to health care reform and to public health responsibilities is the ideological rigidity of business and organized medicine, causing them to discard government-centered solutions out of hand and deliver them up to the managed care solution. Adding to this is the resurgence of the South in American politics and the "Southernization" of the Republican party.[6] This may turn out to be the most potent force behind market populism.

Finally, there is the clear expectation of huge profits, with the opening of a vast new market following in the train of these shifts. The corporate interests in health care, the for-profit health maintenance organizations, the growing chains, the insurance companies, and the Blue Cross plans expect huge profits. Also, the expert and consulting industry, never one to miss an opportunity, has moved in with its vast army of specialists, including academic experts, seeing in the new movement a yet higher level of spending by government and business.

PUBLIC HEALTH AS A PROPHETIC VOICE

How can we live with or reverse these alarming developments? Clearly, it cannot be done exclusively or even mainly by local health departments. In fact, local and state health departments are placed most at risk by the politics of market populism. What is needed is a national campaign, mounted by national public health leadership and its allies, to more broadly counter the emergence of market populism with its deep threat not just to the public's health but to the democratic control over the conditions of the common life.

The first step is to recall that the market prison can be escaped. Lindblom is pessimistic or at least morbidly realistic about the difficulties of escaping the market prison, yet he ignores the experience of the Europeans and Canadians in expanding the scope of communal services, including national health plans, that all share together, making attacks on government by business and other interests more politically risky in those democracies. This should have been the goal of national health care reform in the United States, but it is widely felt that the Clinton plan dynamited this as a possibility.

Also, in the United States we must remember that democratic activism was remarkably successful during the Great Society period in expanding the authority of public health and in creating new public health agencies, which of course formed much of the reaction of business during the 1970s and the Reagan era. Yet these were accomplished despite the market prison.

The second step is for public health to recall its historic role in the health enterprise. Public health is not just a way of discovering the causes of disease or even of advocating prevention by providing conditions that can assure people of maximum health. Public health is also a critique of ongoing societies, including those ideas and structures that produce death, disability, and the destruction of the human community. Public health is also a way of seeing through the world, seeing it at its depths, a social ethic that unmasks the structures and rules that imprison democracy and perpetuate injustice and disease.

The rapid growth of public health during the 1960s was not supposed to happen, at least in American politics. Producer groups tend to outweigh consumer groups or the public in politics, as Lindblom might predict. Public health policies reward consumers or the public in the form of general (albeit small) benefits at a cost to be borne chiefly by a small (and often very influential) part of society.[7] How did public health overcome this?

James Wilson points to the emergence of entrepreneurial politics and "policy entrepreneurs" who "mobilize latent public sentiment (by revealing a scandal or by capitalizing on a crisis), put the opponents of the plan publicly on the defensive (by accusing them of deforming babies or killing motorists), and associating the legislation with widely-shared values (clean air, pure water, health, and safety). The entrepreneur acts as the vicarious representative of groups not directly represented in the legislative process."[7] Policy entrepreneurs are people such as Ralph Nader or legislative aide (and later Federal Trade Commission chairman) Michael Pertschuk.

I would broaden this characterization and say that it is public health's role to speak for the public and the community as a whole and to serve as a prophetic voice representing groups not directly represented in a market-dominated society, including especially the whole community. By "prophetic" I mean to explicitly link public health to the prophetic tradition, and to the role of prophets in speaking out of a position of seeming powerlessness, weakness, and isolation, but of voicing the deep aspirations of the public and the community, aspirations and values that are unarticulated or unheard in routine politics. When Dean Edward McGavran of the University of North Carolina School of Public Health wrote of public health as the physician for the body politic, what he meant was that public health is the body politic's prophet, and that is precisely the idea I am advocating.[8]

William Stringfellow, a public health advocate, comes as close as anyone in articulating what a prophetic ethic might entail.[9] A prophetic ethic is an embodied ethic—a politics of the common body—a body politics exploiting the politics of "hurt and hope."[10] In this politics, death is the master symbol of hurt and the loss of community and alienation, and life the master symbol of health and community. Public health as social justice is minimizing the hurt and death in human communities.[11] When we say that a corporation is practicing the politics of death, we are speaking of more than just the marketing of dangerous or addicting products. We are also speaking of the corporation's drive to loosen and weaken democratic control of the common life.

The idea of markets is a religious one in our society. That is to say, people regard markets as "powers," as institutions that hold great sway on our consciousness, shaping our ideas, our behavior, and our very thoughts, and that have great spiritual sway in our society. The prophets of the Old Testament looked out at the ancient desert tribes and saw a world that was spirit-filled, a world inhabited by gods and powers that people worshipped feverishly, gods usually referred to as Baal. The prophets campaigned ceaselessly against this elemental sin of idolatry. Today we should pay attention to this ancient view and to the world the prophets saw, because it almost certainly has not vanished but has only become disguised in new and more beguiling forms.

PUBLIC HEALTH AS A VOICE FOR THE COMMUNITY

Public health must serve as the voice for the community. Many are concerned that the rapid growth of the managed care industry without appropriate government supervision is a very worrisome development, and they are right. But the most worrisome side of this movement is the loss of the already fragile and frayed sense of community that presently undergirds the health care system. Certainly, the call for the regulation of the managed care industry, including the establishment of federal guidelines, and perhaps federal preemption of regulation, should be considered. The impact of managed care on the poor and the provision of services through the public health sector should also be part of an aggressive new public health campaign.

Public health's basic task is to strengthen community as the most efficacious means for ensuring democratic control of the common life. This means that public health professionals are not simply practitioners of the science of community and the population, but also prophets of and guardians of the community against all of its foes. Public health needs to be relentless in demonstrating how uncontrolled market forces can be destructive of community, can ignore community, and can subordinate the goal of community to the bottom line of profits or market share.

Public health must constantly remind the public and its leaders that the displacement of the goal of national health reform by managed competition has the potential to be a catastrophe, and that the loss of this initiative is not only bad for health care but bad for democratic politics generally. We need national health care reform. We need reform not just because millions are uninsured, nor because costs are still soaring—even the more sober estimates of growth under a market regime predict that costs will be 18% of gross national product by the early part of the 21st century—but because, as a nation, we are deeply divided over issues of race, class, region, and political ideology and because these divisions produce democratic gridlock and the loss of political control by millions of citizens. A national health plan would help create a national institution that extends control over a major domain of the common life, creating loyalties to common practices and institutions. It is like we are a family who has inherited an old house that we must redesign and inhabit, creating a new structure that will enable us to live together in peace under institutional forms that promote common loyalties.[12] Unless we do this, the health care system, especially under market forces that actively promote the philosophy of "the devil take the hindmost" will become a force that divides rather than a force that unites.

The prophets engaged the powers that prevailed, and so must we. This concept might seem familiar, appearing often as "speaking truth to power," but truth to the prophetic imagination means far more than simply announcing the results of the latest survey of teenage pregnancy in the *American Journal of Public Health;* it means naming, identifying, and engaging the powers of this world, the spiritual dimension of power in American life, the "spell" of its major institutions and structures. People in public health must recover and strengthen their own social-justice roots, make sure that they are instilled in students in schools of public health, and encourage practitioners to speak fearlessly on public health's behalf in their communities. The antidote to the spirit-world of Baal is to wait on community and its spirits. Waiting on community means many things. It means placing one's ultimate trust in the power of hope rather than the powers of Baal, or the powers of the modern gods of the market, or money, or expertise. Waiting on community means using hope and other spiritual resources to encounter the ruling powers of this age. This will seem strange to modern secular man and woman, but it may be the key to surviving the captivity that we in public health are entering. Waiting on community means a kind of patience and endurance that enters the fray for the long run. Waiting on community means resisting the temptation of claiming immunity from attack in the powers of science and a neutral method. Public health is not neutral: public health is the struggle for a community based on social justice. Public health is a different kind of ethic from that found typically— a prophetic ethic. By this I mean that public health, like the prophetic tradition of social criticism, is concerned with seeing and naming the powers and with engaging the powers with a radical hope and faith.

We must sound the alarm for the danger to the community and to the nation as a whole from the weakening of the public health infrastructure in the face of a powerful resurgence of epidemic disease, a process that is occurring throughout the world.[13–15] This threat is not occurring because people from the so-called Third World are coming to the United States; it is occurring because of the shrinking of the world generally, the worldwide pace of development and technological change that is destroying or unbalancing vast ecosystems, the resilience of the microbial world in adapting to the use of antibiotics, the movements of whole peoples throughout the world, and the growing permeability of national boundaries. Managed care may provide some increased opportunities for ensuring that enrolled populations are immunized against known epidemics, but as a sentinel and safeguard against threats to communities as a whole, it is hopelessly inadequate. This problem may become known as one of the most serious consequences of wholesale privatization at the public health level.

The focus on privatization diverts us from yet another crisis that threatens to weaken democracy. This is the divide that looms as the next major frontier of public health: the U.S.-Mexican border. It is not simply that the border presents major challenges to the health and safety of the populations on both sides, which of course it does. It is rather that this border and the massive migration that is occurring from Mexico to the United States, the rapidly expanding commerce, and the drug traffic all present great challenges to a democracy already overburdened. The great threat is that the border itself will become not just a national boundary, but a fundamental divide in American politics, one as deep and as threatening to national unity as race and class already are. Indeed, we may already be at that point, and this division will be exploited by the forces of market populism to undermine democracy and the health of the public even more.

Lastly, we need to hold on to our hope, a fundamental aspect of a prophetic ethic. Hope is the faith in the power and efficacy of equality and democracy, and in the value of community in advancing the best interests of people together. When living in the midst of a conservative and market revolution, it is easy to give in to a kind of market individualism that holds that self-interest is the only bedrock of any social experiment. But hope is the reliance on the common good as a unique joining of self-interest and the common interest, and on a resolute refusal to sacrifice that longer view because everyone else has seemingly done so.

In 1988, I left the University of North Carolina at Chapel Hill for Albany, New York, and a job as Deputy Commissioner for Policy and Planning of the New York State Department of Health. My specific assignment was to lead the design of a state universal health care plan, and my clear expectation and that of many others was that this plan would form the platform on which Governor Mario Cuomo, as he then was, would ultimately run for president. The leader of the Department of Health was David Axelrod, a prophetic voice within American public health and its best-known leader apart from Surgeon General Koop. (Axelrod suffered a devastating stroke in 1991 and died July 4, 1994.) Although we based the design of the new plan on single-payer principles, in my mind this choice was not only my public health experience but also the experience of growing up in segregated east and south Texas with the divisions of American life, of which race is the greatest. The plan we set out was deliberately designed to foster community and a new public, one more aware of its power within the body politic. When Cuomo refused to embrace state-level reform, and as the 1992 election loomed, we designed a plan that created a de facto single-payer system by linking private insurance to the Medicare system, a strategy followed by the American Association of Retired Persons and others. Again, our goal was to advance a plan that was premised on creating a stronger national community and body politic, and to make that part of the national debate.

I will never forget the day in May 1992 when Governor Mario Cuomo addressed a large audience of New York University Medical School graduates at Carnegie Hall in a speech that was planned to lay out a blueprint for health reform that Clinton might take heed of. At a critical point, he was to hold up a single card and dramatize the simplicity and public appeal of the plan. When the moment came, Cuomo raised his arm only half-heartedly, and the speech was mostly read and not spoken from the heart. I learned later that Cuomo's press people had privately discouraged the press from attending. In my view, Cuomo had lost hope. Instead of a strong plan that could unite the body politic, we got the Clinton Plan—viewed by many as ill-fated from the start.

I mentioned William Stringfellow earlier as a powerful advocate for a prophetic ethic for the United States. In the mid-1970s he was a guest in our home. We were living in Durham, North Carolina, near Duke University. Stringfellow was the speaker at the graduation ceremonies for the professional schools at Duke—the medical school and the law school, principally. The graduation speech was held in Duke Chapel. What transpired was truly remarkable, probably less so to those who knew him well. Stringfellow was introduced by the president of Duke, Terry Sanford, a former governor and sometime presidential aspirant, who in the 1980s had been a U.S. senator from North Carolina. Stringfellow's talk was a veritable jeremiad against the present state of the professions of medicine and law in the American republic. He left no criticism out, abrasively challenging the pretensions of these two great professions. One could sense the deep unhappiness of the audience of faculty, students, and especially parents who had spent tens of thousands of dollars on their sons' and daughters' education. Afterwards, the chaplain of Duke Chapel and President Sanford seemed delighted to hand Stringfellow over to Bill Smith, the pastor of our church, and he came to supper at our house.

I cannot say that I remember much of what we said; I simply told him how much his work meant to me. Mostly we talked and laughed about his speech in Duke Chapel. He seemed tired and exhausted, and took many pills before sitting down to eat. But the scene that captured everything was Stringfellow walking toward our small group in front of Duke Chapel, with Terry Sanford and the chaplain waiting anxiously, eager to be rid of him. Stringfellow was almost painfully thin and haunted-looking, carrying his things in a shopping bag from a New York City department store.

The two pictures of Cuomo and Stringfellow, both speaking to medical school graduates 20 years apart, are permanently joined in my mind. The image of one of the United States' most powerful politicians, hesitating at a time when everyone knew the health system was in deep crisis and the nation might be poised for its greatest decision (or mistake), his arm half-raised in the air, frozen in indecision, stands beside the image of Bill Stringfellow speaking fearlessly of the shortcomings of medicine years before the "health care crisis" was upon us. After Stringfellow spoke and as he was walking toward our small group from the back of the chapel, carrying his shopping bag, smiling slightly, he seemed to know that his host, a former governor and future senator, was quickly disposing of him, handing him over to a local pastor and a few parishioners. His jaunty step and grim smile seemed to almost perfectly capture the eternal role of the prophet—alone, courageous, seemingly weak and powerless, filled with hope, and serene that in serving the community he would ultimately prevail. And so will we.

REFERENCES

1. Beauchamp D. Public health: alien ethic in a strange land? *Am J Public Health*. 1976; 65:1338–1339.

2. Lindblom C. The market as prison. *J Politics*. 1982;44:324–336.

3. Beauchamp D. *Health Care Reform and the Battle for the Body Politic*. Philadelphia: Temple University Press; 1996.

4. Goodwyn L. *The Populist Moment: A Short History of the Agrarian Revolt in America*. New York: Oxford University Press; 1978.

5. Boyte HC. Beyond politics as usual. In: Boyte HC, Reissman F, eds. *The New Populism: The Politics of Empowerment*. Philadelphia: Temple University Press; 1986:3–15.

6. Lind M. The southern coup. *New Republic*. June 19, 1995:20–29.

7. Wilson J. *The Politics of Regulation*. New York: Basic Books; 1980:357–394.

8. McGavran ES. What is public health? *Can J Public Health*. 1953;44:441–451.

9. Stringfellow W. *An Ethic for Christians and Other Aliens in a Strange Land*. Waco, Tex: Word Press; 1974.

10. Brueggemann W. *Hopeful Imagination: Prophetic Voices in Exile*. Philadelphia: Fortress Press; 1986.

11. Brueggemann W. *The Prophetic Imagination*. Philadelphia: Fortress Press; 1976.

12. Beauchamp D. Public health as social justice. *Inquiry*. 1976;13:3–13.

13. Garrett L. *The Coming Plague: Newly Emerging Diseases in a World Out of Balance*. New York: Penguin; 1994.

14. Brudney K, Dobkin J. Resurgent tuberculosis in New York City. *Am Rev Respir Disord*. 1991;144:745–749.

15. U.S. Department of Health and Human Services, Public Health Service, Centers for Disease Control and Prevention. *Addressing Emerging Infectious Disease Threats: A Prevention Strategy for the United States*. Atlanta, Ga: Centers for Disease Control and Prevention; 1994.

CHAPTER 23

Strategies for Managing the Public's Health: Implications and Next Steps

Paul K. Halverson, Arnold D. Kaluzny, and Curtis P. McLaughlin

Privatization efforts are occurring across a wide range of health care settings, including hospitals, public health clinics, community health centers, nursing facilities, home health services, and mental health facilities. Many of these efforts emerge in response to the growth of managed care plans, which offer government agencies cost containment and clinical accountability in serving patients traditionally cared for in public settings. Privatization also creates opportunities for public sector health care organizations to link with their private sector counterparts in alliances and integrated delivery systems, with the goal of achieving improvements in quality and efficiency.[1]

Whether privatization in health care is viewed as a reaction to changing environments or as a proactive strategy to better manage change, it raises a host of concerns critical to the fundamental principles of public health. Questions about the availability, accessibility, and quality of health services under privatization are paramount, and include:

- Will privatization result in a decline in the availability and accessibility of health services traditionally provided in the public sector?
- Will privatization necessitate a greater role for public agencies in oversight and enforcement in order to ensure availability of services from private providers?

Source: Adapted with permission from P.K. Halverson et al., Privatizing Health Services: Implications for Public Health and Quality Management, *Quality Management in Health Care*, Vol. 5, No. 2, pp. 1–18, © 1997, Aspen Publishers, Inc. and M. Hatcher, P.K. Halverson, and A.D. Kaluzny, Medicaid Managed Care: Lessons and Strategies for Public Health, *Health Care Management: State of the Art Reviews*, Vol. 2, pp. 30–42, © 1996, Hanley and Belfus, Inc.

- Are private sector providers adequately able to assume responsibility for the health care needs of clients traditionally served in the public sector?

- How will privatization impact public sector capacity to serve clients who are unlikely to receive care through private providers, such as the uninsured who are not eligible for public programs like Medicaid?

- Will privatization of personal health services erode funding sources for public health agencies and diminish the ability of these agencies to perform critical nonclinical activities, such as community assessment and policy development?[2,3]

- Will private providers be willing to provide health services that may be unprofitable or require long periods of time to accrue benefits?

These questions strike at the heart of what has been identified as a fundamental public health function—that of ensuring the availability and quality of health services in a community.[4,5] This chapter explores the implications of privatization initiatives for public health and identifies actions that may be taken to manage these processes most effectively.

THE NEW FRONTIER

Privatization has arrived in health care, and in its wake have come the new interests of employers, consumers, and even Wall Street.[6] At the market level, changes in health care financing patterns have created pressure for public providers to reduce operating costs in order to remain financially solvent and competitive with private sector counterparts. The growth of managed care organizations has caused many public providers to serve growing numbers of patients under discounted fee schedules and capitated reimbursement contracts negotiated with managed care plans.[7] Moreover, reimbursement rates for serving Medicaid and Medicare beneficiaries have remained relatively flat in recent years, creating financial pressures for those providers whose patient populations are dominated by these beneficiaries. Federal and state initiatives to enroll these beneficiaries in private managed care plans have forced many public providers to compete with private providers for serving patients who previously would have been served only in the public sector. At the same time, some public providers have experienced reductions in the numbers of privately insured patients they serve, as more of these patients are enrolled in managed care plans that contract with closed panels of private providers.

The market-level pressures facing many public sector providers combine with a range of organization-specific factors to further encourage privatization initiatives. Public providers seek to transfer responsibility for providing a range of services to private providers in order to improve efficiency in delivering these services, or to allow the public agency to specialize in a restricted set of services that are determined to be more central to the organization's core mission. Public providers may also support privatization initiatives as quality improvement strategies, by allowing certain services to be performed by private organizations that offer both expertise and accountability in a given service domain. At the same time, private health care providers may view privatization initiatives as opportunities for market expansion and differentiation. Private hospitals, managed care plans, physicians, and other provider groups may seek to expand their patient base by serving clients traditionally cared for in public settings. These providers may also endeavor to distinguish their services from those of their competitors by tailoring them to the special needs and preferences of clients who traditionally are not served in private settings. Expansion and differentiation efforts represent common organizational responses to increased marketplace competition such as that created by managed care growth and cost-containment initiatives.[8]

Health care privatization efforts are also being encouraged by many of the same factors that are driving privatization and outsourcing in other industries. Many observers of U.S. politics and policy note the rise in American society of "market populism," a general belief that big government is bad and that the free market is an effective policy-generating and self-regulating mechanism.[9] This belief appears to be encouraging the formation of policies at federal, state, and local levels to reduce government involvement in directly providing goods and services and in regulating the activities of private organizations. A related belief among both policy makers and citizens is that the private sector operates more efficiently than the public sector because of the financial incentives created through competition. This belief serves as the rationale for the federal Government Performance and Results Act of 1993, which imposes public sector requirements for strategic management, performance measurement, and accountability mechanisms styled after similar private sector efforts that emerge naturally in response to competition.[10]

Finally, privatization efforts in health care are sustained by the same information and technology explosion that is driving many private corporations to outsource for needed skills and expertise.[11] Observers note that the rapidly expanding body of knowledge and technology in many fields makes it unfeasible and unprofitable to directly acquire all the expertise and capacity organizations may need. Both public and private organizations are realizing that it may often be easier to hire special expertise from flexible, independent contractors.

IMPLICATIONS OF PRIVATIZATION

Privatization efforts are likely to affect the actions and priorities of public health agencies at federal, state, and local levels regardless of the functional and structural models used in these efforts (see Chapter 11 for a discussion of these models). This effect may occur directly through privatization efforts that target services provided by public health agencies, or indirectly through efforts that target health services provided by other public sector institutions, such as hospitals and community health centers. Through both of these pathways, privatization initiatives create a need for heightened federal and state efforts to ensure accountability in the provision of health services and in the use of public funds that support these services. At state and local levels, privatization initiatives create pressures for restructuring health programs and services that traditionally have been organized around categorical funding streams. Privatization initiatives also create the need for effective contract development and enforcement processes at state and local levels. Consequently, health care privatization efforts appear likely to shift the functions and priorities of public health agencies toward greater emphasis on ensuring accountability, restructuring delivery systems, and supporting contract development and enforcement activities.

Ensuring Accountability

Transferring responsibility for health service provision from public institutions to private providers creates concerns about the availability and adequacy of services delivered by private providers and about the appropriate use of public funds supporting these services. Efforts aimed at ensuring accountability in public health care may be complicated by privatization initiatives, however. Multiple private agencies and providers may assume responsibility for a given service originally performed by a single public institution, thereby necessitating more extensive efforts in evaluation and monitoring. Private agencies may show reluctance to release information that is considered proprietary, especially information related to financial performance. These agencies may also use accounting and tracking systems that do not enable the agencies to produce detailed information on services provided and expenditures made specifically through the privatization initiative. Managed care organizations operating under capitated reimbursement often lack this information because fees (and therefore claims) are not generated for each service delivered.

Responsibility for formal accountability systems primarily rests with the federal and state agencies charged with funding health-related programs and services, and with several nongovernmental health care accrediting agencies.[12] Federal funding agencies such as the Health Care Financing Administration (HCFA), the Centers for Disease Control and Prevention (CDC), and the Health Resources and Services Administration face significant challenges in expanding their accountability efforts to encompass the range of private agencies that are assuming responsibility for service provision under privatization initiatives. State health departments face these same challenges with regard to the state funds and federal pass-through funds they administer to public and private health care providers. Federal proposals recently under consideration regarding the establishment of block grants for public health services and Medicaid-funded services may add both urgency and complexity to the task of expanding federal and state roles in ensuring accountability under privatization.[13] In approaching this task, federal and state public health agencies are beginning to examine the efforts of private health care accrediting agencies and trade associations such as the National Committee for Quality Assurance (NCQA), the Joint Commission on Accreditation of Healthcare Organizations, and the Association of Accountable Health Plans (AAHP, formerly Group Health Association of America). Recent collaborative efforts between public health agencies and private accrediting agencies include a Medicaid accountability system developed jointly by HCFA and NCQA,[14] and a working alliance formed between CDC and AAHP to address a wide range of accountability issues within private managed care systems.[15]

To be sure, formal accountability systems are not the only mechanisms for ensuring health care quality, accessibility, and efficiency under privatization. The incentives established through appropriately structured financing and reimbursement systems are perhaps the most effective quality management mechanisms for privatization. Risk-sharing arrangements that make private providers financially accountable for the health status and service needs of their covered population hold great potential as quality management strategies. Performance-based reimbursement mechanisms such as those linked to immunization rates in the United Kingdom[16] or those linked to multiple health status indicators in U.S. health maintenance organizations (HMOs)[17,18] may prove at least as effective as formal accountability systems in ensuring quality and efficiency.

Restructuring Delivery Systems

Many of the health programs and services offered by public sector providers are supported by categorical funding sources administered by federal and state health agencies, and by public health insurance programs such as Medicaid and Medicare. At the federal level, these categorical services include preventive health services, sexually transmitted disease control, childhood immunization, tuberculosis control, cancer prevention and control, diabetes management, tobacco use prevention, disabilities prevention, lead poisoning prevention, breast and cervical cancer prevention and control, and human immunodeficiency virus prevention. Publicly provided services are often organized around these categorical funding sources, with distinct delivery, financing, and management systems established for each funding source. These modular systems of delivery offer effective ways of giving priority to selected services and creating simplicity in accounting and financing tasks, but they also breed duplication and inefficiency within public sector delivery systems.

As health services are transitioned to private sector providers, categorical delivery and financing systems are likely to be dismantled. Private sector providers are most likely to integrate privatized services into their existing delivery and financing systems, thereby offering opportunities for improved efficiency. The move away from a categorical system of service delivery also creates opportunities for certain services to receive less emphasis within the health care delivery system. The role of state and local public health agencies in monitoring these services and in ensuring appropriate access and utilization becomes of heightened importance. One possible solution may be to develop billing and reimbursement systems for the full range of health services provided in the public sector. Like the CPT-4 codes used to denote clinical procedures in medical care settings, these new systems may be used to monitor utilization and performance of services transferred from public to private providers. Developing this system must entail the difficult task of identifying reliable cost estimates for both clinical and nonclinical services that are transitioned to the private sector.

At the same time, public sector providers must face the challenges of reorganizing to best perform new and existing responsibilities that are no longer categorical in their design. A critical component of this reorganization effort involves the identification of funding sources to support noncategorical activities that remain the responsibility of public agencies. Many local public health agencies depend upon revenues generated through categorical programs and services to support delivery of population-based services, such as health assessment, surveillance and research, and policy development. Fees generated from the provision of clinical services to public beneficiaries such as Medicaid and Medicare beneficiaries are another major source of revenue for these population-based services. These fee-based revenues may also be jeopardized under privatization initiatives that transfer responsibility for clinical services provision to private providers. State and local public health agencies may play critical roles in designing and implementing privatization initiatives that include provisions for funding the vital functions that remain in the public domain. These agencies may also lead efforts in restructuring public providers to take advantage of new funding sources and to operate effectively under new priorities and service needs, such as the emphasis on population-based services.

Public providers may also need to restructure their geographic boundaries and service jurisdictions to better correspond with local health care delivery markets. Organizations such as local health departments and county hospitals may improve their abilities to interface with the private health care market by consolidating around metropolitan areas or other geographic regions that define the private market. Consolidation may occur through organizational merger or simply through purchasing and contracting networks. These arrangements may offer managed care plans and other private providers enhanced incentives to work collaboratively with public agencies, since they are able to establish relationships with a single public entity rather than with a diverse collection of small organizations. By pooling their client populations and service capacities through consolidation arrangements, public agencies may also enjoy more leverage in negotiating contracts and agreements with private providers.

Contract Development and Enforcement

An essential public health service within privatization initiatives involves the development and enforcement of contracts with private providers to ensure the quality, accessibility, and cost of services provided by contractors. State and local public health agencies bring three critical assets to this process: (1) a substantive knowledge of the health-related services and practices that private providers should be required to provide under contract, (2) the capacity and expertise to monitor and evaluate the performance of private contractors, and (3) the ability to mobilize community members and political leaders in support of contract enforcement. In states with Medicaid-waiver managed care programs, state health departments are including in their contracts with managed care organizations such provisions as requirements for provision of enabling services such as transportation and language translation; requirements for collection and reporting of quality assurance measures; acceptable criteria for disenrollment of members; allowable methods for marketing to Medicaid beneficiaries; and incentives for contracting with public health providers such as local health departments and community health centers. For programs and services that are privatized at the local level, the responsibility for identifying necessary contract provisions often falls to the local health department.

Under the new health care delivery systems created through privatization, public health agencies at state and local levels need to be able to monitor both their own performance and the performance of private providers along five dimensions: health outcomes; units of service provided; cost; access and demographics of individuals utilizing services; and consumer satisfaction. Contracts established with private providers should support the efforts of public health agencies to obtain information needed to carry out these monitoring activities. These contracts should also include provisions for conducting periodic quality improvement reviews focused on how to improve the outcomes of services provided through privatization initiatives.[19]

Responsibility for contract enforcement may devolve to the local level, even under privatization programs that include substantial state and federal involvement in quality assurance and accountability. Monitoring and evaluation systems are not sensitive to all gaps in performance, and state and federal power to address all identified gaps in private sector performance may be limited. Local health departments are uniquely placed among public health care organizations to detect gaps in performance, and to mobilize community support to encourage private providers to address those gaps. In performing these two core public health functions—assessment and policy development—local public health agencies contribute substantially to the processes of contract development and enforcement under privatization initiatives.

NEXT STEPS

Privatization of health services, and particularly of public health functions, is an unfolding phenomenon that is likely to continue, given the competitive health care environment characterized by increasingly scarce public and private resources. The potentials for damage and for gain in these initiatives are equally possible, and therefore the challenge lies in how best to manage the privatization process. A number of factors appear critical to successful management of this process.[20]

Allow for Proper Timing and Planning

Where privatization has occurred, policy leaders stress the importance of allowing adequate time to plan and implement new service delivery arrangements, to gain support for system change, and to develop organizational and technical capacity.[21] This was especially true in states that developed highly innovative, fully capitated programs for Medicaid recipients. The Arizona Access Program, for example, had major problems because of insufficient time for planning and implementation. Consequently, the program received complaints from participating health plans about failure to provide accurate enrollment data. Enrollees complained because of long waiting periods in physicians' offices and poor health care. Such problems were attributed to "poor management and oversight by the contracting administrative firm, resulting from the state trying to implement the program too quickly."[21]

It is best to plan for a privatization initiative before the proposal is under active consideration by the relevant policy makers. Often, the policy-making process at both local and state levels entails long periods of debate and discussion, which may greatly abbreviate the time available for effective planning. Sometimes, however, substantive policy changes can be made only during periods of budgetary or similar crises when deliberate and careful planning are all but impossible. In fact, almost every state or local government that has implemented significant policy change would probably have desired more time for planning and implementation. By all accounts, privatization as a policy alternative is gaining strength. It is prudent to prepare now for how this alternative may impact the public health system.

There Is No Substitute for Experience: Prototype

If you cannot learn from others—if you are truly on the leading edge—then prototype the service before going into it on a large scale. For example, NC chose to start a fully capitated Medicaid program in only one county, rather than statewide. The volatile processes of health care delivery require risk-averse strategies for change that are grounded in experience-based development and testing. Developing a prototype is a key part of such strategies.

Develop Clear Policy Objectives

The success of a managed care program or any privatization initiative lies in whether or not it meets its policy objectives, not just its Health Plan Employer Data and Information Set standards or its budget. Clearly stated objectives provide the focus for all activity within an uncertain and dynamic environment. For example, TennCare's early experience was disastrous because its implementation was too rapid, but the clear objectives of expanded access allowed the program to move rapidly and effectively in the direction of universal coverage from a starting point of almost no experience in managed care.

Consider the Incentives for Change

Gaining support for policy or system change includes building coalitions and aligning incentives. Creating change through privatization of health services affects many different groups, including providers, insurers, public health and other government agencies, and, most importantly, health care consumers. Even the most obvious technical solutions to public health problems are frequently not implemented for lack of political will to change. To build coalitions for change, opponents and advocates must be identified and their positions and values fully understood. It is unlikely (and undesirable) that any privatization strategy will be adopted solely through the support of either the public or private sector. It is equally unlikely that any one organization acting alone can make the necessary changes to implement such a strategy.

Implementation of privatization initiatives in health care requires cooperation and a relative level of trust. Incentives often win cooperation. Frequently, however, building support for privatization initiatives is accomplished by reducing opposition to a more manageable size and politically dividing the groups into proponents or neutral observers. In Tennessee, for example, the governor received no support for the state's Medicaid managed care program (TennCare) from providers. To gain the passive cooperation or neutrality of hospitals, HMOs, and preferred provider organizations, he "offered to rescind the 6.75% tax on patient revenues earlier than its April 1, 1994, expiration date."[22] Such incentives are effective.

Managed care may offer additional incentives for privatization initiatives. Under managed care arrangements, capitated reimbursement systems that offer a fixed fee per enrollee per period may create financial incentives for plans to maintain and improve health status in their enrolled populations in order to reduce the need for costly health services. Under these incentives, the potential exists for managed care plans and public health agencies to adopt a common emphasis on health promotion and disease prevention. Aligned incentives provide the means to accomplish policy goals oriented toward public health improvement, which may include privatization initiatives. Properly structured, privatization initiatives have the potential to increase the impact of health promotion and disease prevention efforts in the community. For example, Group Health Cooperative of Puget Sound (GHCPS) has demonstrated the value of community-based initiatives through its campaign to reduce head injury. A targeted intervention to promote the use of bicycle helmets—sponsored by GHCPS, the local health department, and other community-based organizations—led to a 67% reduction in the incidence of head injuries.[23] In a managed care environment, health status improvement efforts may be supported by added incentives beyond the fact that they are simply the right thing to do.

Ensure Adequate Capacity Building

Privatization demands a commitment to obtain experienced staff or to train existing staff to manage the transition from public to private provision of services. For private providers who may be assuming new responsibilities under these arrangements, this commitment may involve such activities as acquiring expertise in serving new population groups, providing new health and support services that may be needed by these groups, and redesigning delivery systems to meet the needs of these groups (such as service location and hours of service availability). For public agencies, privatization initiatives may require the acquisition of new skills in contract management, oversight, and regulation.

Measurement of health status becomes increasingly important under privatization initiatives, especially in the context of managed care. This measurement becomes a critical component of the quality management and oversight responsibilities of public agencies, as well as the care management objectives of managed care plans. Health education and community collaboration projects, once viewed as "nice but nonessential," take new meaning and importance under these initiatives as both public and private organizations share the incentives and responsibilities for public health improvement in the community. State and local agencies considering privatization initiatives should begin building the infrastructure necessary for successful implementation long before the initiatives are underway.

Pursue Staged Successes

The capacity to undertake major sustained change, such as capitated Medicaid managed care programs or other privatization initiatives, may be greatly strengthened by a series of "small wins" designed to demonstrate the potential success of a larger strategy.[24] In essence, successful incremental changes that involve elements of privatization may prove helpful when more broad-based change is considered. "Winning" demonstration projects or pilots often go a long way in convincing status quo stakeholders to consider change. This strategy involves two risks: if the pilot is not well implemented, it may fail, but if the pilot is successful, some may think that the problem is now solved. Both reactions are possible and need to be carefully considered and anticipated. "Small wins" through incremental change, however, often demonstrate that change is possible and desirable.

Recognize the "Fuzziness" in Public and Private Health Care Systems

One should never use the descriptors "public" and "private" loosely. Success or failure may well lie in the gradations between public and private organizations. The organizations discussed in this book encompass structures such as state and local governmental agencies; public authorities; quasi-governmental organizations; nonprofit organizations that are donative, entrepreneurial, and membership based; and private companies that have stockholders as well as employee stock ownership plans and individual partnerships. Attention to these differences is clearly warranted. One possible conclusion to draw is that in health care there is no such thing as a purely nonprofit organization.

It is important to be cautious about generalizing the observations from this book to other situations. The case studies in this book make it clear that there is little difference between for-profits and entrepreneurial nonprofits in many situations. A careful study of the motivations, objectives, and internal reward systems of organizations may need to supplant a simple binary classification system based upon type of ownership.

Rethink Accountability Structures

Open-meetings laws need to be revised so that public entities can negotiate with private ones in alliances without having to disclose both parties' trade secrets. At the same time, quasi-public authorities such as local hospital authorities should be required to make their cash and asset positions public knowledge. The community foundations that are developed with the proceeds of hospital privatizations must be made to act more in the interests of the public and less in the interest of board members, many of whom may be former employees.

Emphasize Stability in Privatization Initiatives

Contracts supporting privatization initiatives should be longer than one year, and all parties must be prepared to adjust the terms as real-world issues are encountered. Contracts should become firm only after both parties have prototyped a successful system, which entails testing the system under field conditions rather than in a laboratory microcosm. Therefore, alliances formed under privatization initiatives should be established as learning organizations, rather than only as vehicles for achieving cost minimization and the prevention of fraud and abuse. The objective of these entities must be system evolution, not revolution.

CONCLUSION

Health care privatization initiatives occur in a wide range of service areas, and throughout diverse organizational structures. These initiatives produce concerns about the performance of private providers in addressing health needs in the affected communities, and about the viability of public providers, who may still have roles to serve in these communities after privatization. Given these concerns, public health agencies at all levels of government are needed to play critical roles in designing, implementing, and sustaining these initiatives.

Optimal decision making and management regarding privatization in health services will require additional information in a number of critical areas. First, the critical clinical and nonclinical health services provided by government-owned health care organizations need to be further defined and coded for the purposes of describing units of service, determining the true cost of service units, and delineating new public and private sector roles and responsibilities. Similarly, government agencies undergoing privatization need to be able to define in advance what functions private providers are expected to perform and how much this performance should reasonably cost. Public health agencies at all levels of government need to develop capabilities to measure health services performance both in the public sector and among all private providers across the five dimensions of health outcomes: units of service, cost, access, consumer demographics, and consumer satisfaction. Finally, and perhaps most importantly, additional information is needed regarding how decisions are made to privatize, when privatization is successful, how privatization efforts are sustained and improved over time, and when alternatives to privatization should be considered. As these questions are answered, communities are likely to move closer to the appropriate balance among government and private sector roles in health services delivery, and to sustain this balance by effectively and efficiently managing the public's health.

REFERENCES

1. Zuckerman HS, Kaluzny AD, Ricketts TC. Strategic alliances: a worldwide phenomenon comes to health care. In: Kaluzny AD, Zuckerman HS, Ricketts TC, eds. *Partners for the Dance: Forming Strategic Alliances in Health Care.* Ann Arbor, Mich: Health Administration Press; 1995:1–18.

2. Koeze JS. Paying for public health services in North Carolina. *Popular Government.* 1994;60:11–20.

3. Handler AS, Turnock BJ. Local health department effectiveness in addressing the core functions of public health: essential ingredients. Under review.

4. Institute of Medicine. *The Future of Public Health.* Washington, DC: National Academy Press; 1988.

5. Upshaw VM, Craft EM, Easily AM, Okun M, et al. *Assurance: The Role of Public Health within the Context of Privatization.* Chapel Hill, NC: Public Health Leadership Program, School of Public Health, University of North Carolina at Chapel Hill; 1996.

6. The Advisory Board. *The Rising Tide.* Washington, DC: The Advisory Board; 1996.

7. Kralewski JE, Wingert TD, Feldman R, Rahn GJ, et al. Factors related to the provision of hospital discounts for HMO inpatients. *Health Serv Res.* 1992;27:133–153.

8. Zwanziger J, Melnick GA, Simonson L. Differentiation and specialization in the California hospital industry. *Med Care.* 1996;34:361–372.

9. Beauchamp D. Public health and market populism: a time for reflection. *Qual Manage Health Care.* 1997;5:73–79.

10. U.S. Department of the Treasury, Office of Inspector General. *Government Performance and Results Act of 1993 (GPRA) Implementation Assessment Guide.* Washington, DC: Government Printing Office; 1993.

11. Gingrich N. *To Renew America.* New York: HarperCollins Publishers; 1995.

12. Silberman P. Regulating managed care in a market driven health system: ensuring access and quality. Under review.

13. United States Senate. Public Health Enhancement Act of 1995. *U.S. 104th Congress (1st Session).* Senate Bill 142. Washington, DC: Government Printing Office; 1995.

14. National Committee for Quality Assurance (NCQA). *Medicaid HEDIS 1.0.* Washington, DC: NCQA; 1996.

15. Centers for Disease Control and Prevention. Prevention and managed care: opportunities for managed care organizations, purchasers of health care, and public health agencies. *MMWR*. 1995; 44:1–12.

16. Lynch ML. The uptake of childhood immunization and financial incentives to general practitioners. *Health Economics*. 1994;3:17–25.

17. Kouides RW, Lewis B, Bennett NM, Bell KM, et al. A performance-based incentive program for influenza immunization in the elderly. *Am J Prev Med*. 1993;9:250–255.

18. Schlackman N. Evolution of a quality-based compensation model: the third generation. *Am J Med Qual*. 1993;8:103–110.

19. Speake DL, Mason KP, Broadway TM, Sylvester M, et al. Integrating indicators into a public health quality improvement system. *Am J Public Health*. 1995;85:1448–1449.

20. Hatcher M, Halverson PK, Kaluzny AD. Medicaid managed care: lessons and strategies for public health. *Health Care Manage: State of the Art Rev*. 1995;2:30–42.

21. General Accounting Office (GAO). *Medicaid: States Turn to Managed Care To Improve Access and Control Cost* (GAO/HRD-93-46). Washington, DC: GAO; 1993.

22. Solomon CM, Smith JL. TennCare Up and Running. *Health Syst Rev*. 1994;27:10–13, 16–18, 20.

23. Thompson RF, Taplin SM, McAfee TA, Mandelson MT, et al. Primary and secondary prevention services in clinical practice: twenty years' experience in development, implementation, and evaluation. *J Am Med Assoc*. 1995;273:1130–1135.

24. Weick KE. Small wins: redefining the scale of social problems. *Am Psychol*. 1984;39:40–49.

Medicaid Managed Care Risk Contract Between the State of North Carolina, Division of Medical Assistance, and a Health Maintenance Organization

This Contract is entered into this 1st day of July, 1994, between the State of North Carolina, Division of Medical Assistance, with a principal place of business located at 1985 Umstead Drive, in the City of Raleigh, County of Wake, State of North Carolina and _____ a corporation organized and existing pursuant to laws of the State of North Carolina, which is licensed as a health maintenance organization (HMO), with a principal place of business located at _____ in the city of _____ , County of _____, State of North Carolina.

WHEREAS, the Division of Medical Assistance of the State of North Carolina (the "Division") is charged with the administration of the North Carolina State Plan for Medical Assistance (the "State Plan") in accordance with the requirements of Title XIX of the Social Security Act, as amended, (the "Act") and Articles 67 and 68 of Chapter 58 of the North Carolina General Statutes; and,

WHEREAS, _____ (the "Plan") is an entity eligible to enter into a risk contract in accordance with Section 1903(m) of the Act and 42 CFR, Part 434, and is engaged in the business of providing prepaid comprehensive health care services as defined in 42 CFR Part 434, and is licensed as a health maintenance

Courtesy of the State of North Carolina, Division of Medical Assistance, Raleigh, North Carolina.

organization ("HMO") by the North Carolina Department of Insurance, pursuant to Articles 67 and 68 of Chapter 58 of the North Carolina General Statutes; and,

WHEREAS, the Division desires to contract with health maintenance organizations to obtain services for the benefit of certain Medicaid Recipients residing in the county of _____ ; and,

WHEREAS, the Plan has provided to the Division continuing proof of its capability to provide quality services efficiently, effectively, and economically during the term of this Contract, and continuing proof of its financial responsibility, including adequate protection against the risk of insolvency, upon which the Division relies in entering into this Contract;

NOW THEREFORE, the parties hereby agree as follows:

SECTION 1—GENERAL PROVISIONS

1.1   Definitions and Construction
The terms used in this Contract shall have the definitions set forth in Appendix I, unless this Contract expressly provides otherwise. References to numbered Sections refer to the designated Sections contained in this Contract. Titles of Sections used herein are for reference only and shall not be deemed to be a part of this Contract. In the event of a conflict between this Contract and the documents incorporated into this Contract by reference, the terms of the Contract shall govern.

1.2   Governing Law
In connection with the performance of its obligations under this Contract, the Plan shall comply with all applicable Federal and State regulations and laws (statutory and case law), including Rules of the Division, and of the North Carolina Department of Insurance, and all Federal Medicaid Act provisions which have not been expressly waived by the Health Care Financing Administration.

1.3   Nondiscrimination and Equal Employment Opportunity
The Plan shall comply with all Federal and State laws which prohibit discrimination on the grounds of race, age, creed, sex, religion, national origin, or physical or mental handicap, including Title VI of the Civil Rights Act 42 USC 2000d and regulations issued pursuant thereto; the Americans with Disabilities Act, 42 USC 12101 et seq., and regulations issued pursuant thereto; the Age Discrimination Act of 1975, as amended,

42 USC 6101 et seq., and regulations issued pursuant thereto; the Rehabilitation Act of 1974, as amended, 29 USC §794, and regulations issued pursuant thereto; and Executive Order 11246 "Equal Employment Opportunity" as amended by Executive Order 11375 and regulations issued pursuant thereto.

1.4   Conflict of Interest

No public official of the State of North Carolina and no official or employee of HCFA or any other state or federal agency which exercises any functions or responsibilities in the review or approval of this Contract or its performance shall voluntarily acquire any personal interest, direct or indirect, in this Contract or any subcontract entered into by the Plan. The Plan hereby certifies that no officer, director, employee or agent of the Plan, any subcontractor or supplier, and no person with an ownership or control interest in the Plan, any subcontractor or supplier, is also employed by the State of North Carolina or any of its agencies, the Fiscal Agent or any other agents of the Division, HCFA or any agents of HCFA.

1.5   Reinsurance

The Plan may obtain reinsurance for coverage of Members under this Contract, provided that the Plan remains substantially at risk for providing services under this Contract.

1.6   Force Majeure

Neither party to this Contract shall be responsible for delays or failures in performance resulting from acts beyond the control of such party. Such acts include natural disasters, strikes, riots, acts of war and similar occurrences.

1.7   Disputes

Any dispute arising under this Contract which cannot be disposed of by agreement between the Division and the Plan may be appealed to the Division's Hearing Unit. An appeal must be received in writing by the Division Hearing Unit no later than thirty (30) days from the date of the initial written determination letter from the Managed Care Program Administrator to the Plan. The Plan shall proceed diligently with the performance of this Contract until the final agency decision is rendered by the Division Director based upon findings of facts and conclusions of Law found by the assigned Hearing Officer. The Plan shall be required to bring any and all legal proceedings, including those subsequent to the Division Director's final decision upon an appeal, in North Carolina State courts.

1.8   Disclosure of Information on Ownership and Control

The Plan shall disclose to the Division information on ownership and control of the Plan prior to the beginning of the Contract term, as set forth in Title 42 CFR 455.104.

1.9   Disclosure of Information on Business Transactions

Plans which are not Federally qualified HMOs must disclose to the Division information on certain types of transactions they have with a "party in interest" as defined in the Public Health Service Act. (See Sections 1903(m)(2)(A)(viii) and 1903(m)(4) of the Act.) This requirement is detailed further in Appendix XII.

1.10   Conversion Privileges

The Plan shall offer any Member covered under this Contract the opportunity to convert to a non-group enrollment contract consistent with conversion privileges offered to Members of other groups enrolled in the HMO. Any Member who ceases to qualify as a Member under Section 4.8, Involuntary Disenrollment, is not eligible for conversion privileges.

1.11   Contract Officers

The Managed Care Program Administrator of the Division shall serve as the Contract officer for the State. The Chief Executive Officer of the Health Plan shall serve as the Contract officer for the Plan. Each Contract officer reserves the right to delegate as may be appropriate, such duties to others in the officer's employment.

1.12   Notices

All notices pursuant to this Contract shall be deemed duly given upon the delivery, if delivered by hand (against receipt), or three (3) calendar days after posting, if sent by registered or certified mail, return receipt requested, to a party hereto at the address set forth below or to such other address as a party may designate by notice pursuant hereto.

Plan: _____

_____

Division: _____

_____

SECTION 2—CONTRACT TERM

2.1   Initial Term

The term of this Contract shall begin at 12:01 a.m. on _____ , 1996, and shall continue until the close of the third full fiscal year of the State, at

12:00 midnight on June 30, 1999, subject but not limited to the provisions in Section 13—Default and Termination and Section 10.4—Calculation of Rates.

The Division shall recalculate the capitation rates for each fiscal year of the Contract term, and shall deliver them to the Plan no later than April 1 of each year. In the absence of a notice for nonrenewal, the new capitation rates and maximum enrollment levels shall be deemed to be accepted by both parties, the enrollment status of all Medicaid Members shall continue uninterrupted, and this Contract shall continue in effect through the next fiscal year.

2.2   Renewal Term
This Contract shall be automatically renewed every three years for a three year term beginning on July 1. If either party to this Contract wishes to terminate this relationship at the end of a three year period, a written notice must be delivered to the other party no later than May 1 of the third year.

SECTION 3—MEMBER ELIGIBILITY

3.1   Persons Eligible for Enrollment
To be eligible to enroll in the Plan established pursuant to this Contract, a person must be a Recipient in the North Carolina Medical Assistance (Medicaid) Program in one of the aid categories listed below; and residing in Mecklenburg County; and not eligible for Medicare. The estimated sizes of the eligible aid categories are listed in Appendix II.
a.   Aid to Families with Dependent Children (AFDC)
b.   AFDC-related without Medicaid deductibles (MAF)
c.   Blind and Disabled without Medicaid deductibles (MAB, MAD)
d.   Medicaid Pregnant Women (MPW)
e.   Medicaid for Infants and Children (MIG)
f.   SSI-Medicaid only
g.   Foster Care Children (Eligible at discretion of DSS and guardian.)

3.2   Persons Ineligible for Enrollment
The following categories of Recipients are not eligible to enroll in the Plan:
a.   Medicare Qualified Beneficiaries (MQB)
b.   Medicare/Medicaid Dual Eligibles
c.   Illegal Aliens
d.   Medically Needy (With a Medicaid Deductible)

    e.   Nursing Facility Residents

    f.   Adult Care Home Residents

    g.   Residents of Intermediate Care Facilities for the Mentally Retarded

    h.   Recipients with Presumptive Eligibility

    i.   Refugee Assistance

    j.   Community Alternatives Program (CAP) Recipients

SECTION 4—ENROLLMENT AND DISENROLLMENT

4.1   Plan Selection

Recipients will select and be assigned to a Plan only through an independent Health Benefit Manager (HBM) who will perform this function under separate contract to the Division. The Plan is prohibited from enrolling Recipients directly or conducting any point of sale marketing. The Plan shall provide for a continuous open enrollment throughout the term of this Contract and shall enroll all eligible Recipients without restriction, in the order in which they apply through the HBM; and shall further agree to enroll up to a minimum of 5000 Recipients, subject to the limitations set forth in Sections 4.2 and 6.8.

Eligible family members residing in the same household must select the same Plan. Family members shall be permitted to choose different providers within the same Plan. Eligible Recipients who do not voluntarily select a Plan within 10 business days of the date of interview with the HBM, (30 days for MAD and MAB Recipients), will be assigned to a Plan according to an algorithm approved by the Division.

4.2   Member Composition

No more than seventy-five percent (75%) of a Plan's membership in Mecklenburg County shall be Medicare beneficiaries or Medicaid Recipients, unless a waiver has been granted by the Secretary of the Department of Health and Human Services pursuant to Section 1903 (m)(2) of the Social Security Act. The Division may request a waiver each year for up to three years depending upon the Plan's demonstration of good faith efforts to meet the 75/25 goal.

4.3   Change of Household Composition

The Plan shall report to the County Department of Social Services any change in the household composition of Members, including changes in family size, marital status or residence, within (5) days of such information being known to the Plan.

4.4   Newborns

Newborns of Members shall be automatically enrolled and covered by the mother's Plan, effective from the date of birth. The Plan shall obtain a record of the birth from the hospital in which the birth took place, and shall notify the County Department of Social Services (DSS) of all births to Members within five (5) business days from the date of birth.

4.5   Effective Date of Enrollment/Disenrollment

An enrollment period shall always begin on the first day of a calendar month, except in the case of newborns, and shall end on the last day of a calendar month. Disenrollments and plan transfers shall be effective no earlier than the first of the month following the request or reason for disenrollment or transfer, and no later than the first of the second month following a request or reason for disenrollment or transfer.

4.6   Automatic Re-Enrollment

A Recipient whose membership in the Plan is terminated due to ineligibility as defined in Section 3—Member Eligibility, shall be automatically re-enrolled in the Plan upon resumption of eligibility, unless the Recipient selects a new Plan.

4.7   Automatic Disenrollment

A Recipient shall be automatically disenrolled from the Plan if the Recipient:

a.   no longer resides in the Service Area;
b.   is deceased;
c.   is admitted to a long-term care facility or a correctional facility for more than thirty (30) days;
d.   no longer qualifies for Medicaid or becomes a Recipient ineligible for enrollment as defined in Section 3.2.

4.8   Involuntary Disenrollment

The Plan may request involuntary disenrollment of a Member only for Good Cause, and must submit such request in writing to the HBM. Good Cause is defined as:

a.   Behavior on the part of a Member which is disruptive, unruly, abusive, or uncooperative, to the extent that the ability of the Plan to provide services to the Member or other affected Members is seriously impaired;
b.   Persistent refusal of a Member to follow a reasonable, prescribed course of treatment; or

c.   Fraudulent use of the Medicaid card or the Member ID card issued by the Plan.

Disenrollment of a Member will *not* be approved for reasons such as pre-existing medical conditions; changes in health status; high cost medical needs, or the exercise by a Member of their right to file a complaint, grievance or appeal.

The Plan shall submit to the Division its policies and procedures for assuring that each disenrollment request is consistent with Good Cause, as defined in this Section. The written policies and procedures must include a description of the remedial steps the Plan will take to obtain Member compliance, preceding all requests for involuntary disenrollment.

4.9   Plan Transfers
Members may voluntarily disenroll from the Plan, and transfer to another Plan at any time without cause. The transfer shall be effective the first day of the next calendar month, subject to data processing deadlines, but in no case will it be effective later than the first day of the second month after the transfer is requested.

SECTION 5—MARKETING

5.1   Marketing
The Plan may develop marketing materials in all mediums such as brochures, fact sheets, posters, billboards, radio and television advertising, to solicit eligible Recipients for enrollment; however, the Plan shall obtain the prior written approval of the Division of all marketing plans and materials that will be distributed to, or aimed at Medicaid Recipients, including any material or advertising campaign that mentions Medicaid, Medical Assistance, or Title XIX. The Plan shall have written procedures for monitoring its enrollment practices. All materials must pass current North Carolina readability requirements, G.S. 58-38-1 et seq. and G.S. 58-67-65 (a)(3) and must provide an accurate description of the Plan's rules, procedures, benefits, services, and other information necessary for Recipients to make an informed decision. Any advertisement, solicitation material, member handbook, etc., found to be in conflict with the benefits provided will be interpreted in favor of the Recipient. The Plan must provide materials in English, Spanish and other languages as may be determined necessary by the Division.

The Plan shall be required to participate in County and State-sponsored functions for the purpose of providing consumer education and marketing to potential Members.

The Plan shall reimburse the Division a pro-rata share of the cost of production and supply of (1) A Health Plan Directory—Booklet for Recipients describing each available health plan option; and (2) Enrollment/Disenrollment Forms—For use by the Health Benefit Manager in the enrollment/disenrollment process.

The Plan is prohibited from:
a. door-to-door and other point-of-sale marketing to and solicitation of Recipients;
b. engaging in marketing activities that could mislead, confuse, or defraud Medicaid Recipients, or misrepresent the Plan, its marketing representatives, or the Division; and
c. offering financial incentives to Recipients as an inducement to enroll in the Plan.

SECTION 6—DUTIES AND RESPONSIBILITIES OF THE PLAN

6.1 Performance Standard
The Plan shall perform all duties and responsibilities set forth in this Contract and shall develop, produce and deliver to the Division all of the statements, reports, accountings, claims and documentation described herein, and the Division shall make payments to the Plan in full consideration thereof on a capitated basis as described herein. The Plan agrees that failure to comply with the provisions of this Contract may result in the recoupment of payments, suspension of Member enrollment, assessment of liquidated damages and/or termination of this Contract, in whole or in part. Any payments due hereunder may be withheld until the Division receives from the Plan all written and properly executed documents as required by this Contract.

6.2 Covered Services
The Plan shall provide to Recipients enrolled under this Contract, directly or through arrangements with others, all of the Covered Services identified in Appendix III. Covered services must be medically necessary and provided by, or under the direction of a physician. The Plan shall provide the same standard of care for all Members regardless of eligibility cat-

egory, and shall make all services as accessible in terms of timeliness, amount, duration and scope, to Medicaid Members, as those services are to nonenrolled Medicaid Recipients within the same area. Covered services are defined in the respective Medicaid Provider Manuals and Bulletins which are incorporated by reference (see Appendix IIIA).

6.3   Emergency Medical Services
In accordance with 42 CFR 434.30, the Plan shall arrange for all Medically Necessary medical services which may be required to treat an Emergency Medical Condition 24 hours each day, 7 days a week, either in the Plan's contracted facilities in accordance with the terms of the agreement entered into for services provided to Medicaid Recipients, or through arrangements approved by the Division, with another provider.

Payments for treatment of Emergency Medical Conditions are to be based on the medical signs and symptoms of the condition upon initial presentation to the emergency department. The retrospective findings of a medical work-up may legitimately be the basis for determining how much additional care may be authorized, but will not be used in determining payment for the initial emergency care. The Plan is responsible for educating Members on the appropriate use of emergency services.

6.4   Accessibility of Services
The Plan must establish and maintain provider networks in geographically accessible locations and in sufficient numbers to provide the medically necessary Covered Services for the Plan's Members in a timely and appropriate manner. The Plan shall ensure that all Covered In-Plan Services are as accessible to Members (in terms of timeliness, amount, duration, and scope) as those services are to non-enrolled Medicaid Recipients within the area and that no incentive is provided to providers, monetary or otherwise, for withholding medically necessary services.

Plans shall be required to cooperate with the City of Charlotte to develop the infrastructure necessary to serve those geographic locations most heavily populated by Medicaid Members.

The Plan must provide the Division at least 30 days notice prior to the proposed effective date if it plans to change a location, services, or reduce availability. The Plan must notify in writing those Members affected by such a change at least 15 business days prior to the effective date of such changes, or as soon as possible in the cases of unforeseen circumstances.

The Plan must provide toll-free telephone medical advice by a licensed medical professional, either directly or through its network providers, to Members 24 hours per day, 7 days per week. The Plan shall maintain a record of encounters on the telephone medical advice line, including the date of call, type of call, and resolution. The Plan is responsible for educating Members on medical advice procedures.

The Division shall have the right to review periodically the adequacy of service locations, the hours of operation, and the availability and appropriateness of telephone medical advice. The Division may require the Plan to take corrective action to improve Member access to services based on periodic reviews.

6.5   Appointment Availability
The Plan must ensure that appropriate services are available as follows:
a.   Emergency—immediately upon presentation or notification.
b.   Urgent care—within twenty-four (24) hours.
c.   Routine sick care—within three (3) days.
d.   Regular, non-urgent, well care—within ninety (90) days except in the case of a woman who may be pregnant, then within fifteen (15) business days.
e.   Routine Plan Specialty care—within ninety (90) days.
f.   Telephone medical advice—twenty-four (24) hours a day and return call to Member within one (1) hour.
g.   New Member Health Assessment Encounter—within the first ninety (90) days of enrollment.
h.   Child in DSS custody—within seven (7) days; immediately when child is under age 2 or DSS staff determines the child has chronic and/ or emergent medical need(s).

6.6   Appointment Wait Time
The Plan must agree to provide services within the following wait times:
a.   Scheduled appointment—within one (1) hour.
b.   Walk-in—within two (2) hours or schedule for subsequent appointment.
c.   Life-threatening emergencies—must be managed immediately.

6.7   Member Services
The Plan must staff a Member Services Department to be responsible for:
a.   Explaining the operation of the Plan and answering Member questions.

b.   Assisting Members in making appointments and in obtaining appropriate services.

c.   Assisting Members in securing medically necessary, non-ambulance transportation.

d.   Handling Member complaints and providing information on grievance procedures.

e.   Assisting the HBM with providing appropriate Plan information.

f.   Resolving claim disputes and processing appeals.

g.   Operating a toll-free Member Services telephone line to provide instruction or authorize services 24 hours per day, 7 days a week.

6.8   Choice of Health Professional

The Plan must have written policies and procedures for assigning each of its Medicaid Members to a primary care provider (PCP). To the extent practical, the Plan must offer freedom of choice to Members in selecting or changing to a different PCP within the Plan, in accordance with its policies for other enrolled groups. The Plan must agree to assign no more than 2000 Members to any one full-time-equivalent provider in its network without the written approval of the Division. The Division encourages the Plan to include among its available providers any county, state, and/or federally qualified provider that currently serves Recipients in the service area, including FQHC, school-based health services, and county health departments.

A Member who has received prior authorization from the Plan for referral to a specialist or for inpatient care shall be allowed to choose from among all the available specialists and hospitals within the Plan, to the extent reasonable and appropriate.

6.9   Member Identification Card

The Plan must issue identification cards to Medicaid Members within 7 days after the effective date of enrollment. The card may identify the holder as a Medicaid Member through an alpha or numeric indicator, but should not be different in design and/or color than the card issued to its commercial Members. The card must include the twenty-four (24) hour medical advice telephone number and the toll-free Member services number.

6.10   Facilities and Resources

The Plan must provide directly or by contract the following:

a.   Specialists for adult and pediatric care, including care appropriate to the elderly, disabled, and adolescent enrollees;

b. Experienced and qualified care management staff;
c. One fully-accredited general acute care hospital bed per 727 enrollees;
d. A designated emergency service facility providing care 24 hours a day, 7 days a week;
e. Facilities at all service locations which meet the applicable Federal, State, and local requirements, pertaining to health care facilities and laboratories;
f. Telecommunications system sufficient to meet the needs of the Members;
g. A qualified Plan Administrator;
h. Sufficient support staff;
i. A licensed physician to serve as medical director to oversee and be responsible for the proper provision of Covered Services to Members;
j. A qualified quality assurance director;
k. A data processing person qualified to provide necessary and timely reports to the Division.

6.11 Orientation of New Members

The Plan shall provide each new Member, within fourteen (14) days from enrollment, written information on the Plan. All new Member Plan material must be approved by the Division prior to its release, and shall include at least the following information:

a. List of Primary Care Providers and the procedures for selecting an individual physician and scheduling an initial health assessment encounter within ninety (90) days from enrollment;
b. Each service location, including the address, telephone numbers, office hours, and procedures for scheduling appointments;
c. Benefits and services provided and any limitations or exclusions applicable to In-Plan Services;
d. Procedures for notifying Members affected by the termination or change in any benefits, services, service delivery, or office site;
e. Member rights and responsibilities, including the right to voluntarily change health plans;
f. Referral policy for specialty care and a current list of specialty care providers;
g. Provisions for after-hour and emergency care;
h. Role of primary care providers (PCPs);
i. How to access services;
j. The right to formulate Advance Directives;
k. Procedures for obtaining out of area coverage or services;

l. The right to receive family planning services and supplies from Out-of-Plan Providers;

m. Policies regarding the treatment of minors;

n. Any limitations that may apply to services obtained from Out-of-Plan Providers, including a disclosure of the responsibility of Members to pay for unauthorized health care services obtained from Out-of-Plan Providers, and the procedures for obtaining authorization for such services;

o. Circumstances under which a Member may transfer or be involuntarily disenrolled from the Plan;

p. Procedures for voicing complaints and grievances or recommending changes in policies and services;

q. Procedures for appealing adverse determinations affecting coverage, benefits or enrollment, including the right to appeal directly to the Division;

r. Process for accessing the Health Benefits Manager;

s. Information about the Plan's ability to make reasonable accommodations for people with physical accessibility difficulties;

t. Information concerning transportation arrangements offered by the Plan.

6.12   Care Management

The Plan shall be responsible for the management and continuity of medical care for all Members through the following minimum care management functions:

a. Appropriate referral and scheduling assistance for Members needing specialty health care services, including those needing referrals for additional Health Check Services, mental health services, nutritional referrals (WIC), or coordinated medical/social services;

b. Documentation of referral services in each Member's medical record;

c. Monitoring and treatment of Members with ongoing medical conditions according to appropriate standards of medical practice;

d. Documentation in each medical record of all emergency encounters and any medically indicated follow-up care;

e. Coordination of hospital and institutional admissions and discharges, including discharge planning;

f. Coordination of home-based care and home health services;

g. Determination of the need for Out-of-Plan services and referral of Members to the appropriate service setting, utilizing assistance as needed from the Division;

h. The use of multidisciplinary teams to assist in diagnosis and treatment of Members with complex medical needs.

6.13 New Member Health Assessments

The Plan shall provide a face to face initial health assessment visit to all new Members within the first ninety (90) days of enrollment. The Plan shall document its efforts to contact each new Member within the first forty-five (45) days of enrollment to schedule the health assessment. For Members known or appearing to be pregnant or suspected of being pregnant, an initial assessment shall be provided to the Member within 15 business days of enrollment.

The Division shall review the Plan's success in providing initial face-to-face health assessments within 90 days of enrollment. Should the Division find that the Plan has been unable to meet its obligation, the Plan will develop a written corrective action plan to identify strategies to increase the number of new Member health assessments.

6.14 Family Planning Services

Each Member shall have the right to freely choose a provider or providers of Family Planning Services. Such services may be obtained from Out-of-Plan Providers without a referral or prior authorization from the Plan. Family Planning Services and supplies provided by Out-of-Plan Providers shall be covered by the Plan at fees set by the provider not to exceed the Medicaid allowable rates.

6.15 Health Check (EPSDT) Services

The Plan must have written policies and procedures for providing Health Check (EPSDT) services and immunizations to Members under twenty-one (21) years of age. The Plan must comply with all Health Check (EPSDT) regulations set forth in 42 USC §1396 d(r)(5) and 42 USC §1396 d(a). The Plan must assure the provision of periodic health screens, including health education; and the provision of any treatment or services covered by the State's Medicaid program, necessary to correct or ameliorate defects and physical or mental illnesses and conditions discovered during screening services. The Scope of Health Check (EPSDT) Services is included in Appendix IV, and the Medicaid Special Bulletin for Health Check Providers, May, 1994, is included in the set of Provider Manuals.

The Plan must comply with the Health Check and immunization reporting requirements in Appendix V. The Plan has the option of providing Health Check services directly or contracting with the County Health Department, School Based Health Centers, or other qualified providers. The Plan must track and monitor the need for and completion of all Health Check services provided to each Member under age 21.

6.16   Health Education Services

The Plan shall make available on an on-going basis the following health education services at convenient times, in accessible locations, and at no cost to Medicaid Members:

Childbirth Education Classes: Offer parents the opportunity to develop knowledge and skills about the maternity cycle, delivery process, and initial information about newborn care.

Parenting Classes: Provided to expectant and new parents. The classes will provide general information about parenting skills and care of infants and children. Classes should include topics such as bathing, feeding (including breast feeding), injury prevention, sleeping, illness, preventive care, screening recommendations, and when to call a medical provider.

Child Development Classes: Provide parents the opportunity to learn about the normal stages of child growth and development.

Diabetes Self-Care Instruction: The Plan must provide for the assessment of skills, knowledge, and attitude for all Members who have been diagnosed with either type I or II diabetes. The Plan must develop a plan of care that addresses the specific and unique health care needs of the diabetic Member, including the need for specific training and education in the management of diabetes and the possible need for referral.

Smoking Cessation Classes: Provide information and offer support to Members who need education and assistance in smoking cessation.

Nutrition Services: The Plan must agree to incorporate comprehensive nutrition assessments, education, and counseling for all Members. The Plan must provide follow-up and/or referral to any Member who has a diagnosis or risk factors for which nutrition therapy is a critical component of medical management.

6.17   Support Services

The Plan shall develop strategies for addressing the special needs of the Medicaid population. Strategies should incorporate the use of staff training to increase awareness and sensitivity to the needs of persons who may be disadvantaged by low income, disability and illiteracy, or who may be non-English speaking. Staff training should include topics such as sensitivity to different cultures and beliefs, the use of bilingual interpreters, overcoming barriers to accessing medical care, understanding the role of substandard housing, poor diet, and lack of telephone and transportation in health and health care.

The Plan shall provide the following services as necessary to ensure Member access to and appropriate utilization of medically necessary services covered under this Contract:

Transportation: The Plan will assist with the arrangement of non-emergency transportation for its Members through available public and private services. The Plan will provide Members with written information concerning transportation arrangements offered by the Plan. The Plan shall document the provision of transportation services to any Member requiring such assistance.

Interpreter Services: Interpreter services shall be made available by telephone, and/or in-person to ensure that Members are able to communicate with the Plan and providers.

Coordination and Referral to Community Resources: The Plan shall provide referral to available community services, including but not limited to those identified in Appendix VII. The Plan shall have staff who are familiar with these resources and shall maintain a written description of appropriate referral procedures.

Referral to the WIC Program: Pursuant to Public Law 103-448, 204(e), the Plan shall ensure coordination with the WIC Program, described in Appendix VII. This coordination should include the referral of potentially eligible women, infants, and children to the WIC Program and include the provision of medical information from the Plan provider to the WIC Program.

6.18   Referrals for Out-of-Plan Services

The Plan shall ensure that Members are referred for all medically necessary services, both in-plan and out-of-plan. The Plan must consult with the County DSS when referring Members to long term institutional services such as those provided by nursing facilities, hospital swing bed units, intermediate care facilities for the mentally retarded or mentally ill, or to the Community Alternatives Program, as described in Appendix VI. The Plan shall have written policies and procedures for the referral of Members for Out-of-Plan services. These procedures shall be applicable to the appropriate referral of Members upon disenrollment from the Plan, regardless of the reason for disenrollment.

6.19   Payment to Out-of-Plan Providers

The Plan shall reimburse Out-of-Plan Providers for Covered Services which may be obtained by Members without prior authorization from the Plan for the following:

a.   Emergency medical services which could not be provided by the Plan because the time to reach the Plan Provider capable of providing such services would have meant risk of serious damage or injury to the Member's health. The Plan shall consider each claim for reimbursement for emergency medical services provided to Members by Out-of-Plan Providers based upon its own merits and the requirements of this Section, and shall not routinely deny such claims based upon failure to obtain prior authorization.

b.   Medicaid covered family planning services and supplies.

c.   Services provided by a Public Health Department for the screening, diagnosis, counseling, or treatment of STD's, TB, HIV, or family planning services. In the absence of a contractual arrangement with the Public Health Department, the Plan must pay for the service at fees set by the provider not to exceed the Medicaid allowable rates.

The Member may be required to complete an Out-of-Plan claim form to assist in proper and prompt payment of services. The Plan shall describe in writing the procedures whereby Out-of-Plan Providers can appeal claims denied by the Plan.

6.20   Advance Directives

The Plan shall maintain written policies and procedures concerning Advance Directives, and shall meet State and federal requirements as outlined in *Medicaid Special Bulletin on Advance Directives*, November 1991.

6.21   Payments from Members

The Plan may not require copayments, deductibles, or other forms of cost sharing from Members for services covered under this Contract, nor may the Plan charge Members for missed appointments. Members who obtain services from Out-of-Plan Providers without Plan authorization, except those services specified in Sections 6.3, 6.14 and 6.19, shall be responsible for payment of costs associated with such services. The Plan shall include on all Member identification cards a Member Services telephone number which may be used by Out-of-Plan Providers to obtain referral and billing information.

6.22   Inpatient Hospital Services

The Division shall be responsible for reimbursement of inpatient hospital services provided to Recipients who are inpatients prior to the effective date of their enrollment in the Plan, until such Recipient is discharged from the hospital. The Plan shall provide all other Covered Services to hospitalized Members commencing on the effective date of enrollment. The Plan shall provide all Covered Services (including inpatient hospital services) to newborn infants of female Members until such infant is discharged from the hospital, and shall continue to provide all inpatient hospital services to

Members who are hospitalized on the effective date of disenrollment (whether voluntary or involuntary) until such Member is discharged from the hospital.

SECTION 7—QUALITY ASSURANCE AND QUALITY IMPROVEMENT

7.1   Internal Quality Assurance/Quality Improvement System

The Plan shall establish and maintain an internal quality assurance system consistent with 42 CFR 434.34, that:

- is consistent with the utilization control program required by the HCFA for the State's overall Medicaid program, as described in 42 CFR 456
- provides for review by appropriate health professionals of the process followed in providing health services
- provides for systematic data collection of performance and patient results
- provides for interpretation of these data to the practitioners
- provides for making needed changes

a.   The Plan shall have a written description of its Quality Assurance (QA)/Quality Improvement (QI) program. The description shall contain QA/QI objectives with timetables for implementing and accomplishing objectives. The scope of the QA program shall be comprehensive, addressing both the clinical and non-clinical aspects of service, and shall assure that all demographic groups, care settings, and types of services are included in the scope of the review. (This review of the entire range of care is expected to be carried out over multiple review periods.)

b.   The Plan shall objectively and systematically monitor and evaluate the quality and appropriateness of care and services to Members through focused quality of care studies and other related activities, and shall pursue opportunities for improvement on an ongoing basis. This process shall provide feedback to health professionals and other Plan staff regarding performance and patient results.

The Plan shall perform focused care studies of health care services each year. Such studies shall be performed in accordance with the Division's guidelines described in Appendix VIII. The Division shall designate specific focused care studies to be undertaken by the Plan. The number of State required focused care studies will not exceed 2 (two) topics in any given year.

c. The Plan shall conduct an annual Member Satisfaction Survey. A description of the methodology to be used in conducting the survey, the percentage of Members to be surveyed, and a sample questionnaire shall be submitted to the Division for prior approval. The Survey will include questions about access to care (routine, urgent, and emergent), timeliness of care, availability of providers, wait times for appointments, time in the office to be seen, Member education, technical quality of care and communication. The results of the survey must be filed with the Division within 90 days of completion.

d. The Plan shall maintain an active QA/QI committee or other structure which shall be responsible for carrying out the planned activities of the QA/QI program. This committee shall have regular meetings, shall document attendance by providers, and shall be accountable and report regularly to the governing board or its designee concerning QA/QI activities. The Plan shall maintain records documenting the committee's findings, recommendations, and actions.

e. The Plan shall designate a senior executive who shall be responsible for program implementation. The Plan's Medical Director shall have substantial involvement in the QA/QI activities. The Plan shall remain accountable for all QA/QI program functions, such as credentialing and utilization review and review and monitoring of its subcontractors.

7.2   Health Check Reviews

A sample of medical records of Members under age 21 will be reviewed periodically by the Division to determine the percentage of Health Check Screenings completed by the Plan. The evaluation shall be based upon the documentation present in the medical record, claims information, and other factors such as age of the Member, length of Member enrollment, and provider attempts to provide Health Check Services.

If the audited sample reflects eighty percent (80%) or more of Members under age 21 have received all appropriate immunizations and Health Check services, no further Plan action shall be required.

If the review indicates compliance of at least sixty percent (60%), but less than eighty percent (80%), the Plan shall be required to:

a. submit a written corrective action plan outlining strategies it will employ to increase the completion rate for Health Check screenings and immunizations; and

b. the Plan's Quality Improvement/Quality Assurance Committee shall be required to address and track the progress of Health Check Services.

If the compliance rate is at least forty percent (40%), but less than sixty percent (60%), the Plan shall be required to comply with requirements a. and b. above, and

c. the Plan's Quality Assurance Director shall be required to attend quarterly Division-sponsored Health Check Improvement meetings.

If the review indicates a compliance rate below 40%, the Plan shall be required to comply with requirements a., b. and c., above, and the Division will withhold 1% of each subsequent months' capitation payments until the Plan's Health Check completion rate is at least 40%. Withheld payments will be refunded when the completion rate is 40% or above.

7.3 Medical Audits

Pursuant to 42 CFR 434.53, the Division shall conduct annual medical audits to ensure the provision of quality, accessible health care; identify and collect management data for use by medical audit personnel, and provide that the data include information on use of services and reasons for enrollment and termination. In addition, the Division shall contract with a utilization and quality control peer review organization or private accreditation body to conduct an annual independent external review of the quality of services furnished under this Contract.

7.4 Inspection and Monitoring

The Division shall monitor the Plan's enrollment and disenrollment practices and shall insure the proper implementation of the Plan's grievance procedures, in accordance with 42 CFR 434.63.

Pursuant to 42 CFR 438.38, the Division, the United States Department of Health and Human Services (HHS) and any other authorized federal or state personnel or their authorized representatives may inspect and audit any financial records of the Plan or its subcontractors relating to the Plan's capacity to bear the risk of potential financial losses.

Pursuant to 42 CFR 434.6(a)(5), and as otherwise provided under this Contract, the Division, HHS and any other authorized federal or state personnel or their authorized representatives shall evaluate through inspection or other means, the quality, appropriateness and timeliness of services performed under this Contract.

Such monitoring activities may include on-site inspections of all service locations and health care facilities; financial and medical audits; review and reproduction of any records developed under this Contract; review of management systems, policies and procedures; and review of any other areas or materials relevant to or pertaining to this Contract. The Division shall retain the right to develop monitoring tools to carry out inspections. The Division will provide the Plan with a report of its findings and recommendations, and may require the Plan to develop corrective action plans as appropriate.

7.5   Utilization Management
The Plan shall have a written utilization management program that is consistent with 42 CFR 456 and includes mechanisms to detect underutilization as well as overutilization of services. The written description shall address procedures to evaluate medical necessity, criteria used, information sources, and the process used to review and approve the provision of medical services.

7.6   Grievance/Complaint Procedure
The Plan shall have a timely and organized system with written policies and procedures for resolving internal grievances in accordance with 42 CFR 434.32, and the requirements set forth in Appendix IX, that:
a.   Is approved in writing by the Division;
b.   Provides for prompt resolution; and
c.   Assures the participation of individuals with the authority to require corrective action.

Tracking and analysis of transfers, complaints, and grievance data shall be used by the Plan for quality improvement. A summary of the complaints and grievances data shall be submitted to the Division for review on an annual basis.

7.7   Credentialing
The Plan shall have written policies and procedures for provider credentialing and recredentialing to identify providers who fall under its scope of authority and action. The Plan shall meet all credentialing requirements as determined by the North Carolina Department of Insurance.

SECTION 8—RECORDS

8.1   Medical Records
The Plan shall set standards for medical records which reflect all aspects of patient care, including ancillary services. These standards, at a minimum, shall provide for the following:

a.   Each page or electronic file in the record contains the patient's name or patient ID number;

b.   Personal and biographical data is recorded and includes age, sex, address, employer, home and work telephone numbers, and marital status;

c.   All entries are dated;

d.   All entries are identified as to the author;

e.   Medication allergies and adverse reactions are prominently noted and easily identifiable as well as the absence of allergies;

f.   Past medical history is easily identified including serious accidents, operations, illnesses. For children, past medical history relates to prenatal care and birth;

g.   The record is legible to someone other than the writer;

h.   There is a completed immunization record. For pediatric records (ages 12 and under) there is a completed record or notation that immunizations are up to date;

i.   Diagnostic information, medication, medical conditions, significant illnesses, and health maintenance concerns are recorded in the medical record;

j.   Notation concerning smoking, alcohol, and other substance abuse is present for patients age 12 and over at the first routine visit;

k.   Notes from consultations are in the record. Consultation, lab, and X-ray reports filed in the chart have the ordering provider's initials or other documentations signifying review. Consultation and significantly abnormal lab and imaging results have an explicit notation in the record of the follow-up plans;

l.   Emergency care is documented in the record;

m.   Discharge summaries are included as part of the medical record for all hospital admissions which occur while the patient is enrolled in the Plan; and

n.   Documentation of individual encounters which provide adequate evidence of appropriate history, physical examination, diagnosis, diagnostic tests, therapies, and other prescribed regimens, follow-up care, referrals and results thereof, and all other aspects of patient care, including ancillary services.

8.2   Confidentiality of Records

The Plan shall comply with the requirements of 42 CFR 431 Subpart F, to restrict the use or disclosure of information concerning Members to purposes directly related to the performance of its duties and securement of its rights under this Contract. The Division, the State Attorney General's

Office, the State Audit Department, authorized federal or state personnel, or the authorized representatives of these parties including, without limitation, any employee, agent, or contractor of the Division, HCFA, and the Department of Human Resources, shall have access to all confidential information in accordance with the requirements of this Contract and state and federal law and regulations pertaining to such access.

8.3   Access to Records

Any records requested pursuant to monitoring, audit or inspection as called for in this Contract shall be produced immediately for on-site review or sent to the requesting authority by mail within 14 days following the request. All records shall be provided at the sole cost and expense of the Plan. The Division shall have unlimited rights to use, disclose, and duplicate information and data developed, derived, documented, or furnished by the Plan and in any way relating to this Contract.

8.4   Maintenance of Records

The Plan and/or Plan Providers shall maintain detailed records of the administrative costs and expenses incurred pursuant to this Contract including provision of Covered Services and all relevant medical information relating to individual Members, for the purpose of audit and evaluation by the Division and other federal or state personnel. All records shall be maintained and available for review by authorized federal and state personnel during the entire term of this Contract and for a period of five (5) years thereafter, unless an audit is in progress. When an audit is in progress or audit findings are unresolved, records shall be kept until all issues are finally resolved.

SECTION 9—REPORTS AND DATA

9.1   Enrollment Report

The Division shall provide to the Plan an Enrollment Report, on or before the first (1st) day of each month, listing all Recipients who are Members of the Plan for that month. All enrollments and disenrollments shall be effective on the first day of the calendar month for which the enrollment or disenrollment is listed on the Enrollment Report. The Enrollment Report shall serve as the basis for capitated payments to the Plan for the ensuing month. The Plan shall reconcile the Enrollment Report against its internal records within ten (10) business days and shall notify the Division of any discrepancies. Adjustments will be made to the next enrollment report reflecting corrections reported to the Division on or before the fifteenth (15th) day of each month.

9.2   Encounter Data

The Plan must submit to the Division one hundred percent (100%) encounter data within ninety (90) days from the end of the month in which the service was rendered. The data must be submitted electronically according to ANSI standards using the HCFA 1500, UB-92, and American Dental Association claim formats. Refer to Appendix X for Encounter Data minimum reporting elements. The Division will conduct validation studies of encounter data, testing for timeliness, accuracy and completeness.

9.3   Reporting Recruirements

The Plan shall comply with the reporting requirements set forth by the Division. The Division shall furnish the Plan with timely notice of reporting requirements, including acceptable reporting formats, instructions, and timetables for submission and such technical assistance in filing reports and data as may be permitted by the Division's available resources. The Division reserves the right to modify from time to time the form, content, instruction, and timetables for collection and reporting of data. The Plan shall send a representative to Data Advisory Meetings sponsored by the Division, held no more often than quarterly. The Division agrees to involve Plans in the decision process prior to implementing changes in format, and will request Plans to review and comment on format changes before they go into effect. Plans will be given sixty (60) days to comply with new requests. In the event that the Plan fails to submit any data or report required pursuant to this Section, the Division shall have the right to withhold up to ten percent (10%) of the subsequent months' capitation payments, pending receipt of the respective data or report by the Division. The Division may reduce the requirement from quarterly to yearly reporting when the Plan submits three consecutive quarterly reports that are complete, valid, accurate, and timely.

SECTION 10—PAYMENTS TO THE PLAN

10.1   Monthly Payment

In full consideration of all services rendered by the HMO under this Contract, the Division shall remit to the Plan the capitation rate specified in Appendix XI for each Member listed on the Enrollment Report issued for that month, on or before the tenth (10th) day of each month. The payment is contingent upon satisfactory performance by the Plan of its duties and responsibilities as set forth in this Contract. All payments shall be made by electronic funds transfers. The Plan shall set up the necessary bank accounts and provide written authorization to the Division's Fiscal Agent to generate and process monthly payments through the internal billing methods, in form and substance designated by the Division.

10.2   Payment in Full

The Plan shall accept the capitation rate paid each month by the Division as payment in full for all services to be provided pursuant to this Contract, including all administrative costs associated therewith. A minimum of eighty-five percent (85%) of all the Plan's income generated under this Contract, including but not limited to Third Party Recoupments and Interest, shall be expended on the medical and related services required under this Contract to be provided to the Plan's Medicaid Members. If the Plan does not expend a minimum of eighty-five percent (85%) on medical and related services of the Contract, the Division will withhold an amount so that the Plan's ratio for service expenditures is eighty-five percent (85%). Administrative costs and other financial information will be monitored on a regular basis by the Division.

Members shall be entitled to receive all Covered Services for the entire period for which payment has been made by the Division. Any and all costs incurred by the Plan in excess of the capitation payment will be borne in full by the Plan. Interest generated through investment of funds paid to the Plan pursuant to this Contract shall be the property of the Plan.

10.3   Payment Adjustments

Monthly capitation payments will be adjusted to reflect corrections to the Enrollment Report issued for the preceding month, provided the Division is notified of discrepancies by the fifteenth (15th) day of the current month. Payments will also be adjusted to reflect the automatic re-enrollment of reopened AFDC cases and the automatic enrollment of eligible newborns. Failure to request a payment adjustment within the time limit specified in this Section shall not relieve the Plan of its obligations to provide coverage pursuant to this Contract.

Payment adjustments may be initiated by the Division when keying errors and/or system errors affecting correct capitation payments to the Plan occur.

Each payment adjustment transaction will be included on the remittance advice in the month following the correction. Each transaction will include identifying Member information and the payment adjustment amount.

10.4   Calculation of Rates

Consistent with 42 CFR 434.61 and 447.361, capitation rates have been computed on an actuarially sound basis, and shall not exceed the upper payment limit defined as the projected cost of providing the same services covered under this Contract to a comparable Medicaid population on a fee-for-services basis. The capitation rate shall be a percentage of the upper payment limit. Capitation rates will be calculated according to category of enrollees, which shall be determined by the Division and may be adjusted by the Division prior to each fiscal year.

The upper payment limit for each group shall be calculated each fiscal year (July 1–June 30) by determining the historical costs incurred by the Division in providing Covered Services (excluding expanded services) on a fee-for-service basis to nonenrolled Recipients in each eligibility group, for each Medicaid HMO program area, during one or more fiscal years ending one year prior to the first day of the next fiscal year (base period), deducting amounts recovered from third party resources, adjusting costs to account for changes in benefits and payment levels subsequent to the base period and applying appropriate trend factors (to be determined by the Division) to project base period costs into the renewal term. Appendix XI indicates projected and maximum authorized enrollment levels and the capitation rates applicable to each Member group for the initial fiscal year of this Contract. Using this methodology, rates will be recalculated each fiscal year and the Plan will be notified by April 1 of the new rates to be effective July 1 of the next fiscal year.

10.5   Rate Adjustments

The Plan and the Division acknowledge that the capitation rates and calculation methodology are subject to approval by HCFA. Prospective adjustments to the rates may be required. The rate of payment and total dollar amount shall be adjusted pursuant to a properly executed amendment when Medicaid fee-for-service expenditure changes have been established through the appropriations process, and subsequently identified in the Division's operating budget. Legislatively mandated changes will take effect on the dates specified in the legislation.

10.6   Recoupment

If the Plan fraudulently reports, knowingly fails to report, or errs intentionally or unintentionally in reporting information regarding payments, the Division will request a refund of, or it may recoup from subsequent payments, any payment previously made to the Plan.

The Division may recoup payments made to the Plan when keying errors and/or system errors affecting correct capitation payments occur.

Each recoupment transaction will be included on the remittance advice in the month following the correction. Each transaction will include identifying Member information and the recoupment amount.

10.7   Third Party Resources

The capitated rates set forth in this Contract have been adjusted to account for the primary liability of third parties to pay such expenses. The Plan shall be responsible for making every reasonable effort to determine the legal liability of third parties, including casualty and other tort liability claims, to pay for services rendered to Members pursuant to this Contract. All funds recovered by the Plan from third party resources shall be treated as income to the Plan.

The Plan may delay payment to a subcontractor or Out-of-Plan Provider for up to sixty (60) days following the date of service in the event that a third party resource is identified from which the subcontractor or Out-of-Plan Provider is obligated to collect payment. If payment is not made by the third party within such sixty (60) day period, the Plan must pay the subcontractor or Out-of-Plan Provider and obtain a refund of any subsequent payments made by the third party. The Plan may not withhold payment from a subcontractor or Out-of-Plan Provider for services provided to a Member due to the existence of third party resources, because the liability of a third party resource cannot be determined, or because payment will not be available within sixty (60) days. The Plan shall comply with provisions of 42 CFR 433.139 (b) (2) and (3) in payment of claims for services furnished to certain Medicaid Recipients (e.g., children and pregnant women).

SECTION 11—INDEMNIFICATION

11.1   State's Indemnity

In no event will the State, the Division, or any Recipient be liable for the payment of any debt or fulfillment of any obligation of the Plan or any subcontractor, supplier, Out-of-Plan Provider or any other party, for any reason whatsoever, including the insolvency of the Plan or any of its subcontractors.

The Plan agrees to indemnify, defend, save and hold harmless the Division, its officers, agents, and employees, and each and every Member, from all claims, demands, liabilities, suits, judgments, or damages, including court costs and attorney fees, arising out of the performance of this Contract by the Plan, its officers, agents, employees, suppliers, subcontractors or Out-of-Plan Providers, of the covenants and agreements of the Plan set forth herein, including without limitation any claim attributable to:

a. The improper performance of any service, or improper provision of any materials or supplies, irrespective of whether the Division knew or should have known such service, supplies or materials were improper or defective;

b. The erroneous or negligent acts or omissions, including without limitation, disregard of federal or State law or regulations, irrespective of whether the Division knew or should have known of such erroneous or negligent acts;

c. The publication, translation, reproduction, delivery, collection, data processing, use, or disposition of any information to which access is obtained pursuant to this Contract in a manner not authorized by this Contract or by federal or State law or regulations, irrespective of whether the Division knew or should have known of such publication, translation, reproduction, delivery, collection, data processing, use, or disposition; and

d. Any failure to observe federal or State law or regulations, including but not limited to, insurance and labor laws, irrespective of whether the Division knew or should have known of such failure.

The Division shall give the Plan written notice within fifteen (15) days of receipt of any claim or demand made against the Division for which it is entitled to indemnification hereunder (claim); and shall give the Plan an opportunity to appear and defend such claim. Under no circumstances shall the Plan be deemed to have the right to represent the State of North Carolina in any legal matter.

The Plan, its subcontractors, agents, officers, and employees shall act in an independent capacity in the performance of this Contract and not as officers or employees of the Division or of the State of North Carolina. This Contract shall not be construed as a partnership or joint venture between the Plan or any Plan subcontractor and the Division or the State of North Carolina.

SECTION 12—SUBCONTRACTS

12.1   Requirements

The Plan may enter into subcontracts for the performance of its administrative functions or for the provision of various Covered Services to Members. Each subcontract, and any amendment to a subcontract, shall be in writing and approved in writing by the Division. All subcontracts must fulfill the requirements of 42 CFR 434.6 that are appropriate to the service or activity delegated under the subcontract. All subcontractors must be eligible for participation in the Medicaid program and are bound to all the terms of this Contract and applicable federal and state laws and regulations. No subcontract shall in any way relieve the Plan of any responsibility for the performance of its duties pursuant to this Contract. The Plan shall notify the Division in writing of the termination of any approved subcontract within ten (10) days following termination. All subcontracts shall:

a.   Identify the population covered by the subcontract;

b.   Specify the amount, duration and scope of services to be provided by the subcontractor;

c.   Specify procedures and criteria for extension, re-negotiation and termination;

d.   Make full disclosure of the method and amount of compensation or other consideration to be received from the Plan;

e.   Provide for monitoring by the Plan of the quality of services rendered to Members;

f.   Contain no provision which provides incentives, monetary or otherwise, for the withholding from Members of medically necessary services;

g.   Contain a prohibition on assignment or any further subcontracting without the prior written consent of the Division; and

h.   Incorporate all provisions of this Contract to the fullest extent applicable to the service or activity delegated pursuant to the subcontract, including without limitation, the obligation to comply with all applicable federal and State laws and regulations, all rules, policies and procedures of the Department, and all standards governing the provision of Covered Services and information to Members; all quality assurance requirements; all record keeping and reporting requirements; the obligation to maintain the confidentiality of information; all rights of the Division and other officials to inspect, monitor and audit operations; all indemnification and insurance.

12.2   Remedies

The Division shall have the right to invoke against any subcontractor, any remedy set forth in this Contract, including the right to require the termination of any subcontract, for each and every reason for which it may invoke such a remedy against the Plan or require the termination of this Contract.

SECTION 13—DEFAULT AND TERMINATION

13.1   Severability

In the event that any provision of this Contract (including items incorporated by reference) is found to be unlawful or unenforceable, then both the Department and the Plan shall be relieved of all obligations arising under such provision. If the remainder of this Contract is capable of performance, then this Contract shall continue in full force and effect, and all remaining provisions shall be binding upon each party of this Contract. If the laws and regulations governing this Contract should be amended or judicially interpreted so as to render the fulfillment of this Contract impossible or economically infeasible, as determined jointly by the Division and the Plan, then both the Division and the Plan shall be discharged from any further obligations created under the terms of this Contract.

13.2   Plan Breach, Remedies

If the Plan fails to fulfill its duties and obligations pursuant to this Contract, the Division may issue a written notice to the Plan indicating the violation(s) and requiring the submission of a corrective action plan that is subject to the approval of the Division; or depending upon the nature of the deficiency, the Division shall be entitled to exercise any other right or remedy available to it, whether or not it issues a deficiency notice or provides the Plan with the opportunity to take corrective action. Failure to correct the violation(s), to the satisfaction of the Division may lead to the imposition of all or some of the sanctions listed below:
a.   Suspension of further enrollment for a defined time period;
b.   Suspension, recoupment or withholding up to ten percent (10%) of monthly capitation payments;
c.   Termination of this Contract.

13.3   Option To Terminate

This Contract may be terminated without cause by either party upon sixty (60) days prior written notice to the other party. Termination shall be effective only at midnight of the last day of a calendar month. The option of the Plan to terminate this Contract prior to the end of the initial term or any renewal term shall be contingent upon the payment of liquidated damages pursuant to Section 13.6, performance of all obligations upon termination, pursuant to Section 13.5, and payment in full of any refunds or other sums due the Division pursuant to this Contract.

13.4   Grounds for Immediate Termination

The Division shall have the right to immediately terminate this Contract upon the occurrence of any of the following events:

a.   The Plan, its subcontractors or suppliers violate or fail to comply with any applicable provision of Federal or State law or regulations;

b.   The conduct of the Plan, any subcontractor or supplier, or the standard of services provided by or on behalf of the Plan threatens to place the health or safety of any Member in jeopardy;

c.   The Plan becomes subject to exclusion from participation in the Medicaid program pursuant to Section 1902 (p)(2) of the Act (42 USC 1396 a(p));

d.   The Plan or any subcontractor provides fraudulent, misleading, or misrepresented information to any Member;

e.   Gratuities of any kind were offered to or received by any public official, employee or agent of the State from the Plan, its agents, employees, subcontractors or suppliers, in violation of Section 1.4;

f.   Either of the sources of reimbursement for Medical Assistance, appropriations from the General Assembly of the State or from the Congress of the United States, no longer exists, or in the event that the sum of all obligations of the Division incurred pursuant to this Contract and all other Contracts entered into by the Division, including without limitation, all Statements of Participation entered into pursuant to the State Plan, equals or exceeds the balance of such sources available to the Division for "Medical Assistance Benefits" for the fiscal year in which this Contract is effective, less One Hundred Dollars ($100.00), then this Contract shall immediately terminate without further obligations of the Division as of that moment.

Certification by the Director of the Division of the occurrence of any of the events stated above shall be conclusive. The Division will attempt to provide the Plan with ten (10) days notice of the possible occurrence of events described in Subsection f of this Section.

13.5   Obligations upon Termination

Upon termination of this Contract, the Plan shall be solely responsible for the provision and payment for all Covered Services for all Members for the remainder of any month for which the Division has paid the monthly capitation rate. Upon final notice of termination, on the date, and to the extent specified in the notice of termination, the Plan shall:

a.   Continue providing Covered Services to all Members until midnight on the last day of the calendar month for which a capitated rate payment has been made by the Division;

b.   Continue providing all Covered Services to all infants of female Members who have not been discharged from the hospital following birth, until each infant is discharged;

c.   Continue providing inpatient Hospital Services to any Members who are hospitalized on the termination date, until each Member is discharged;

d.   Arrange for the transfer of patients and medical records to other appropriate providers;

e.   Promptly supply to the Division information on all outstanding claims and arrange for the payment of such claims within the time periods provided herein;

f.   Take such action as may be necessary, or as the Division may direct, for the protection of property related to this Contract, which is in the possession of the contractor and in which the Division has or may acquire an interest; and

g.   Provide for the maintenance of all records for audit and inspection by the Division, HCFA and other authorized government officials, in accordance with Section 8; the transfer of all data and records to the Division or its agents as may be requested by the Division; and the preparation and delivery of any reports, forms or other documents to the Division as may be required pursuant to this Contract or any applicable policies and procedures of the Division.

The covenants set forth in this Section shall survive the termination of this Contract and shall remain fully enforceable by the Division against the Plan. In the event that the Plan fails to fulfill each covenant set forth in this Section, the Division shall have the right, but not the obligation, to arrange for the provision of such services and the fulfillment of such covenants, all at the sole cost and expense of the Plan and the Plan shall refund to the Division all sums expended by the Division in so doing.

13.6   Liquidated Damages

The Plan acknowledges and agrees that the Division has incurred substantial expense in connection with the preparation and entry into this Contract, including expenses relating to training of staff, data collection and processing, actuarial determination of capitated rates for the initial term and each renewal term, and ongoing changes to the Medicaid Management Information System (MMIS). The Plan further acknowledges and agrees that in the event this Contract is terminated prior to the end of the initial term or any renewal term, due to the actions of the Plan or due to the Plan's failure to fully comply with the terms and conditions of this Contract, the Division will incur substantial additional expense in processing the disenrollment of all Members and mass MMIS changes, in effecting additional staffing changes, in procuring alternative health care arrangements for Members and in modifying any Member service materials identifying the Plan; and that such expense is difficult or impossible of accurate estimation.

Based upon the foregoing, the Plan and the Division have agreed to provide for the payment by the Plan to the Division of liquidated damages equal to ten thousand ($10,000) plus one percent (1%) of the maximum monthly capitation payment for each month of the Contract term remaining after the effective date of termination, such payment to be made no later than thirty (30) days following the date of termination. The Division and the Plan agree that the sum set forth herein as liquidated damages is a reasonable pre-estimate of the probable loss which will be incurred by the Division in the event this Contract is terminated prior to the end of the Contract term or any renewal term.

13.7   Third Party Beneficiaries

Medicaid Members are the intended third party beneficiaries of contracts between the Division and the Plan and any subcontractors or provider agreements entered into by the Plan. Members are entitled to the remedies accorded to third party beneficiaries under the law. This provision is not intended to provide cause of action against the Division or the State of North Carolina by Members beyond any that may exist under State or Federal law.

SECTION 14—ENTIRE AGREEMENT

This Contract and Appendices, and the Application Form represent the entire agreement between the Plan and the Division with respect to the subject matter stated herein and supersedes all other contracts and agreements between the parties. No modification or change to any provision of this Contract shall be effective unless it is in writing and signed by a duly authorized representative of the Plan and the Division, and without the prior approval of HCFA, provided however that this Contract shall be amended whenever and to the extent required by changes in federal or State law or regulations.

IN WITNESS WHEREOF, the parties have caused this Contract to be executed by their duly authorized representatives.

Attest: [PLAN]

_____   By _____
Title: Corporate Secretary   Name:
                                              Title: Chief Executive Director

                                              STATE OF NORTH CAROLINA
                                              DIVISION OF MEDICAL ASSISTANCE

_____   By _____
Managed Care Director   Barbara D. Matula, Director

APPENDIX I
DEFINITION OF TERMS

1.1   **AFDC**—Aid to Families with Dependent Children.

1.2   **ANSI**—American National Standards Institute.

1.3   **Applicant**—Any person who has signed an application for enrollment in an HMO and whose enrollment certification is pending.

1.4   **Attending Physician**—The participating or referral physician in whose immediate care a Member may be for a particular illness, injury or condition.

1.5   **Capitation Rate**—The amount to be advanced monthly to a Plan for each Member enrolled in the Plan's Health Benefit Plan based on the Member's aid category, age, gender and HMO program area.

1.6   **Care Management**—Services providing assistance in gaining access to and coordination of needed social, educational, and other medically necessary services regardless of the source of the funding for the needed service.

1.7   **CFR**—Code of Federal Regulations.

1.8   **Contract Term**—The initial term of this Contract or any renewal term. Coincides with the State's fiscal year beginning on July 1 and ending on June 30.

1.9   **Covered Services**—The services identified in Appendix III, which the Plan agrees to provide to all Members pursuant to the terms of this Contract.

1.10   **DHHS**—United States Department of Health and Human Services.

1.11   **Days**—Except as otherwise noted, refers to calendar days. "Working day" or "business day" means day on which the Division is officially open to conduct its affairs.

1.12   **Disenrollment**—Action taken by the Division to remove a Member's name from the monthly Enrollment Report following a Division's receipt and approval of a request for disenrollment or a determination that the Member is no longer eligible for enrollment in the Plan.

1.13   **Division**—The State of North Carolina, Division of Medical Assistance.

1.14   **DSS**—Department of Social Services.

1.15   **Eligible Recipient**—Recipients who are eligible to elect HMO coverage.

1.16   **Emergency Medical Condition**—
    (A) A medical condition manifesting itself by acute symptoms of sufficient severity (including severe pain) such that the absence of immediate medical attention could reasonably be expected to result in:
        (1) placing the health of the individual (or with respect to a pregnant woman, the health of the woman or her unborn child) in serious jeopardy,
        (2) serious impairment to bodily functions, or
        (3) serious dysfunction of any bodily organ or part; or

(B) With respect to a pregnant woman who is having contractions:
    (1) that there is inadequate time to effect a safe transfer to another hospital before delivery, or
    (2) that transfer may pose a threat to the health or safety of the woman or the unborn child.

1.17 **Encounter Data**—a record of a medically related service or visit rendered by a provider to a Member who is enrolled in the Plan during the date of service. It includes all services for which the Plan incurred any financial responsibility.

1.18 **Enrollees**—The entire membership in the Plan, including all of the Members and all persons, other than recipients, who are enrolled in the Plan.

1.19 **Enrollment**—Action taken by the Division to add a Member's name to the monthly Enrollment report following the receipt and approval by the Division of an enrollment application from an eligible Recipient.

1.20 **Enrollment Period**—The time span during which a recipient is enrolled with a Plan.

1.21 **Expanded Services**—Services included in Covered Services which are in addition to the minimum coverage required by the Division and which the Plan agrees to provide throughout the term of this Contract in accordance with the standards and requirements set forth in this Contract.

1.22 **Facility**—Any premises (a) owned, leased, used or operated directly or indirectly by or for the Plan or its affiliates for purposes related to this Contract; or (b) maintained by a subcontractor to provide services on behalf of the Plan.

1.23 **Family Planning**—Services, procedures, and supplies which enable individuals of child bearing age, including minors considered to be sexually active, to freely determine the size of their families and/or to space their children.

1.24 **Fee-for-Service**—A method of making payment directly to health care providers enrolled in the Medicaid program for the provision of health care services to Recipients based on the payment methods set forth in the State Plan and the applicable policies and procedures of the Division.

1.25 **Fiscal Agent**—An agency that processes and audits Medicaid provider claims for payment and performs certain other related functions as an agent of the Division.

1.26 **FQHC**—A Federally Qualified Health Center.

1.27 **FTE**—Full time equivalent, based on forty (40) hours worked per week.

1.28 **Grievance Procedure**—The written procedures pursuant to which Members may express dissatisfaction with the provision of services by the Plan and the methods for resolution of Member complaints by the Plan.

1.29 **Health Benefits Manager (HBM)**—Third Party Contractor who will enroll Recipients in a Plan.

1.30 **HCFA**—Health Care Financing Administration.

1.31   **Health Assessment**—The systematic collection of subjective and objective information used to determine the client's health status and need for medical care in relation to developmental, physiological, preventive, and psychological life processes.

1.32   **Health Check**—A child health program for recipients through the age of 20 designed to improve the availability and accessibility of preventive and primary health care services. It is sponsored by the Division.

1.33   **Hearing**—A formal proceeding before an Office of Administrative Hearing Law Judge in which parties affected by an action or an intended action of the Division shall be allowed to present testimony, documentary evidence and argument as to why such action should or should not be taken.

1.34   **Insolvency**—The inability of the Plan to pay its obligations when they are due, or when its admitted assets do not exceed its liabilities plus the greater of: (i) any capital and surplus required by law for its organization; or (ii) the total par or stated value of its authorized and issued capital stock. "Liabilities" shall include, but not be limited to, reserve required by the Department of Insurance pursuant to Chapter 58 Articles 67 of the North Carolina General Statutes.

1.35   **Marketing**—Any activity conducted by or on behalf of the Plan, in which information regarding the services offered by the Plan is disseminated in order to encourage eligible Recipients to enroll in the Plan.

1.36   **Medicaid HEDIS**—Standardized performance measurements for states and plans to use to promote the standardization of information systems and data collection to improve the quality of care.

1.37   **Medicaid Identification (MID) Card**—The Medical Assistance Eligibility Certification card issued monthly by the Division to Recipients.

1.38   **Medicaid for Infants and Children (MIC)**—A program for medical assistance for children under the age of 19 whose countable income falls under a specific percentage of the Federal Poverty Limit and who are not already eligible for Medicaid in another category.

1.39   **Medicaid for Pregnant Women (MPW)**—A program for medical assistance for pregnant women whose income falls under a specified percentage of the Federal Poverty Limit and who are not already eligible in another category.

1.40   **Medical Assistance (Medicaid) Program**—The Division's program to provide medical assistance to eligible citizens of the State of North Carolina, established pursuant to Chapter 58, Articles 67 and 68 of the North Carolina General Statutes and Title XIX of the Social Security Act, 42 USC §1396 et seq.

1.41   **Medical Record**—A single complete record which documents all of the treatment plans developed for, and medical services received by, the Member including inpatient, outpatient, referral services and emergency medical services whether provided by Plan Providers or Out-of-Plan Providers.

1.42   **Medically Necessary Services**—Those services which are, in the opinion of the treating physician, reasonable and necessary in establishing a diagnosis and providing palliative, curative or restorative treatment for physical and/or mental health conditions in accordance with the standards of medical practice generally accepted at the time the services are rendered. Each service must be sufficient in amount, duration, and scope to reasonably achieve its purpose; and the amount, duration, or scope of coverage, may not arbitrarily be denied or reduced solely because of the diagnosis, type of illness, or condition (42 CFR 440.230). Medicaid EPSDT coverage rules (42 USC §1396 (r)(5) and 42 USC§1396 d(a)).

1.43   **Member**—An eligible Recipient who is enrolled in the Plan.

1.44   **Out-of-Plan Services**—Health care services which the Plan is not required to provide under the terms of this Contract which are Medicaid covered services but are covered by Medicaid on a Fee-for-Service basis.

1.45   **Out-of-Network Provider**—Any person or entity providing services who is not directly employed by or through the Plan or any of its subcontractors.

1.46   **Plan**—An HMO licensed by the North Carolina Department of Insurance which has signed a Contract with the Division to provide and manage the health care needs of enrolled Members on a prepaid basis.

1.47   **Plan Benefits**—The prepaid health care benefits offered by the Plan for the provision of Covered Services pursuant to this Contract.

1.48   **Plan Provider**—Any person or entity providing Covered Services on behalf of the Plan that is directly employed by or through the Plan or any of its subcontractors.

1.49   **Primary Care Provider (PCP)**—A licensed medical practitioner responsible for supervising, coordinating and providing initial and primary care to a Member, for initiating referrals for specialist care, and for maintaining the continuity of patient care; a General Medical Practitioner, an Internist, a Pediatrician, an Obstetrician/Gynecologist, a Family Practitioner, a Physician's Assistant, or a Family Nurse Practitioner.

1.50   **Prior Authorization**—The act of authorizing specific services before they are rendered.

1.51   **Provider**—Any person or entity approved by the Division which renders health care services to Recipients.

1.52   **QARI**—Also referred to as a health care quality improvement system for states; a framework for a health care quality improvement system for Medicaid managed care; recommends evaluation procedures to be used by states to evaluate a Plan's internal quality improvement system.

1.53   **Quality Assurance/Quality Improvement**—The process of assuring that health care services provided to Members are appropriate, timely, accessible, available and medically necessary.

1.54   **Recipient**—Any person certified by the Division as eligible to receive services and benefits under the North Carolina Medicaid Program.

1.55   **Reconsideration Review**—An informal session before a Division Hearing Officer wherein a Member or the Plan, affected by an action or an intended action by the Division and the Managed Care Director shall be allowed to present and discuss information as to why such action should or should not be taken, and described more specifically in NCAC T10:26I (for Members) and NCAC T10:26K (for the Plan). The decision of the Hearing Officer is subject to appeal through the Office of Administrative Hearings (OH).

1.56   **Reinsurance**—Insurance purchased by a Plan from insurance companies to protect against part of the costs of providing Covered Services to Members.

1.57   **Reopened (Administratively) AFDC Case**—A terminated AFDC case may be administratively reopened with no loss of coverage if certain eligibility criteria are met within specified time frames.

1.58   **Risk**—A significant chance of loss assumed by the Plan which arises if cost of providing Covered Services to Members exceeds the capitation rate paid by the Division to the Plan.

1.59   **Service Area**—Any defined geographic area within which the Plan and the Division have agreed to make Covered Services available and readily accessible to the Members.

1.60   **Service Location**—Any location at which a Member may obtain any Covered Services from a Plan Provider.

1.61   **State**—State of North Carolina.

1.62   **State Plan**—The "State Plan" submitted under Title XIX of the Social Security Act, Medical Assistance Program for the State of North Carolina and approved by HCFA.

1.63   **Subcontract**—An agreement approved in writing by the Division which is entered into by the Plan in accordance with Section 12.

1.64   **Subcontractor**—Any person or entity which has entered into a subcontract with the Plan.

1.65   **Third Party Resource**—Any resource available to a Member for payment of expenses associated with the provision of Covered Services, other than those which are exempt under Title XIX of the Act, including but not limited to, insurers, tortfeasors, and worker's compensation plans.

1.66 **Urgent Conditions**—A medical condition that warrants medical attention and intervention within 12–24 hours. If medical care is not rendered, the "urgent" condition could seriously compromise the patient's condition and outcome for a full recovery.

APPENDIX II
ELIGIBILITY GROUPS

Enrollment in Durham County for the Month of October 1996

Category	Enrollment
Aid to Families with Dependent Children (AFDC)	10,582
Family and Children's Medicaid without Medicaid deductible	89
Medicaid for Infants and Children (MIC)	3,388
Foster Care Children	110
[with SSI]	[24]

Enrollment in Orange County for the Month of October 1996

Category	Enrollment
Aid to Families with Dependent Children (AFDC)	1,707
Family and Children's Medicaid without Medicaid deductible	79
Medicaid for Infants and Children (MIC)	1,195
Foster Care Children	23
[with SSI]	[14]

Enrollment in Wake County for the Month of October 1996

Category	Enrollment
Aid to Families with Dependent Children (AFDC)	11,915
Family and Children's Medicaid without Medicaid deductible	148
Medicaid for Infants and Children (MIC)	6,866
Foster Care Children	194
[with SSI]	[86]

APPENDIX III
SCHEDULE OF BENEFITS (In-Plan and Out-of-Plan)

In-Plan Benefits

Abortion
Adult Health Screening
Ambulance
Chiropractic Services
Clinical Services—Except for Mental Health
    and Substance Abuse
Diagnostic Services
Dialysis
Durable Medical Equipment
Emergency Room
EPSDT/Health Check
Eye Care
Family Planning Services and Supplies
Hearing Aids
Home Health
Home Infusion Therapy
Hospice
Inpatient Hospital—Except for Mental
    Health and Substance Abuse

Laboratory Service
Midwife
Occupational Therapy
Optical Supplies
Outpatient Hospital
Physical Therapy
Physician Services, Including Physician
    Assistants and Family Nurse
    Practitioners—Except for Mental Health
    and Substance Abuse
Podiatry
Private Duty Nursing
Prosthetics/Orthotics
Radiology Services
Speech Therapy
Sterilization
Total Parenteral Nutrition

Out-of-Plan Benefits

CAP Services
Carolina Alternatives
Case Management DDS
Child Service Coordination
Dental
DHHS Immunization
Domiciliary Care
Head Start
HIV Case Management

ICF/MR
Maternity Care Coordination
Mental Health and Substance Abuse
Mental Health—Inpatient and Outpatient
Non-Emergency Transportation
Nursing Home
Personal Care Services
Prescription Drugs
School-Related Health Services

APPENDIX IIIA
PROVIDER MANUALS AND BULLETINS

Ambulance Services Manual

Abortion Bulletin

CRNA Special Bulletin

Chiropractic Services Manual

Community Care Manual

Durable Medical Equipment Manual

Health Check (EPSDT) Special Bulletin

Hearing Aid Services Manual

Hospital Services Manual

Nurse Practitioners Special Bulletin

Physician Services Manual

Planned Parenthood Special Bulletin

Podiatry Information Sheet

Sterilization Special Bulletin

Transportation

Vision Care Services Special Bulletin

APPENDIX IV
SCOPE OF HEALTH CHECK/EPSDT SERVICES

42 USC §1396d(r)(5); 42 USC §1396d(a)

The Plan must assure the provision of any treatment or services covered by the State's Medicaid program necessary to correct or ameliorate defects and physical or mental illnesses and conditions discovered during screening services.

- inpatient or outpatient hospital
- laboratory and X-ray
- EPSDT
- family planning
- physician's services
- medical care, or any other type of remedial care recognized under State law, furnished by licensed practitioners within the scope of their practice as defined by State law
- home health services
- private duty nursing services
- physical therapy and related services
- prescribed prosthetic devices
- eyeglasses
- other diagnostic, screening, preventive, and rehabilitative services, including any medical or remedial services recommended by a physician or other licensed practitioner of the healing arts within the scope of their practice under State law, for the maximum reduction of physical or mental disability and restoration of an individual to the best possible functional level
- services furnished by a nurse-midwife
- hospice care
- case management services
- respiratory care services
- services furnished by a certified pediatric nurse practitioner or certified family nurse practitioner
- any other medical care, and any other type of remedial care recognized under state law, and/or as specified by the Secretary of HHS

APPENDIX V
STATISTICAL REPORTING REQUIREMENTS*

The Plan will be provided with the necessary information and forms to be used in meeting the statistical and other reporting requirements of this Contract at the first meeting of the Data Advisory Committee Meetings. Described below are the reports the Plan is required to complete on a quarterly basis, unless another timeframe is specified by the Division. The Plan must follow Medicaid HEDIS collection and reporting instructions for those items below that have been identified as Medicaid HEDIS measures. The Plan may provide feedback regarding reporting requirements through Data Advisory Committee Meetings.

A. **Medicaid Members Enrolled in the Plan**
1. Data will be reported on the number of member months of enrollment from all payers (Medicaid and non-Medicaid). Data will be stratified by number of member months of Medicaid enrollment by age, gender, and type of Medicaid eligibility and the number of member months of enrollment from all payers (Medicaid HEDIS).
2. Data will be reported on the number of Medicaid beneficiaries by age, gender, and type of Medicaid eligibility enrolled in the Plan during the reporting period (Medicaid HEDIS).
3. Data will be reported on the distribution of Medicaid Members enrolled in the Plan at any time during the reporting period according to race, Hispanic origin, and primary language (Medicaid HEDIS).
4. Stage of Pregnancy—(Medicaid HEDIS) Data will be reported on the number and percentage of pregnant women enrolled according to their weeks of pregnancy at the time of enrollment into the health Plan using the following categories:
   • prior to pregnancy
   • during the first 12 weeks of pregnancy
   • during the 12–27 weeks of pregnancy
   • the 28th week or later

B. **Utilization Measures**
1. Data will be reported on the frequency of selected procedures and reported by age categories, totals and rate per 1,000 member months for cholecystectomy, hysterectomy, tonsillectomy/adenoidectomy and myringotomy (Medicaid HEDIS).

---

*Statistical reporting requirements are drawn from Medicaid HEDIS, 1996, and Draft HEDIS 3.0, 1996.

2. Data will be reported on inpatient utilization (for general hospital/acute care) by age and aid categories for inpatient experience for which the Plan is financially responsible (Medicaid HEDIS).
   a. number of discharges and rate per 1,000 Members
   b. number of days of inpatient care and rate per 1,000 Members; and
   c. average length of stay.
3. Data will be reported on face-to-face encounters between provider and Member for all outpatient visits by total number of visits by age and visits per 1,000 member months (Medicaid HEDIS).
4. Data will be reported on the number of emergency room visits that do not result in an inpatient stay. Data is recorded by total number of ER visits by age and by visits per 1,000 member months (Medicaid HEDIS). Data will be reported on the number of ER claims filed and the number and percent of ER claims denied (rejected).
5. Data will be reported on the total number of ambulatory surgical procedures performed by age and aid categories and by the number of procedures performed per 1,000 member months (Medicaid HEDIS).
6. Data will be reported on the number and rate of discharges for deliveries resulting in a live birth; the number and rate of maternity inpatient days; the average length of stay for all discharges for deliveries resulting in a live birth; the number of C-section deliveries; and the discharge rate per 1000 female member months (Medicaid HEDIS). Data will be reported on the ratio of expected to received prenatal care visits for females who had a live birth in the reporting period.
7. Data will be reported on the number of newborns (both well and complex), the number of newborns per 1000 female member months from age 10–40; the average length of stay of the newborn. This information should be provided separately for each aid category (Medicaid HEDIS). Data will be reported on the number and rate of low birthweight newborns weighing equal to or less than 1500 Grams and the number and rate of those weighing between 1501 to 2000 Grams (Medicaid HEDIS).
8. Outpatient Drug Utilization—Data will be reported on the total cost of prescriptions per member per month and on the annual total of prescriptions per member per month (Medicaid HEDIS).
9. Within 45 days of the end of each calendar year quarter, financial data shall be reported on total revenue, expenses, overall loss ratio, medical loss ratio, gross margin, administrative loss ratio, operating profit after corporate expenses for most recent completed quarter and forecasted quarters (modified HEDIS).

The Plan shall within 10 days of filing the National Association of Insurance Commissioners (NAIC) Annual Statement, HMO Edition, with the North Carolina Department of Insurance, file a copy of said statement with the Division. The Plan shall within 10 days of filing the NAIC Quarterly Statement with the North Carolina Department of Insurance, file a copy of said document with the Division of Medical Assistance. The Plan shall file within 60 days of the end of each calendar quarter, the North Carolina Quarterly Statement of Revenues and Expenses. This form may be obtained from the Division.

10. The Plan will report by age the number of Members screened and the total number of Health Check Screens provided. The Plan will provide a count of the number of Health Check Members referred for diagnostic/treatment services, and the number of Members receiving vision, preventive dental, and hearing services (modified HEDIS).

11. The Plan shall report all Medicaid Member grievances, complaints, and appeals. The report must contain the number and type of complaints and action taken for each. Reports must be submitted to the Division no later than 45 days after the end of the calendar quarter.

The Plan will provide a count of the number of Members receiving specific immunizations by age (DPT, MMR, HIB, DTaP, Hepatitis B, DTP/HIB, measles, polio, tetanus toroid) (modified HEDIS).

C. Quality of Care Core Concerns

With further direction and instructions from the Division, the Plan will be required to submit data and measurements on a yearly basis for core concern measures. Some core concern measures will be phased-in during consecutive Contract years at the discretion of the Division. Required and Phased-In measures are listed below.

1. *Required Core Measures*
   a. number and percent of cervical cancer screenings (Medicaid HEDIS)
   b. asthma inpatient admission rate (Medicaid HEDIS)
   c. number and percent of diabetics receiving a biyearly glycohemoglobin level (Medicaid HEDIS)
   d. Plan performed provider profiling information (written summary and examples)

2. *Phased-In Reporting Measures*
   a. annual rate of diabetic retinal exams completed for type I and type II diabetics (Medicaid HEDIS)
   b. mammography screenings for female Members age 50–64 (Medicaid HEDIS)

　　c.　number and rate of family planning services utilized by females age 10–49 and describe in a written summary the network of family planning providers available to members

　　d.　number and percent of adult health screenings by age

　　e.　availability and utilization of Primary Care Providers (modified HEDIS)

　　f.　estimated number of referrals within and out of Plan for Medicaid members

　　g.　estimated number and percent of Medicaid members enrolled at least 12 consecutive months who have not had an encounter service

APPENDIX VI
LONG TERM CARE SERVICES (USE OF AN FL-2)

The Long Term Care Services form (FL-2) should be completed by the attending physician with the assistance of the county department of social services, in conjunction with the facility or responsible party when it is known that the patient is to be referred to a nursing facility or CAP. All copies of the form must be submitted when requesting prior approval. Assure that the form contains sufficient data for patient identification and medical condition to allow medical review consultants to render an appropriate decision as to the level of care required by the patient. All FL-2s requesting prior approval (except request for retroactive approval) should be sent through the county department of social services.

The following chart describes when to submit an FL-2 for prior approval:

	To Hospital	To ICF (Facility)	To SNF (Facility)	To ICF (CAP)	To SNF (CAP)
From home	No FL-2	Approved FL-2	Approved FL-2	Approved FL-2	Approved FL-2 (SNF)
From hospital	No FL-2	Approved FL-2	Approved FL-2	Approved FL-2	Approved FL-2 (SNF)

APPENDIX VII
COMMUNITY RESOURCES

Carolina Alternatives: Carolina Alternatives is a coordinated-care system for the delivery of child mental health and substance abuse services. Under Carolina Alternatives, mental health and substance abuse services for children aged 0–17 who are eligible for Medicaid must be approved by the local Area Mental Health, Developmental Disabilities, and Substance Abuse Program (Area Program). Providers must have a Contract with the Area Program, which will authorize and directly reimburse all mental health and substance abuse services. Durham, Orange, and Wake Counties are all Carolina Alternative counties. Children whose eligibility for Medicaid is established in one of the counties will be automatically enrolled in Carolina Alternatives.

Through Carolina Alternatives, Plans are required to refer children who need mental health and substance abuse services to the Area Program for treatment. Exception: Primary Care Providers can continue to bill EDS directly for routine office visit codes, even when treating children whose diagnoses fall in the range covered by Carolina Alternatives. For example, a pediatrician who is treating a child with Attention Deficit Hyperactivity Disorder may continue to monitor the child's medication. The physician may also refer the child to the Area Program for additional services. Any billing for psychiatric/psychological treatment codes, such as CPT codes in 908 series, must be done through a Contract with the Area Program. For more information, see the North Carolina Medicaid Special Bulletins describing Carolina Alternatives (December 1993 and June 1995).

School Health Services: School-based health services can be an effective means of making primary and preventive health care available to children, and in particular to adolescents, who may not otherwise receive these services. Health plans are encouraged to enter into agreements or subcontracts for the provision of services at school-based health centers. Plans must establish written policies and procedures for the coordination of services delivered at school-based sites.

Maternity Care Coordination (MCC): In 1987, the Baby Love Program was introduced to improve access to health care and support services for low-income pregnant women and young children. Key features of the Baby Love Program include:
- expansion of Medicaid eligibility to 185% of the federal poverty level (FPL) for pregnant women and infants
- outreach and program promotion to increase participation rates in Medicaid

- implementation of presumptive eligibility and other measures to reduce red tape in the application process
- implementation of a statewide Maternity Care Coordination system to enhance local recipient advocacy, eliminating barriers to utilization of services

The care coordination system is designed to:
- ensure that eligible women receive all health care services necessary for positive pregnancy outcomes
- facilitate integrated service delivery among the various health and social service providers
- monitor the effectiveness of care coordination services in meeting the recipient's medical, nutritional, psychosocial. and resource needs

MCCs are located in all 100 county health departments, most rural and community health centers, and the Cherokee Health Delivery System. MCCs work in concert with the recipient's medical provider to assist women in the Medicaid eligibility process, to arrange transportation to medical appointments, to make referrals to appropriate community agencies, and to provide follow-up in any of these areas as needed.

Child Service Coordination: The Child Service Coordination Program was introduced in October of 1990 to enhance services to children and their families. Since its inception, the CSC Program has worked to improve and enhance health care to children during their first years of life. CSC involves teams of parents, professionals and agencies working collaboratively to enhance the health care delivery system. The CSCs are based in the local health departments.

Women, Infants, and Children (WIC) Program: Congress created this Special Supplemental Food Program in 1972 to meet the special nutritional needs of pregnant, breastfeeding and postpartum women, infants and children up to age five (5). Currently, WIC operates through State health departments. The supplemental foods provided by WIC contain nutrients often lacking in diets of the target population. The WIC program provides information and education emphasizing the relationship between nutrition and good health. In addition, WIC offices make referrals to health and social services to help clients access Health Check Screenings, drug and alcohol use counseling, family planning, Food Stamps, migrant services, Head Start, Even Start, and child abuse counseling.

Developmental Evaluation Centers: The Developmental Evaluation Centers Program (DEC) consists of a statewide network of 18 regional centers with a team of professionals with specialities in pediatrics, social work, psychology, speech and language, hearing, physical/occupational therapy, special education and nursing. Service priorities are directed to young children having or suspected of having multifaceted, severe conditions and lacking access to other care providers. These children may have physical, psychological, neuromotor, socio-emotional, speech, language, hearing, or learning problems. The services offered are:

- individual assessment/evaluation and diagnosis
- treatment and client instruction
- service coordination
- screening
- technical assistance to other providers

Through a state interagency agreement, DECs are the lead agency under Public Law 99-457 for evaluation of children under 5 years of age. DECs also serve as coordinator/host of regional genetics clinics. Any child under age 21 and/or his family may apply for services. Anyone may refer a client with the family's consent.

Community Alternatives Program for Persons with Mental Retardation/ Developmental Disabilities (CAP-MR/DD): CAP-MR/DD provides an alternative to care in an ICF/MR. The program is available statewide to individuals of all ages. Each CAP-MR/DD client has a case manager designated by the Area Program. This case manager arranges, coordinates and monitors CAP-MR/DD services as well as other aspects of the client's care in the community.

HIV Case Management Services (HIV CMS): HIV CMS assist Medicaid-eligible recipients who have a diagnosis of HIV seropositivity to access needed medical, social, educational and other services. Case managers evaluate a recipient's situation; develop and implement an individualized plan of care to meet the recipient's service needs; assist in locating and contacting providers, programs and local resources; coordinate the delivery of services when multiple providers or programs are involved; and monitor to ensure that the services received meet the recipient's needs and are consistent with quality care.

Community Alternatives Program (CAP): CAP provides an alternative to nursing facility and hospital care for children and adults who have complex medical needs. This is a statewide program with certain enrollment limits. The Health Care Financing Administration (HCFA) allows the State to serve a specific number of individuals each year. The Division allots a portion of the State's limit to each CAP county. Each county program is administered by a lead agency selected by the county commissioners.

Nursing Facility Care (Skilled and Intermediate Care Nursing): A nursing facility is licensed and certified by Division of Facility Services to provide both skilled and intermediate nursing care. All Medicaid certified beds are inter-changeable as skilled or intermediate beds based on the level of care needed by the patient.

Other Community Resources include:
1. Planned Parenthood
2. Teen Health Connection
3. Local Transportation Options

APPENDIX VIII
DIVISION GUIDELINES FOR FOCUSED CARE STUDIES

Focused quality of care studies are detailed investigations of certain aspects of healthcare services which are designed to answer defined questions about the quality and appropriateness of care and offer direction in improving that care. Through focused quality of care studies, the organization can reasonably expect to improve care and service.

A focused study may be conducted by reviewing medical records, claims, or other administrative data, or by conducting special surveys. All well designed studies have the following components:

1. A clearly defined study question which focuses on relevant areas of concern specific to Members in the organization. A study question may be narrowly focused or broad and more complex. The study area selected should reflect the organization's Medicaid enrollment in terms of demographic characteristics and the prevalence of risk and/or disease;
2. Well defined clinical or quality indicators help answer the study question. Indicators are measurable variables relating to a specified clinical or health services delivery area, which are reviewed over a period of time to monitor the process or outcomes of care delivered in that area. Quality indicators are objective, measurable, and based on current knowledge and clinical experience. Practice guidelines or health service standards should be used in the development of indicators;
3. A standard or standards against which the organization compares itself;
4. Methods to collect sufficient data in a timely and appropriate manner to detect problem areas;
5. A method for analyzing the results; and
6. A system to develop, implement, and evaluate improvement strategies.

Possible Clinical Areas of Concern:
childhood immunizations
prenatal care
pregnancy prevention
sexually transmitted diseases
smoking prevention and cessation
cervical cancer screening
lead toxicity
health checks
asthma
diabetes
hypertension

ETOH and other substance abuse
sickle cell anemia
prescription drug abuse
adult health screenings

Possible Health Services Delivery Areas of Concern:
access to care
coordination of services
telephone medical advice
use of emergency services
health education
continuity of care
utilization of services

Resources for developing Focused Care Studies:
1. *Health Care Quality Improvement Studies in Managed Care Settings: A Guide for State Medicaid Agencies,* National Committee for Quality Assurance, 1994.
2. *A Healthcare Quality Improvement System for Medicaid Managed Care: A Guide for States,* Medicaid Bureau, HCFA, 1993.

APPENDIX IX
GRIEVANCE PROCEDURES

The Plan shall have a timely and organized internal grievance system with written policies and procedures (42 CFR 434.32). The Plan shall establish an internal grievance process to resolve complaints from Members whose claims for medical assistance are denied, terminated, reduced, inappropriate to needs, or not acted upon promptly. A denial includes any instance in which a request for a medical service has been made in which a Member has been told "no". The process will be available for disputes between the Plan and the Member concerning disenrollments.

A. Through the internal grievance process, Members can seek to resolve disputes with the Plan. The Plan's internal grievance procedures are not a substitute for the State appeal procedures, set forth in 10 North Carolina Administrative Code, Chapter 26, Subchapter I (10 NCAC 26I), which shall be available to Medicaid applicants/recipients at any time.

B. The Plan shall develop written policies and procedures which detail the operation of the internal grievance process and which shall:
    1. be approved by the Plan's governing body and be the direct responsibility of the governing body;
    2. be approved by the Division prior to implementation;
    3. be distributed to all Members upon enrollment, and to all subcontractors at time of subcontract;
    4. inform Members and applicants about the internal Plan grievance process and state appeals process set forth in 10 NCAC 26I in writing, through a State developed or approved description of the grievance process, at: 1) the time of enrollment; 2) each time a service is denied/reduced; 3) and when a patient is billed for service because the Plan has denied payment for a covered Medicaid service provided by an out-of-network provider;
    5. name specific individuals in the Plan who have authority to administer the internal grievance policy;
    6. include an adequately staffed consumer relations or member services office which can receive telephone calls and meet personally with Members and which Members can use to ask questions and resolve problems. This aspect of the internal grievance process will be informal and operate through verbal communication. The consumer relations/member services office will maintain records that include a short, dated summary of each question or problem, name of the Member, date of contact, the response, and the resolution. If the Plan does not have a

separate log for Medicaid recipients, the log shall distinguish Medicaid recipients from other Plan enrollees;

7. include an internal grievance process through which Members can complain directly to the Plan's governing body. The governing body may delegate this authority to an internal grievance committee, but the delegation must be in writing. Grievances are to be filed in writing either by the Member or Member's representative, stating the reason for the grievance. The Plan will maintain records that include a copy of the original grievance, the response, and the resolution. This system shall distinguish Medicaid recipients from other Plan Members and identify the grievant and the date of complaint;

8. provide for retention of the records described in subparagraphs 6 and 7, above, for five (5) years following a final decision or close of the grievance. If any litigation, claims negotiation, audit, or other action involving the records has been started before the expiration of the five (5) year period, the records shall be retained until completion of the action and resolution of issues which arise from it or until the end of the regular five-year period, whichever is later;

9. resolve all emergency (as defined in Appendix I.1.16) complaints within 24 hours and resolve all urgent (as defined in Appendix I.1.66) complaints within 48 hours. All other complaints shall be resolved by the Plan within thirty (30) days of the date of the grievance;

10. assure that Plan executives with the authority to require corrective action are involved in the internal grievance process.

C. When a Plan denies, reduces or terminates a Member's request for service or requests the Division to disenroll a Member, a written notice to the Member (or the Member's authorized representative) must explain:

1. that Member has a right to a second opinion if medically necessary, at the Plan's expense and how to exercise that right;

2. how to contact the consumer relations or member services office and how to file an internal grievance with the Plan;

3. the right to file an informal or formal appeal with the State pursuant to 10 NCAC 26I and how to obtain more information about those procedures;

4. that filing or resolving a grievance through the Plan's internal grievance mechanism is not a prerequisite to filing an informal or formal appeal with the State pursuant to 10 NCAC 26I;

5. the circumstances under which health services must be continued pending resolution of the internal grievance or state appeal (see section D, below);

6. the circumstances that will cause an expedited hearing;

7.   the right to be advised or represented by a lay advocate or attorney and of the potential availability of free legal services;

8.   the right to enroll in another Plan if the Member is not satisfied at the end of the internal grievance or State appeal process;

9.   that the Health Benefits Manager is available to the Member/Applicant, at any time, to provide assistance during the internal plan grievance process or the State appeal process under 10 NCAC 26I.

D.   If a Member files an internal grievance with the Plan or appeals to the State pursuant to 10 NCAC 26I on or before the tenth day after a decision is communicated in writing to the Member to reduce, suspend, or terminate services the Member had been receiving from the Plan on an ongoing basis, or before the date of the proposed action, whichever is later, and the treating Plan physician or another Plan physician has ordered the services at the present level and is authorized by the Contract with the Plan to order the services, the Plan will continue to provide services at a level equal to the level ordered by the Plan physician until a final decision is made by the Plan and/ or the State. If the resolution by the Plan is adverse, in whole or part, to the Member, the Member must be notified again of the right to a State appeal pursuant to 10 NCAC 26I and to continued services pending the appeal. If the Member appeals a Plan's written resolution within ten (10) days after it is issued, or before the date of the proposed action, whichever is later, services must be continued pending a final state-level decision. A resolution is made or issued on the date it is mailed or the date postmarked, whichever is later.

E.   The Plan must make the information and notices described in this addendum readily available orally and in writing in the recipient's primary language.

F.   Information regarding the nature of internal grievances and resolution may be publicly disclosed by the State in consumer information materials.

G.   The Plan's final written decision upon completion of the internal grievance shall be delivered by certified mail to the Member and it will contain the information set forth in section C.3 and C.5–9, above.

H.   If the Plan's decision is appealed under 10 NCAC 26I, all supporting documentation must be received by the State no later than five (5) working days from the date the Plan receives the appeal or notice from the State that an appeal has been filed. The appeal file must include:

1.   written request of the grievant asking for appeal;

2.   copies of the entire file that include investigation material, medical records, the Plan's decision(s), and the Member's response;
3.   any information used by the Plan to reach its decision.

APPENDIX X
ENCOUNTER DATA MINIMUM REQUIREMENTS

Element	*Definition*
Physician and other providers	
Beneficiary ID	a number that uniquely identifies an individual eligible for benefits
Beneficiary Name	name of the beneficiary
Beneficiary Date of Birth	beneficiary date of birth
Beneficiary Gender	beneficiary gender
EPSDT Indicator	indicator that procedure was performed as part of an EPSDT program
Facility ID	unique number assigned to the facility where the service was provided
First Date of Service	first date procedure was rendered
Last Date of Service	last date procedure was rendered
Other Diagnosis Code (take maximum possible)	diagnosis code of any condition other than the principal condition
Physician/Provider ID	unique number assigned to each physician or other provider of service
Place of Service	code indicating type of facility in which a service was rendered by a provider
Plan ID	number assigned to the Plan with which the beneficiary is associated
Principal Diagnosis Code	diagnosis code for the principal condition
Procedure Code (take maximum possible)	code identifying the medical procedure performed (outpt); principal procedure related to the principal diagnosis (inpt)
Provider Location Code	code for the geographic or geopolitical subdivision in which the service is rendered
Record Format	code indicating record type, e.g. physician, hospital
Specialty Code	identification of medical specialty or classification of the provider
Unit of Service/Quantity	quantitative measure of service (e.g., days, visits, miles, injections
Hospital	
Beneficiary ID	a number that uniquely identifies an individual eligible for benefits

Beneficiary Name	name of the beneficiary
Beneficiary Date of Birth	beneficiary date of birth
Beneficiary Gender	beneficiary gender
Attending/Referring Physician ID	unique number assigned to the attending or referring physician
Date of Service	date of the procedure/date a prescription was filled
Discharge Patient Destination	code indicating patient's destination upon discharge or death
Facility ID	unique number assigned to the facility where the service was provided
From Date of Service	first date covered by this encounter period
Length of Stay	number of inpatient hospital days
Other Diagnostic Code (take maximum possible)	diagnosis code by any condition other than the the principal condition
Performing Provider ID	unique number assigned to provider performing the major procedure
Plan ID	number assigned to the Plan with which the beneficiary is associated
Principal Diagnosis Code	diagnosis code for the principal condition
Procedure Code (take maximum possible)	code identifying the medical procedure performed (outpt); principal procedure related to the principal diagnosis (inpt)
Provider Location Code	code for the geographic or geopolitical subdivision in which the service is rendered
Provider Type	code indicating the classification of the facility providing the service
Record Format	code indicating record type, e.g. physician, hospital
Revenue Code	code which identifies a specific accommodation, ancillary service or billing center
Through Date of Service	inpatient release date/last treatment date
Type of Record	code indicating inpatient, outpatient, etc.
Unit of Service/Quantity	measure of service quantity (days, visits)

Long-term care

Beneficiary ID	unique individual identification number
Beneficiary Name	name of the beneficiary
Beneficiary Date of Birth	beneficiary date of birth
Beneficiary Gender	beneficiary gender

Date of Service	date of procedure/date prescription filled
Days Since Admission	number of days patient in LTC facility
Discharge Patient Destination	patient's destination upon discharge or death
Facility ID	unique facility identification number
From Date of Service	first date covered by this encounter period
National Drug Code	code assigned to all drugs by the FDA
Physician/Provider ID	unique number assigned to physician/provider
Plan ID	number assigned to the Plan with which the beneficiary is associated
Procedure Code (take maximum possible)	code identifying the medical procedure performed (outpt); principal procedure related to the principal diagnosis (inpt)
Provider Location Code	code for the geographic or geopolitical subdivision in which the service is rendered
Record Format	record type, e.g. physician, hospital
Revenue Code	code identifying specific accommodation, ancillary service or billing center
Specialty Code	identification of medical specialty or classification of the provider
Through Date of Service	inpatient release date/date of last treatment
Unit of Service/Quantity	quantitative measure of service (e.g. days, visits, miles, injections)

Drugs

Beneficiary ID	unique individual beneficiary identification
Beneficiary Name	name of the beneficiary
Beneficiary Date of Birth	beneficiary date of birth
Beneficiary Gender	beneficiary gender
Date of Service	date of procedure/date prescription filled
National Drug Code	code assigned to all drugs by the FDA
Physician/Provider ID	unique number assigned to each physician or other provider of service
Plan ID	number assigned to the Plan with which the beneficiary is associated
Provider ID	unique number assigned to each pharmacy provider of service/dental provider
Provider Location Code	code for the geographic or geopolitical subdivision in which the service is rendered

Quantity	number of units of the drug dispensed (e.g. cc, capsule, tablet)
Record Format	code indicating record type, e.g. physician, hospital
Unit of Measure	unit in which a drug is dispensed (e.g. cc, capsule, tablet)
Unit of Service/Quantity	quantitative measure of service (e.g. days, visits, miles, injections)

Dental

Beneficiary ID	a number that uniquely identifies an individual eligible for benefits
Beneficiary Name	name of the beneficiary
Beneficiary Date of Birth	beneficiary date of birth
Beneficiary Gender	beneficiary gender
Date of Service	date of the procedure/date a prescription was filled
Dental Quadrant	code identifying the quadrant of the mouth in which service was rendered
EPSDT Indicator	indicator that procedure was performed as part of an EPSDT program
Physician/Provider ID	unique number assigned to each physician or other provider of service
Place of Service	code indicating type of facility in which a service was rendered by a provider
Plan ID	number assigned to the Plan with which the beneficiary is associated
Provider ID	unique number assigned to each pharmacy provider of service/dental provider
Provider Location Code	code for the geographic or geopolitical subdivision in which the service is rendered
Record Format	code indicating record type, e.g. physician, hospital
Tooth Number	code identifying the specific tooth being treated
Unit of Service/Quantity	quantitative measure of service (e.g. days, visits, miles, injections)

APPENDIX XI
RATE SHEET

Medicaid PEPM rates, March 1996

Covered population	C&L Projected FFS upper limit (no pharmacy)	Projected FFS upper limit (no pharmacy; no GME)	Final revised rate (no pharmacy; no GME)	Effective discount
Aid to Families with Dependent Children-CN Newborns <Age 1	$392.21	$367.47	$311.72	15.2%
Aid to Families with Dependent Children-CN Ages 1–5	$51.16	$50.28	$45.74	9.0%
Aid to Families with Dependent Children-CN Ages 6–13	$26.38	$25.88	$25.00	3.4%
Aid to Families with Dependent Children-CN Females 14–20	$142.92	$138.55	$126.08	9.0%
Aid to Families with Dependent Children-CN Males 14–20	$33.12	$32.35	$28.53	11.8%
Aid to Families with Dependent Children-CN Ages 21 and Over	$134.81	$130.96	$117.86	10.0%
Aid to Families with Dependent Children-MN Newborns <Age 1	$315.57	$297.68	$255.40	14.2%
Aid to Families with Dependent Children-MN Ages 1–5	$104.30	$101.13	$95.00	6.1%
Aid to Families with Dependent Children-MN Ages 6–13	$71.02	$68.43	$62.27	9.0%
Aid to Families with Dependent Children-MN Females 14–20	$148.55	$143.51	$130.59	9.0%
Aid to Families with Dependent Children-MN Males 14–20	$127.13	$121.23	$103.74	14.4%
Aid to Families with Dependent Children-MN Ages 21 and Over	$218.71	$210.36	$189.32	10.0%
Medicaid for Infants and Children Newborns	$372.55	$349.47	$297.59	14.8%
Medicaid for Infants and Children Females 1–5	$79.07	$77.23	$70.38	8.9%
Medicaid for Infants and Children Males 1–5	$99.01	$96.71	$88.20	8.8%
Medicaid for Infants and Children Females 6–13	$45.40	$44.36	$40.07	9.7%
Medicaid for Infants and Children Males 6–13	$73.33	$57.75	$52.20	9.6%
Medicaid for Infants and Children Females 14–20	$137.81	$132.93	$116.13	12.6%
Medicaid for Infants and Children Males 14–20	$78.82	$76.03	$66.58	12.4%
Medicaid for Pregnant Women	$436.17	$422.13	$405.64	3.9%
Blind and Disabled <1	$1203.24	$1148.74	$1033.75	10.0%
Blind and Disabled 1–20	$351.35	$337.55	$305.25	9.6%
Blind and Disabled 21–44	$462.37	$441.97	$388.44	12.1%
Blind and Disabled 45 and over	$561.48	$536.17	$472.96	11.8%

Note: CN = categorically needy; MN = medically needy.

APPENDIX XII
BUSINESS TRANSACTIONS

All HMOs which are not Federally qualified must disclose to the Division information on certain types of transactions they have with a "party in interest" as defined in the Public Health Service Act. (See Sections 1903(m)(2)(A)(viii) and 1903(m)(4) of the Act.)

A.   Definition of a Party in Interest—As defined in Section 1318(b) of the Public Health Service Act, a party in interest is:

  (1)   Any director, officer, partner or employee responsible for management or administration of an HMO and HIO; any person who is directly or indirectly the beneficial owner of more than 5% of the equity of the HMO; any person who is the beneficial owner of more than 5% of the HIO; or, in the case of an HMO organized as a nonprofit corporation, an incorporator or member of such corporation under applicable State corporation law;

  (2)   Any organization in which a person described in subsection 1 is director, officer or partner; has directly or indirectly a beneficial interest of more than 5% of the equity of the HMO; or has a mortgage, deed of trust, note, or other interest valuing more than 5% of the assets of the HMO;

  (3)   Any person directly or indirectly controlling, controlled by, or under common control with an HMO; or

  (4)   Any spouse, child, or parent of an individual described in subsections 1, 2, or 3.

B.   Types of Transactions Which Must Be Disclosed—Business transactions which must be disclosed include:

  (1)   Any sale, exchange or lease of any property between the HMO and a party in interest;

  (2)   Any lending of money or other extension of credit between the HMO and a party in interest; and

  (3)   Any furnishing for consideration of goods, services (including management services) or facilities between the HMO and the party in interest. This does not include salaries paid to employees for services provided in the normal course of their employment.

The information which must be disclosed in the transactions listed in subsection B between an HMO and a party in interest includes:

(1) The name of the party in interest for each transaction;
(2) A description of each transaction and the quantity or units involved;
(3) The accrued dollar value of each transaction during the fiscal year; and
(4) Justification of the reasonableness of each transaction.

If this HMO contract is being renewed or extended, the HMO must disclose information on these business transactions which occurred during the prior contract period. If the contract is an initial contract with Medicaid, but the HMO has operated previously in the commercial or Medicare markets, information on business transactions for the entire year preceding the initial contract period must be disclosed. The business transactions which must be reported are not limited to transactions related to serving the Medicaid enrollment. All of these HMO business transactions must be reported.

Sample Contract Between a Local Health Department and a Health Maintenance Organization

PUBLIC HEALTH DEPARTMENT AGREEMENT

This PUBLIC HEALTH DEPARTMENT AGREEMENT ("this Agreement") is dated as of this _____ day of _____, _____, by and between _____, a Tennessee corporation ("HMO"), and _____, ("HEALTH DEPARTMENT"). This Agreement will be effective the later of _____, or the effective date of TennCare as defined herein.

RECITAL

WHEREAS, _____ operates a health maintenance organization and provides or arranges for the provision of hospital and medical services, through contractual arrangements with physicians and hospitals, to be delivered to persons eligible for such services under its Subscription Agreements ("Members"). HEALTH DEPARTMENT desires to enter into this Agreement pursuant to which HEALTH DEPARTMENT will undertake to provide certain medical services to Members on the basis of the terms and conditions set forth in this Agreement. It is the objective of the parties to develop a medical services program that is of high quality, utilizes well-coordinated clinical case management and strives to minimize service expenses.

THEREFORE, in consideration of the mutual covenants and agreements herein contained, and for other good and valuable consideration, the receipt and sufficiency of which are hereby acknowledged, the parties hereto agree as follows:

Courtesy of Memphis-Shelby County Department of Health, Memphis, Tennessee.

1. RELATIONSHIP OF PARTIES.

1.1 RELATIONSHIP OF THE ENTITIES. HMO and HEALTH DEPART-MENT are independent entities, and neither party is the agent, employee, or servant of the other.

2. HEALTH DEPARTMENT-PATIENT RELATIONSHIP.

2.1 AGREEMENT TO ACCEPT MEMBERS. At the time of enrollment, a Member shall be entitled to select from the list of Participating Physicians, including clinics of the HEALTH DEPARTMENT, that Participating Primary Care Provider from which the Member wishes to receive the Medical Services covered by the Subscription Agreement pertaining to the Member, subject to the ability of such Primary Care Provider to accept additional Members under this Agreement between the HEALTH DEPARTMENT and HMO. If a clinic of the HEALTH DEPARTMENT is so selected by a Member to provide medical services, HEALTH DEPARTMENT shall not refuse to offer medical services to the Member, provided the Member has been certified by HMO as being eligible and provided the maximum number of Members set forth in the appendix (not shown) has not been exceeded. HEALTH DEPARTMENT has the option of refusing to accept more Members than set forth or, if HEALTH DEPARTMENT is already treating more Members than the maximum set forth, of refusing to accept additional Members, provided HEALTH DEPARTMENT shall have given HMO thirty (30) days' prior written notice of such refusal.

2.2 TRANSFER OF MEMBERS. Because the Primary Care Provider-patient relationship is a personal one and may become unacceptable to either party, HEALTH DEPARTMENT may request, in writing, to HMO that a Member be transferred to another Participating Primary Care Provider. HEALTH DEPART-MENT shall not, however, seek to have a Member transferred because of the amount of medical services required by the Member or because of the physical condition of the Member. HEALTH DEPARTMENT acknowledges that Members have a contractual right with HMO to request to be transferred to another Participating Primary Care Provider. All such transfers subsequently approved shall become effective as soon as administratively feasible, but, in any event, within 60 days from the date of request.

3. FINANCIAL CONSIDERATIONS.

3.1 ALLOCATION OF PAYMENTS FOR MEDICAL SERVICES.

3.1.1 CAPITATION AND MEDICAL MANAGEMENT FUNDS. Each month, HMO shall make a monthly payment in an amount as set forth in the appendix (not shown) in the form of a Primary Care Provider Capitation to HEALTH DEPART-MENT. In addition, each month HMO shall credit the amount set forth into a Medical Management Fund for each Member enrolled with a clinic of the HEALTH DEPARTMENT to provide payment for medical services.

This capitation amount and fund are specific to HEALTH DEPARTMENT's practice, and the fund is more fully described in section 3.3.

3.2 PRIMARY CARE PROVIDER CAPITATION.

3.2.1 PRIMARY CARE PROVIDER CAPITATION. HMO shall make monthly payments to HEALTH DEPARTMENT based on the age, sex, and number of Members enrolled in HEALTH DEPARTMENT's practice, as specified in the appendix (not shown). Payments shall be made to HEALTH DEPARTMENT no later than the fifteenth (15th) business day of the month for which services are made available under this Agreement.

3.2.2 SERVICES COVERED BY PRIMARY CARE PROVIDER CAPITA-TION. The Primary Care Provider Capitation is payment for professional services available on a 24-hour per day basis, including but not limited to, preventive health care services, health appraisals, laboratory services, medical supplies dispensed from HEALTH DEPARTMENT's office, injectibles, preventive care, or other services provided by HEALTH DEPARTMENT's staff covering Primary Care Providers, on-call partners at the office, hospital, skilled nursing facility, patient's home, or any other location where primary care is provided. Examples of services covered by the Primary Care Provider Capitation are listed in the appendix (not shown). In no case will HEALTH DEPARTMENT be required to pay for Referral Services from Primary Care Provider Capitation.

3.3 MEDICAL MANAGEMENT FUND.

3.3.1 MEDICAL MANAGEMENT FUND. HMO shall establish a Participating Primary Care Provider's Medical Management Fund ("Medical Management Fund") to recognize the importance of efficiently managing the entire treatment process for HMO Members. Each Month, HMO shall credit the Medical Management Fund in an amount as set forth for each member. The amount per Member per month ("PMPM") to be credited to the Medical Management Fund may be adjusted from time to time at the discretion of HMO.

3.3.2 ELIGIBILITY FOR DISTRIBUTIONS. If HEALTH DEPARTMENT meets the eligibility criteria established from time to time, HEALTH DEPART-MENT will participate in the distribution from the Medical Management Fund pursuant to Section 3.3.4. Only those HEALTH DEPARTMENT practices serving at least 400 HMO Members are eligible to participate in the Medical Management Fund. In addition, eligibility to receive the maximum distributions shall be conditioned upon the HEALTH DEPARTMENT practice remaining open to accept new HMO Members during a specific period of the year.

3.3.3 COST TARGETS. For purposes of evaluating the efficiency of Participating Primary Care Providers' treatment patterns, HMO shall, on a quarterly basis, prepare a written report which shall include information relating to: (1) the utilization of all medical services provided for Members enrolled in each Participating Primary Care Provider Practice, including but not limited to, hospital, hospital emergency department, referral and ancillary services, and (2) amounts paid by HMO for claims for such medical services in accordance herewith.

HMO shall then establish budgeted cost targets based on the actual costs of the above medical services provided by all Participating Primary Care Providers engaged in Family Practice, Internal Medicine, and Pediatrics Practices.

3.3.4 ACCOUNTING AND DISTRIBUTION. On a quarterly basis, HMO will provide HEALTH DEPARTMENT an accounting of its eligibility to receive a distribution from the Medical Management Fund with such accounting to be provided no later than one hundred and twenty (120) days from the close of the previous accounting period. Distributions shall then be made to each primary care provider practice experiencing a favorable variance in net PMPM costs of medical services provided by that practice compared to the budgeted PMPM cost targets established by HMO. The amount of the distribution will be determined by HMO based on the size of the variance, with a maximum distribution of one hundred percent (100%) of the amount credited to the Medical Management Fund for that practice for the quarter.

3.3.5 PER MEMBER MAXIMUM. The maximum aggregate medical expenses to be tabulated against the targeted medical expenses shall be twenty-five thousand ($25000) dollars per Member per year, exclusive of prescription drug costs.

3.4 MEDICAL EXECUTIVE COMMITTEE AND MEDICAL MANAGE-MENT REVIEW COMMITTEE.

3.4.1 MEDICAL EXECUTIVE. HMO shall establish a Medical Executive Committee consisting of selected Participating Primary Care Providers, medical professionals, and HMO management staff. Voting members of the Committee shall be Primary Care Providers. The Medical Executive Committee will advise HMO senior management in all matters pertaining to the professional health care of Members based upon reports and recommendations from the appropriate staff, care providers, departments, and/or committees. The Medical Executive Committee's responsibilities will include, but not be limited to, credentialing of Participating

Providers, initiation of or participation in the corrective action process or review of measures to ensure ethical conduct and competent clinical care and to ensure the coordination and implementation of clinical protocols and guidelines for the provision of medical services to Members.

3.4.2 MEDICAL MANAGEMENT REVIEW COMMITTEE. HMO shall establish a Medical Management Review Committee (the "Committee"), consisting of selected Participating Primary Care Providers, medical professionals, and HMO management staff. The Medical Management Review Committee will review on a periodic basis, but not less than annually, the practice of any Participating Primary Care Provider whose utilization of Individual Referral Services or Hospital Services results in a negative variance or an unusual surplus balance when compared to budgeted PMPM costs. In addition, the Medical Management Review Committee shall review any other matters agreed upon by HMO and HEALTH DEPARTMENT.

3.4.3 REVIEW OF PARTICIPATING PRIMARY CARE PROVIDERS WITH DEFICITS OR UNUSUAL SURPLUSES IN UTILIZATION PRACTICES. The Medical Management Review Committee shall review on a periodic basis, but not less than annually, prior to March 31, the practice of each Participating Primary Care Provider whose Individual Referral Services and/or Hospital Services utilization has a negative variance or an unusual surplus variance at year end when compared to budgeted PMPM cost targets. If the Committee determines that the unusual surplus variance in either or both of those categories of utilization resulted from inappropriate management of services rather than factors outside the control of the Participating Primary Care Provider, the Committee shall have the right to institute a Variable Rate Withhold Program as described in 3.4.4. If the Committee determines that the unusual surplus variance in either or both of those categories of utilization resulted from inappropriate underutilization of services rather than factors outside the control of the Participating Primary Care Provider, the Committee shall recommend the appropriate action to HMO.

3.4.4 VARIABLE RATE WITHHOLD PROGRAM. If HEALTH DEPART-MENT fails to maintain a surplus variance in its Individual Referral categories of utilization and/or Hospital Services categories of utilization at the end of any calendar year, HEALTH DEPARTMENT may, at the discretion of HMO, be subject to a Variable Rate Withhold Program ("Withhold Pool") for all future primary capitation payments made pursuant to Section 3.2. The Withhold amount may at each subsequent review, and subject to the Plan's Corrective Action Plan, increase or decrease in 10% increments. HEALTH DEPARTMENT's fund will be monitored quarterly after an initial 180 days in the program and adjustments made quarterly thereafter. A specific percentage of the monthly capitation will be deducted from HEALTH DEPARTMENT's Primary Care Provider Capitation, and placed in the Withhold Pool. Participating Primary Care Providers who are subject to the Withhold Pool and who have less than 100 Members assigned will initially be reimbursed at 90% of the capitation rate set forth in the appendix (not shown). HEALTH DEPARTMENTS who are subject to the Withhold Pool and who have 100 Members will initially be reimbursed at 80% of the capitation rate set forth.

3.5 RETROACTIVE MEMBER CANCELLATIONS AND ADDITIONS.

3.5.1 CANCELLATIONS. If a Member's eligibility has been canceled retroactively, HMO may deduct up to three months' Primary Care Provider Capitation payments to HEALTH DEPARTMENT and credits to the Medical Management Fund previously made with respect to such Member from the current payments to, and credits on behalf of, HEALTH DEPARTMENT. HMO shall pay HEALTH DEPARTMENT for Medical Services provided by HEALTH DEPARTMENT during the period for which payments were deducted, the Primary Care Primary Care Provider Capitation amounts applicable to the Member for the period in question. This activity does not constitute a violation of the provisions of Section 5.3 hereof.

3.5.2 ADDITIONS. If a Member's eligibility has been added retroactively for more than three months, HMO will make capitation payments to HEALTH DEPARTMENT and credit the Medical Management Fund for a period not to exceed three months. HMO shall pay HEALTH DEPARTMENT for the Medical Services provided by HEALTH DEPARTMENT during the eligibility period but prior to the period for which retroactive payment was made by paying HEALTH DEPARTMENT an amount equal to the Primary Care Provider Capitation amount applicable to the Member for the period in question.

4. HEALTH DEPARTMENT SERVICES TO MEMBERS.

4.1 SERVICES PROVIDED AND CARE ARRANGED BY HEALTH DE- PARTMENT. HEALTH DEPARTMENT shall provide or arrange for and authorize as set forth herein, those services covered in the HMO Subscription Agreement to Members at all HEALTH DEPARTMENT location(s) including but not limited to locations described in the appendix (not shown). In addition, HEALTH DEPARTMENT agrees to use generic substitution under the Drug Formulary developed for HMO as amended from time to time, and attached hereto (not shown) and incorporated herein by reference, for those prescriptions where a generic is available unless HEALTH DEPARTMENT indicates that a generic is not medically appropriate. Final determination of Member eligibility and payment for services shall be made at the sole discretion of HMO. HEALTH DEPARTMENT shall abide by all provisions of the HMO Subscription Agreement, which may be amended from time to time, and which is incorporated herein by reference. HEALTH DEPARTMENT agrees to implement peer review and credentialing of nurse practitioners, physician assistants, and other ancillary personnel who provide services to HMO members.

4.2 NATIONAL ASSOCIATION OF INSURANCE COMMISSIONERS SOLE SOURCE OF PAY CLAUSE. HEALTH DEPARTMENT agrees and warrants that in no event, including, but not limited to, nonpayment, HMO's insolvency, or breach of this Agreement, shall HEALTH DEPARTMENT bill; charge; collect a deposit from; seek compensation, remuneration, or reimbursement from; or have any recourse against Members or persons acting on their behalf for services listed in this Agreement. This provision shall not prohibit collection of supplemental charges or copayments on HEALTH DEPARTMENT's behalf made in accordance with the terms of the HMO Subscription Agreement pertaining to the Member. HEALTH DEPARTMENT further agrees that: (1) the hold-harmless provisions and warranty herein shall survive the termination of this Agreement, regardless of the cause giving rise to the termination, and that (2) this hold-harmless provision and warranty supersedes any oral or written contrary agreement heretofore entered into between HEALTH DEPARTMENT and Members or persons acting on their behalf. Any modification, addition, or deletion to the provisions of this section shall become effective on a date not earlier than thirty (30) days after the Tennessee Commissioner of Insurance has received a report of such proposed changes.

4.3 MEDICARE ENROLLMENT OF MEMBERS. If HEALTH DEPARTMENT provides services to a Member who is a Medicare enrollee, HEALTH DEPARTMENT shall accept the Primary Care Provider Capitation payment from HMO plus payment from Medicare as complete payment for all Medical Services to the Member for services that are the responsibility of HEALTH DEPARTMENT under this Agreement.

4.4 CHARGES FOR EXCLUDED AND/OR NON-COVERED SERVICES. HEALTH DEPARTMENT may charge Members for medical services excluded from the Subscription Agreement, or determined by HEALTH DEPARTMENT and HMO to be medically unnecessary.

4.5 PREFERRED PROVIDER. HEALTH DEPARTMENT shall refer Members to the approved Preferred Providers specified (not shown), as amended by

HMO from time to time. In particular cases, other providers may be used with the prior approval of the HMO Medical Director. In cases where the Member is admitted to a nonpreferred hospital due to an emergency, HEALTH DEPART-MENT shall participate in arranging for transfer of the Member to a Preferred Provider once the Member's condition is considered stable.

4.6 CONSIDERATION OF REFERRAL SPECIALISTS. HEALTH DE-PARTMENT shall routinely use referral specialists who agree:
- not to bill Member and to send bills for authorized services to HMO
- to cooperate with the HMO Utilization Review and Quality Assurance programs
- to cooperate with HMO Consumer Affairs Department in resolving Member problems
- to accept payments by HMO as payment in full for covered services
- to accept responsible and competitive fees for their services
- to agree to use HMO Preferred Providers as specified in a list published and amended by HMO from time to time
- to permit use of generic substitution under the Drug Formulary as amended from time to time, developed for HMO and attached hereto (not shown) for those prescriptions where a generic is available unless the referral specialist specifically indicates that a generic is not medically appropriate

5. INSPECTION.

5.1 INSPECTION OF SERVICES AND FACILITIES. HEALTH DEPART-MENT shall permit authorized representatives of HMO, given reasonable notice when possible, and/or authorized representatives of any state or federal supervisory authority or agency to inspect HEALTH DEPARTMENT's facilities and to review the records of Medical Services provided to Members.

6. RECORDS.

6.1 HEALTH DEPARTMENT RECORDS AND PROCEDURES. HEALTH DEPARTMENT shall maintain, at its sole expense, up-to-date records in accordance with accepted professional standards and sound internal control practices. Medical records, subject to all applicable privacy and confidentiality requirements, shall be made available upon request by any proper committee of HMO to determine whether content and quality are acceptable, as well as for peer review or grievance or complaint review or for corrective action, for administration of the plan for other lawful purposes, and by authorized government officials. HEALTH

DEPARTMENT shall retain and provide access to HMO and any governmental agency to said records for not less than seven (7) years after the expiration of this Agreement. HEALTH DEPARTMENT shall, upon reasonable notice, provide HMO with any such data as may be requested. HMO may provide forms for keeping certain records, which shall be submitted to HMO on a monthly basis.

6.1.1 RECORDS AFTER TERMINATION. It is understood that in the event of termination of this Agreement, regardless of the cause, HEALTH DEPART-MENT shall cooperate in the orderly transfer of a copy of medical records of Members to HMO and Participating Primary Care Providers. Such transfer of records shall not exceed thirty (30) days from the date HEALTH DEPARTMENT receives instructions regarding where to send the records. HMO shall pay HEALTH DEPARTMENT its actual cost for copying such information.

6.1.2 MEMBER REQUEST FOR RECORDS. At such time as a Member leaves the care of HEALTH DEPARTMENT hereunder for another Participating Primary Care Provider for reasons other than the termination of this Agreement, HEALTH DEPARTMENT will provide, upon request, such physician(s) assuming the responsibility for medical care with copies of the medical records and ancillary records such as X-rays, etc., maintained by HEALTH DEPARTMENT at no cost, within thirty (30) days of any such request.

6.2 HMO REPORTING TO HEALTH DEPARTMENT. HMO shall provide quarterly reports to HEALTH DEPARTMENT regarding the utilization/medical management of services provided by HEALTH DEPARTMENT to Member.

6.3 HEALTH DEPARTMENT REPORTING. HEALTH DEPARTMENT shall use HMO Encounter Forms and submit such forms to HMO weekly; use HMO authorization procedures for consultant referrals; provide telephone or written confirmation to HMO about all authorized hospital admissions prior to or on the day of admission; and use such other forms or systems as may be developed by HMO.

6.4 QUALITY ASSURANCE AND UTILIZATION REVIEW. HEALTH DEPARTMENT shall participate in the HMO Quality Assurance/Utilization Review Process, including prior review by the HMO Medical Director or his designee of all elective admissions and elective surgeries, monitoring for appropriate length of stay, discharge planning, and the use of appropriate alternatives for hospitalization and shall attend, or cause a physician associated with HEALTH DEPARTMENT to attend, HMO quarterly Advisory Medical Management Committee meetings.

7. STANDARDS.

7.1 STANDARDS OF CARE. HEALTH DEPARTMENT shall cooperate with HMO in developing written reports on the quality of medical services rendered by HEALTH DEPARTMENT, including various techniques developed by HEALTH department and HMO to ensure high-quality, comprehensive, continuous, accessible, and cost-effective medical services emphasizing preventive care and health maintenance. HEALTH DEPARTMENT, together with other physicians associated with HMO and/or an outside professional medical organization, society, or university, will establish a mechanism to provide for an external audit of HEALTH DEPARTMENT. The finding regarding HEALTH DEPARTMENT shall be confidential between HMO and any supervisory authority or agency and HEALTH DEPARTMENT. Such external audits are not intended to be punitive, but are to provide a means of ensuring the quality of medical care. HEALTH DEPARTMENT will have the responsibility of implementing any needed changes cited in such audits. The cost of such audits shall be borne by HMO; any time spent by HEALTH DEPARTMENT in complying herewith shall not be reimbursed. HMO and HEALTH DEPARTMENT further agree to jointly develop methods, procedures, and techniques designed to educate all Members receiving health care hereunder regarding the proper utilization of medical services.

7.2 PRINCIPLES OF PRACTICE. HEALTH DEPARTMENT shall abide by the Principles of Practice as adopted and amended by HMO and as incorporated herein by reference.

7.3 HIGH-QUALITY COST-EFFECTIVE CARE. HEALTH DEPARTMENT shall provide and arrange for high-quality, cost-effective medical care in accordance with HMO policies.

7.4 SERVICE STANDARDS. HEALTH DEPARTMENT shall treat Members with the same levels of courtesy and respect accorded all other patients of HEALTH DEPARTMENT, and comply with the Member Service Standards set forth in the HMO Principles of Practice. HEALTH DEPARTMENT shall at all times ensure that the medical services are rendered in a dignified, exemplary, and nondiscriminatory manner.

8. REPORTING REQUIREMENTS.

8.1 REPORTING REQUIREMENTS OF HEALTH DEPARTMENT. HEALTH DEPARTMENT shall give notice to HMO of any action involving HEALTH DEPARTMENT's Primary Care Provider's hospital privileges or conditions relating to its ability to admit patients to any hospital or inpatient facility; any situation that develops regarding HEALTH DEPARTMENT when notice of that situation has been given to the appropriate Health-Related Board or any other licensing agency or board, or any situation involving an investigation complaint filed by the appropriate Health-Related Board or any other licensing agency or board regarding a complaint against the Health Care Provider's license; when a change in the HEALTH DEPARTMENT's Health Care Provider's license to practice is affected or any form of reportable discipline is taken against HEALTH DEPARTMENT and/or one of its Primary Care Providers alleging professional malpractice, regardless of whether the lawsuit or claim involves a Member.

In any such instance described above, HEALTH DEPARTMENT must notify HMO in writing within ten (10) days from the date it first receives notice, whether written or oral, with the exception of those lawsuits or claims that do not involve a Member, with respect to which HEALTH DEPARTMENT has thirty (30) days to notify HMO.

8.1.1 CONFLICT OF INTEREST. HEALTH DEPARTMENT shall report to HMO any transactions in connection with HEALTH DEPARTMENT's obligations under this Agreement, with any provider or entity in which HEALTH DEPARTMENT has a financial interest. HEALTH DEPARTMENT's contracting with a competitor managed care organization is not deemed to be a conflict of interest.

9. INSURANCE.

9.1 LIABILITY INSURANCE REQUIREMENTS. HEALTH DEPARTMENT shall ensure that HEALTH DEPARTMENT and each Primary Care Provider associated with HEALTH DEPARTMENT who provides services under this Agreement to HMO Members carries at his/her own expense, or is covered under policies provided by HEALTH DEPARTMENT at its sole expense, liability insurance of at least one million dollars ($1000000) per person per occurrence and at least three million dollars ($3000000) in the annual aggregate insuring against professional errors and omissions (malpractice) in providing medical services under the terms of this Agreement; HEALTH DEPARTMENT at its sole expense, if any, shall cause certificates of insurance or verifications of required coverages for professional liability to be mailed to HMO for all coverages listed herein and for subsequent renewals of all required coverages. The primary care provider is self-insured for all liability, except professional liability subject to the limits of liability as set forth in the Tennessee Government Liability Act T.C.A. 29-20-1 et seq.

9.2 TAIL COVERAGE. If any of the insurance coverage described in Section 9.1 is provided through "claims made" rather than "occurrence" forms, then HEALTH

DEPARTMENT shall provide, or ensure that the Primary Care Providers associated with it provide, "tail coverage" in the amounts described in Section 9.1 upon the termination or expiration of this Agreement or the termination or expiration of such Primary Care Providers' association with HEALTH DEPARTMENT.

9.3 INDEMNIFICATION. Each party to this Agreement agrees that if either of them is without fault and is held liable for the acts of the other arising out of the rendering or failure to render professional services, their rights of indemnity or contribution as provided by the applicable laws for the state of Tennessee may be pursued in accordance with such laws.

10. SOLICITATION OF MEMBERS.

10.1 SOLICITATION OF MEMBERS TO CHANGE. During the term of this Agreement or any renewal thereof, and for a period of one year from the date of termination, neither HEALTH DEPARTMENT nor any employee or agent of HEALTH DEPARTMENT, nor any Primary Care Provider associated with HEALTH DEPARTMENT shall, within the Service Area of the Plan, advise or counsel any HMO Member to end enrollment with HMO and will not solicit any such Member to become enrolled with any other health maintenance organization or other hospitalization or medical payment plan or insurance policy.

11. TERM AND TERMINATION.

11.1 NOTICE REQUIRED TO TERMINATE AGREEMENT. This Agreement will commence on the date set forth in the Preamble of this Agreement and shall continue in effect indefinitely unless or until either party notifies the other in writing not less than ninety (90) days prior to the anniversary of the effective date that it desires to terminate the Agreement on such anniversary date. This Agreement may be terminated at any time upon the mutual consent of the parties. In addition, under the circumstances specified in Section 13.3, HEALTH DEPARTMENT may terminate this Agreement upon the effective date of any proposed amendment to this Agreement provided HEALTH DEPARTMENT shall have given HMO at least sixty (60) days' prior written notice of such termination.

11.2 TERMINATION OF AGREEMENT FOR CAUSE. Either party may terminate this Agreement at any time for cause upon delivery of written notice at least sixty (60) days prior to the proposed termination date in the event of the following:

11.2.1 MATERIAL DEFAULT. The other party shall materially default on the performance of a provision of this Agreement or any other agreements referred to herein, and such default shall continue for a period of thirty (30) days after the mailing of written notice to the defaulting party stating the specific default.

11.2.2 BANKRUPTCY AND INSOLVENCY. The other party shall apply for or consent to the appointment of a receiver, trustee, or liquidator of all or a substantial part of its assets; file a voluntary petition in bankruptcy or admit in writing its inability to pay its debts as they become due; make a general assignment for the benefit of creditors; file a petition or an answer seeking reorganization or arrangement with creditors or to take advantage of an insolvency law; or, if an order, judgment, or decree shall be entered by a court of competent jurisdiction, on the application of a creditor, adjudicating such a party a bankrupt or insolvent or approving a petition seeking reorganization of the party or appointment of a receiver, trustee, or liquidator of all or a substantial part of its assets.

11.2.3 LOSS OF LICENSE. The other party loses its state license to operate a HMO or to practice medicine or osteopathy.

11.2.4 DANGER TO HEALTH OR SAFETY OF MEMBERS. HMO may suspend this Agreement immediately whenever HMO believes that there is clear and convincing evidence that the health or safety of HMO Members is endangered by actions of the HEALTH DEPARTMENT or agents or employees of the HEALTH DEPARTMENT. In the event that such condition is continuing and remains unresolved with reasonable satisfaction to HMO for a period of thirty (30) days, HMO may terminate this Agreement effective immediately upon notification to HEALTH DEPARTMENT. HEALTH DEPARTMENT shall have the right to have said adverse decision considered under the provisions of HMO's Corrective Action Plan. Notwithstanding, this Agreement shall remain terminated until the conclusion of HEALTH DEPARTMENT's appeal of HMO's actions regarding the original determination to suspend this Agreement.

11.3 NOTICE TO MEMBERS ABOUT TERMINATION OF AGREEMENT. HMO shall be solely responsible for notifying Members that this Agreement has been terminated by HEALTH DEPARTMENT or HMO.

11.4 RIGHTS OF PARTIES UPON TERMINATION OF THIS AGREEMENT. Upon the expiration or termination, HEALTH DEPARTMENT shall turn over to HMO and shall make available to HMO such information and records as may be requested. HEALTH DEPARTMENT shall transfer copies of HMO Member records to Participating Primary Care Providers subsequently chosen by Members transferring out of HEALTH DEPARTMENT's practice. HEALTH

DEPARTMENT shall remain obligated to provide Medical Services to any Member who is at the time of said expiration or termination a registered bed patient at a hospital until such Member's discharge from the hospital and HMO will reimburse HEALTH DEPARTMENT for such medical services at the fee schedule being used by HMO at the time of service.

12. ASSIGNMENT.

12.1 ASSIGNMENT OF AGREEMENT. This Agreement, being intended to secure the personal services of HEALTH DEPARTMENT, shall not be assigned or transferred by HEALTH DEPARTMENT. HEALTH DEPARTMENT must give prior written consent to the Assignment of this Agreement by HMO to a Primary Care Provider Office Network, which may be created after the effective date of this Agreement and which may consist, in whole or in part, of Participating Primary Care Providers affiliated with HMO.

13. AMENDMENTS.

13.1 AMENDMENT BY MUTUAL WRITTEN AGREEMENT. This Agreement may be amended at any time by the mutual written agreement of HEALTH DEPARTMENT and HMO. This Agreement is subject to all rules and regulations promulgated at any time by any state or federal regulatory agency or authority having supervisory authority over HMO, and this Agreement shall be deemed to be amended to conform therewith at all times.

13.2 SUBSCRIPTION AGREEMENT. If any provision of this Agreement is inconsistent, or in conflict with, any Subscription Agreement in effect from time to time that sets forth the rights of Members, the Subscription Agreement then in effect shall take precedence.

13.3 AMENDMENTS. HMO shall have the right to promulgate amendments to this Agreement and the appendices to this Agreement by notifying HEALTH DEPARTMENT at least ninety (90) days prior to the effective date of the amendment. If HEALTH DEPARTMENT does not provide notice of intent to terminate this Agreement within said ninety-day period, it will be deemed to have accepted said amendment and will be bound by it.

14. SEVERABILITY.

14.1 SEVERABILITY. If any one or more of the provisions contained in this Agreement shall for any reason be held to be invalid, illegal, or unenforceable in any respect, such invalidity, illegality, or unenforceability shall not affect any other provisions of this Agreement, and this Agreement shall be construed as if such invalid, illegal, or unenforceable provision had never been contained herein.

15. DEFINITIONS.

15.1 DEFINITIONS. As used in this Agreement, the following terms shall have the meanings set forth below. Any terms not defined in this Agreement that are defined in the Subscription Agreement shall have the meaning set forth in the Subscription Agreement.

15.1.1 COORDINATION OF BENEFITS OR COB. "Coordination of Benefits" or "COB" means the procedures set forth in the Subscription Agreement to determine which coverage is primary for payment of benefits to Members with duplicate coverage.

15.1.2 DEPENDENT. "Dependent" means an individual who qualifies as a Dependent under the terms of the Subscription Agreement.

15.1.3 DRUG FORMULARY. "Drug Formulary" means the listing of prescription medications that are approved for use by HMO and that will be dispensed through a Participating Provider to a Member. When designated by HMO, a generic equivalent shall be dispensed. Generic substitution shall not be required (a) when the generic product is not commercially available, or (b) in such instances when HMO and Participating Primary Care Provider agree that substitutions are not medically advisable, or (c) where generic substitution is not permitted by applicable law. This list shall be subject to periodic review, modification and approval by HMO. To be classified as a prescription medication the drug must have been approved by the Food and Drug Administration for the use for which it has been prescribed, and under Federal or State law, can be dispensed only pursuant to a prescription order.

15.1.4 ENCOUNTER FORM. "Encounter Form" means the form provided to HEALTH DEPARTMENT by HMO for the reporting of medical services delivered by HEALTH DEPARTMENT.

15.1.5 HEALTH DEPARTMENT. "Health Department" means the party named in the Preamble to this Agreement whose individual physicians and other health care professionals are appropriately licensed based upon the laws of the state of Tennessee.

15.1.6 HOSPITAL SERVICES. "Hospital Services" means: (a) medical services provided under the Subscription Agreement by an entity that is licensed, certified, and operates as a hospital, (b) medical services for chemical dependency, (c) medical services outside the Plan Service Area, and (d) any other medical services not specifically included as services covered by HEALTH DEPARTMENT Capitation or as Referral Services.

15.1.7 MEDICAL DIRECTOR. "Medical Director" means that Primary Care Provider designated by HMO to perform the duties of Medical Director as set forth in this Agreement and in accordance with the policies of HMO.

15.1.8 MEDICAL MANAGEMENT FUND. "Medical Management Fund" means the fund established for the purpose of sharing the savings resulting from efficiently managing the entire treatment process as reflected by HEALTH DEPARTMENT's performance compared to established cost targets.

15.1.9 MEDICAL SERVICES. "Medical services" means those professional, emergency, hospital, and referral services furnished to a Member pursuant to the Subscription Agreement incorporated herein by reference and attached hereto in the appendix (not shown).

15.1.10 MEMBER. "Member" means an eligible subscriber or Dependent as defined in the applicable Subscription Agreement who has elected coverage through HEALTH DEPARTMENT.

15.1.11 PARTICIPATING PRIMARY CARE PROVIDER. "Participating Primary Care Provider" means a Primary Care Provider practicing in the Service Area who has entered into a contract substantially similar to this Agreement and who is not employed by or otherwise affiliated with HEALTH DEPARTMENT.

15.1.12 PARTICIPATING PROVIDER. "Participating Provider" means any duly licensed hospital, skilled nursing facility, home health agency, or other institutional provider that has contracted with, or on whose behalf a contract has been entered into with HMO to provide certain medical services that are plan benefits to Members. A list of Participating Providers is attached hereto in the appendix (not shown) and incorporated herein by reference. Said list is subject to amendment from time to time by HMO.

15.1.13 PER-MEMBER MAXIMUM. "Per-Member Maximum" means the per-Member per-year limitations on referral or hospital charges as established by HMO from time to time.

15.1.14 HMO. "HMO" is a corporation licensed as a health maintenance organization that has contractually agreed to provide or arrange for the provision of health care services for the Medicaid-eligible members of TennCare.

15.1.15 PHYSICIAN. "Physician" means the party who is licensed to practice either medicine or osteopathy in the state of Tennessee.

15.1.16 PRIMARY CARE PROVIDER OFFICE NETWORK. "Primary Care Provider Office Network" means a Primary Care Provider network, an individual practice association, or a medical group that has entered into an agreement with HMO to provide health care services to HMO Members, has as its primary purpose the delivery or arrangement for delivery of health care services, and has entered into written service agreements or other arrangements with health care professionals, the majority of whom are licensed to practice medicine or osteopathy.

15.1.17 PLAN. "Plan" means the health maintenance organization operated by HMO in the Service Area.

15.1.18 PLAN BENEFITS. "Plan Benefits" means the covered medical services, hospital services, and other health care services to which a Member is entitled under the Subscription Agreement, and any applicable supplemental benefit riders when such services are medically necessary and are provided in such a manner consistent with the most appropriate supply or level of service that can be provided to a Member. Such benefits may be modified from time to time as required by changes in the statutes or regulations or otherwise provided by this Agreement.

15.1.19 PMPM. "PMPM" means per Member per month.

15.1.20 PREFERRED PROVIDER. "Preferred Provider" means providers approved and designated by HMO as Preferred Providers from time to time.

15.1.21 PRIMARY CARE PROVIDER. A "Primary Care Provider" means a primary care physician or registered professional nurse or physician assistant practicing in accordance with state law who is responsible for supervising, coordinating, and providing initial and primary care to patients; for initiating referrals for specialist care; and for maintaining the continuity of patient care.

15.1.22 PRIMARY CARE PROVIDER CAPITATION. "Primary Care Provider Capitation" means the amount paid to HEALTH DEPARTMENT monthly for services based on the age, sex, and number of Members selecting HEALTH DEPARTMENT Clinics.

15.1.23 REFERRAL SERVICES. "Referral Services" means covered medical services arranged by HEALTH DEPARTMENT and provided outside HEALTH DEPARTMENT's office other than Hospital Services.

15.1.24 SERVICE AREA. "Service Area" means the area described in the appendix (not shown).

15.1.25 SUBROGATION. "Subrogation" means the recovery of the cost of services and benefits provided to Members by HMO for which other parties are liable.

15.1.26 SUBSCRIBER. "Subscriber" means the employee or individual with whom HMO enters into, or who is the direct beneficiary of, a Subscription Agreement.

15.1.27 SUBSCRIPTION AGREEMENT. "Subscription Agreement" means both group and individual contracts between HMO and an employer or individual pursuant to which HMO provides covered medical and hospital services, as such agreement may be amended from time to time.

15.1.28 TENNCARE. "TennCare" means the alternative health care plan provided by the State of Tennessee to the Medicaid population and the uninsured sector of the population. TennCare was formulated on the basis of global budgeting, a capitated managed care delivery system with emphasis on preventive care and reasonable cost-sharing requirements for the purpose of extending quality health care to the eligible covered individuals in the State of Tennessee.

16. MISCELLANEOUS.

16.1 BINDING EFFECT AGREEMENT. This Agreement shall inure to the benefit of and be binding upon the parties hereto, their employees, successors, and permitted assigns. Except with respect to Section 4.3, this Agreement is not intended to be for the benefit of a third person.

16.2 NOTICE. Any notice required by this Agreement shall be given by registered or certified mail, addressed to the party to whom such notice is intended to be given, at the last known address of that party's principal place of business.

16.3 GOVERNING LAW. All matters affecting the interpretation of this Agreement and the rights and obligations of the parties hereto shall be governed by and construed in accordance with the laws of the State of Tennessee.

16.4 WAIVER. The failure of any party to insist upon the strict performance of any provision of this Agreement shall not be deemed to be a waiver of any breach of this Agreement or of the right to insist upon strict performance of such provision at any future time.

16.5 ENTIRE AGREEMENT. This Agreement and the appendices and attachments hereto, as modified by the Subscription Agreement from time to time, is the entire Agreement between the parties and supersedes any and all prior agreements between HMO and HEALTH DEPARTMENT or any predecessor of either party.

16.6 AUTHORITY TO SIGN AGREEMENT. The person signing this Agreement on behalf of HEALTH DEPARTMENT represents and warrants that such person is duly authorized and empowered to execute this Agreement on behalf of the HEALTH DEPARTMENT.

INDEX

453